Guidelines for Chiropractic Quality Assurance and Practice Parameters

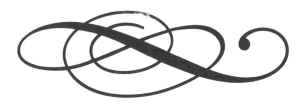

Proceedings of the Mercy Center Consensus Conference

Edited by
Scott Haldeman, DC, MD, PhD
Commission Chairman

David Chapman-Smith, LLB
Commission Counsel

Donald M. Petersen, Jr., BS
Commission Secretary

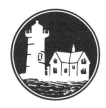

JONES AND BARTLETT PUBLISHERS

Sudbury, Massachusetts

BOSTON   TORONTO   LONDON   SINGAPORE

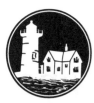

World Headquarters
Jones and Bartlett Publishers
40 Tall Pine Drive
Sudbury, MA 01776
978-443-5000
info@jbpub.com
www.jbpub.com

Jones and Bartlett Publishers Canada
2406 Nikanna Road
Mississauga, ON L5C 2W6
CANADA

Jones and Bartlett Publishers International
Barb House, Barb Mews
London W6 7PA
UK

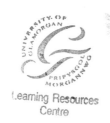

ISBN: 0-7637-2921-3

Production Credits
Executive Editor: Jack Bruggeman
Production Manager: Amy Rose
Associate Production Editor: Karen C. Ferreira
Media Services Specialist: Colleen Halloran
Editorial Assistant: Kylah McNeill
Manufacturing and Inventory Coordinator: Amy Bacus
Printing and Binding: PA Hutchison
Cover Printing: PA Hutchison

Printed in the United States of America
08 07 06 05 04   10 9 8 7 6 5 4 3 2 1

Guidelines for Chiropractic Quality Assurance and Practice Parameters

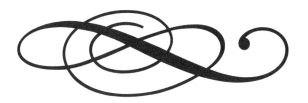

Proceedings of a Consensus Conference
Conference Commissioned by the Congress of Chiropractic State Associations
Held at the Mercy Conference Center
Burlingame, California, USA
January 25-30, 1992

Edited by

Scott Haldeman, DC, MD, PhD
Commission Chairman

David Chapman-Smith, LLB
Commission Counsel

Donald M. Petersen, Jr., BS
Commission Secretary

GENERAL DISCLAIMER

This document contains guidelines or parameters for the practice of chiropractic developed by a commission of thirty-five (35) chiropractors established by the Congress of Chiropractic State Associations (COCSA). It provides part of an ongoing effort by the chiropractic profession to provide practitioners with improved guidelines for practice.

These guidelines, which may need to be modified, are intended to be flexible. They are not standards of care. Adherence to them is voluntary. The Commission understands that alternative practices are possible and may be preferable under certain clinical conditions. The ultimate judgment regarding the propriety of any specific procedure must be made by the practitioner in light of the individual circumstances presented by each patient.

It is not the purpose of this document, which is advisory in nature, to take precedence over any federal, state or local statute, rule, regulation or ordinance which may affect chiropractic practice, or over a rating or determination previously made by judicial or administrative proceeding.

This document may provide some assistance to third party payers in the evaluation of care, but is not by itself a proper basis for evaluation. Many factors must be considered in determining clinical or medical necessity. Further, guidelines require constant re-evaluation as additional scientific and clinical information becomes available.

This document does not necessarily reflect the consensus of all members of COCSA, nor is it intended to be an official policy statement of COCSA.

DISCLAIMER ON USE OF EXTRACT

Disclaimer to be used when quoting an extract or part only of these proceedings:

The reader is warned that the following is an extract or part only of a major publication suggesting guidelines for the practice of chiropractic.

Any part of the publication is likely to be confusing and/or misinterpreted unless read in the context of the full document, which includes detailed commentary, definitions, and explanation of rating systems used.

It is recommended that you obtain a copy of the full publication.

EFFECTIVE DATE

It is anticipated that those wishing to incorporate these guidelines in their practices would be aware of them and have had an opportunity to adopt them by July 1, 1993.

PROFESSIONAL TITLE

The use of professional title is governed by law and individual preference, and varies according to jurisdiction. Common titles used for the general practice of chiropractic include "chiropractor," "chiropractic physician," and "doctor of chiropractic."

Throughout this document, for reasons of uniformity and clarity, the word "practitioner" is used. This has the additional benefit of being inclusive, and denoting chiropractic and medical practitioners where the context requires.

Specialties exist in chiropractic in areas such as orthopedics, radiology, and sports chiropractic. Specialist practitioners are given their common and usual titles (e.g., chiropractic radiologist).

Conference for the Establishment of Guidelines for Chiropractic Quality Assurance and Standards of Practice

Mercy Center • San Francisco, California • January 25-30, 1992

A united effort by the chiropractic profession to establish its own practice guidelines, using accepted consensus methods.

Principal Sponsoring Agencies

Congress of Chiropractic State Associations

*

American Chiropractic Association

Canadian Chiropractic Association

International Chiropractors Association

*

Association of Chiropractic Colleges

Federation of Chiropractic Licensing Boards

Foundation for Chiropractic Education and Research

Commission Chairman
Scott Haldeman, D.C., M.D., Ph.D.

Commission Counsel
David Chapman-Smith, L.L. B. (Hons)

Commission Secretary
Donald M. Petersen Jr., H.C.D. (hc)

P.O. Box 6070
Huntington Beach,
California 92615
Tel: (714) 536-6557
Fax: (714) 536-1482

July 1, 1992

Robert Dark, D.C.
President
Congress of Chiropractic State Associations
1996-1998 "D" Street
San Bernardino, CA 92401 U.S.A

Dear Dr. Dark:

We are pleased to submit the final recommendations of the Commission for the Establishment of Guidelines for Chiropractic Quality Assurance and Practice Parameters.

In keeping with the Commission's mandate, the Guidelines have been developed pursuant to a formal consensus process, and by a representative group comprising 35 members of the chiropractic profession.

Respectfully submitted,

Scott Haldeman, DC, MD, PhD
Chairman, Steering Committee

Alan Adams, DC, MS
Member

Gerard W. Clum, DC
Member

Daniel T. Hansen, DC
Member

William Meeker, DC, MPH
Member

Reed Phillips, DC, PhD
Member

John J. Triano, DC, MA
Member

David Chapman-Smith
Commission Counsel

Donald M. Petersen, Jr., BS
Commission Secretary

Table of Contents

The dissemination of the *Guidelines for Chiropractic Quality Assurance and Practice Parameters* to their policyholders has been made possible by the generous donation of:

National Chiropractic Mutual Insurance Company

1441 29 Street, West Des Moines, Iowa 50265-1309
515-222-1736   WATS 800-247-8043   Fax 515-222-2999
Mailing Address: P.O. Box 9118 Des Moines, Iowa 50306-9118

Malpractice Insurance *Plus*

Board of Directors:

Phil L. Aiken, D.C.   Jerome McAndrews, D.C.
Arnold E. Cianciulli, D.C.   Stephen E. Owens, D.C.
Jerilynn Kaibel, D.C.   Louis Sportelli, D.C.
Don Krogh, D.C.

Executive Vice President
Larry Rister

*   *   *   *

OUM Group

11100 NE 8th Street, #90
Bellevue, WA 98004-4441

Professional Liability Insurance

*   *   *   *

In addition, the dissemination of the *Guidelines for Chiropractic Quality Assurance and Practice Parameters* has been made possible by generous donations from:

National Chiropractic Mutual Insurance Company
Foot Levelers, Inc.
OUM Group
California Chiropractic Association
Leander Health Technologies
Activator Methods
The Practice Resource Group
Motion Palpation Institute
Parker Chiropractic Resource Foundation
Synergy
Visual Odyssey

The above companies and institutions have all made substantial contributions to help defray the costs of dissemination of this important document to every licensed doctor of chiropractic within the United States. These contributors deserve our thanks and support for their dedication to the chiropractic profession. Distribution to all U.S. chiropractors without charge would not have otherwise been possible. The contributions are not, however, considered an endorsement nor have any of the above contributors passed upon the accuracy or adequacy of these practice guidelines.

Steering Committee

Chairman/Editor
Scott Haldeman, DC, MD, PhD
Chairman, Research Council, World Federation of
    Chiropractic
Associate Clinical Professor, Department of Neurology,
University of California, Irvine

Counsel/Editor
David Chapman-Smith, LLB (Hons)
Secretary-General, World Federation of Chiropractic,
Editor/Publisher, *The Chiropractic Report*

Secretary/Editor
Donald M. Petersen, Jr., BS
Editor/Publisher, *Dynamic Chiropractic*

Alan Adams, DC, MSEd, DACBN
Vice President of Chiropractic Education,
Los Angeles College of Chiropractic

Gerard W. Clum, DC
President, Life Chiropractic College West
President, Association of Chiropractic Colleges

Daniel T. Hansen, DC, FICC
Postgraduate Faculty,
Los Angeles College of Chiropractic
Private practice

William Meeker, DC, MPH
Dean of Research, Palmer College of Chiropractic West
President, Consortium for Chiropractic Research

Reed Phillips, DC, PhD, DACBR
President, Los Angeles College of Chiropractic
Vice President, Association of Chiropractic Colleges

John J. Triano, DC, MA
Director, Joint Ergonomics & Research Laboratory,
National College of Chiropractic

Commission Members

Alan Adams, DC, MSEd, DACBN
Vice President of Chiropractic Education
Professor, Clinical Science Division,
Los Angeles College of Chiropractic

Meredith H. Bakke, BA, DC
Chair, Professional Standards Committee,
Federation of Chiropractic Licensing Boards
Chair, Wisconsin Chiropractic Examining Board
Currently in practice

Ralph Boone, PhD, DC
President, Southern California College of Chiropractic

Linda Bowers, DC, BS, MT(ASCP), DABCO, DABCI,
   DACBN
Professor, Northwestern College of Chiropractic
Currently in practice

Gerard W. Clum, DC
President, Life Chiropractic College West
President, Association of Chiropractic Colleges

Tammy DeKoekkoek, DC, DABCO
Associate Professor, Dept. of Diagnosis, Principles &
   Practice, Los Angeles College of Chiropractic
Currently in practice

Robert Francis, DC
Dean of Clinical Sciences, Texas Chiropractic College
Currently in practice, with hospital appointments

Arlan W. Fuhr, DC
President, National Institute of Chiropractic Research
Postgraduate Faculty, Logan College of Chiropractic
Currently in practice

R. James Gregg, DC, FICA
President, International Chiropractors' Association
Currently in practice, with hospital appointments

Daniel T. Hansen, DC, FICC
Postgraduate Faculty, Los Angeles College of Chiropractic
Currently in practice

Donald Henderson, DC, BSc, FCCS(C), DACBR, FCCR, FICC
Vice President, Canadian Chiropractic Association
Chairman, CCA Standards of Practice Committee
Currently in practice

John Hsieh, DC, MS, RPT, LicA
Assistant Professor, Research Department,
Los Angeles College of Chiropractic
Currently in practice

Thomas Hyde, DC
President, ACA Council Sports Injuries and Physical Fitness
   Postgraduate Faculty, Logan College of Chiropractic
Currently in practice

Donald Kern, DC
President, Palmer College of Chiropractic
Secretary/Treasurer, Association of Chiropractic Colleges

Sponsoring Organizations

For the Consensus Conference

CHIROPRACTIC ORGANIZATIONS AND AGENCIES

Congress of State Chiropractic Associations
American Chiropractic Association
International Chiropractic Association
Canadian Chiropractic Association
Federation of Chiropractic Licensing Boards
Association of Chiropractic Colleges
Southeastern Chiropractic Federation
Texas Chiropractic Association
Foundation for Chiropractic Education and Research
National Upper Cervical Chiropractic Association

INDUSTRIAL SPONSORS

Activator Methods
The Chiropractic Report
Foot Levelers, Inc.

Leander Technologies
Motion Palpation Institute
National Chiropractic Mutual Insurance Company
Nutri-West
OUM Group Inc.
Superfeet
World Wide Chiropractic Placement Service

For distribution of the Guidelines to all members of the chiropractic profession

National Chiropractic Mutual Insurance Company
Foot Levelers, Inc.
OUM Group
California Chiropractic Association
Leander Health Technologies
Activator Methods
The Practice Resource Group
Motion Palpation Institute
Parker Chiropractic Resource Foundation
Synergy
Visual Odyssey

The above sponsors have all made substantial contributions to ensure that this document is distributed without charge to every licensed doctor of chiropractic in the United States. Such distribution would not have otherwise have been possible. The contributions are not, however, considered an endorsement nor have any of the above contributors passed upon the accuracy or adequacy of the practice guidelines.

Consultants

Thomas J. Allenburg, DC
Eden Prairie, MN

Herberto M. Alves, DC
San Leandro, CA

James Antos, DC
Ormond Beach, FL

Rand Baird, DC, MPH, RRA
Torrance, CA

Gregg N. Bakke, BS, DC
DeForest, WI

Howard A. Balduc, DC
Arlington, VA

Scott D. Banks, DC
Virginia Beach, VA

David J. Beneliyahu, DC, CCSP,
  DNBCT
Selden, NY

Thomas F. Bergmann, D.C.
Mendota Heights, MN

Grant Bjornson, DC
Bobcaygeon, Ontario, Canada

Raymond E. Breitbach, DC
Kaukauna, WI

Michael Buehler, DC, DACBR
Lake Zurich, IL

G. Curtis Casey, DC
Hayward, CA

Donald Cassata, PhD
Bloomington, MN

Mark G. Christensen, PhD
Greeley, CO

Arnold E. Cianciulli, BS, DC, MS,
  FICC, FACC
Bayonne, NJ

Timothy Conwell, DC, DABCO
Lakewood, CO

Jeffrey R. Cooley, DC, DACBR
Fullerton, CA

Michael Coon, DC, DAAPM
Charleston, SC

Robert Cooperstein, DC
Oakland, CA

Ian Coulter, PhD
Los Angeles, CA

John J. DeMatte, DC
Lehighton, PA

Frank DiGiacomo, DC
Seneca Falls, NY

Phillip S. Ebrall, BAppSc
  (Chiropractic)
Northcote, Victoria, Australia

Shelby Elliott, DC
Dayton, TX

Edward J. Farinelli, DC
Fort Collins, Colorado

Leonard J. Faye, DC
Los Angeles, CA

Edward Feinberg, DC
Santa Clara, CA

Richard A. Flaherty
Port Orchard, WA

Franklin W. Forman, DC
Gibson City, IL

Robert S. Francis, DC
Pasadena, TX

Robert Frewing, JD
Bellevue, WA

John H. Gantner, DC, DABCO
Medina, NY

Steven L. Gardner, DC
Portland, OR

Meridel I. Gatterman, MA, DC
Toronto, Ontario, Canada

David F. Gendreau, DC
Long Beach, CA

George A. Goodman, DC, FICC
St. Louis, MO

Adrian Grice, MSC, DC, FCCS
Weston, Ontario, Canada

John Grostic, DC
Kennesaw, GA

Martin I. Gruder, DC, FACO,
 DACAN
Foxboro, MA

Gary M. Guebert, DC, DACBR
Maryland Heights, MO

Warren I. Hammer, MS, DC, DABCO
Norwalk, CT

James D. Harrison, LLB, JD
Indianapolis, IN

Brad M. Hayes, DC
Tulsa, OK

Kurt Hegetschweiler, DC
Palos Verdes, CA

Ronald M. Hendrickson, MA, MSc
Arlington, VA

Samuel Homola, DC
Panama City, FL

Brian A. Howard, DC, MD, FACR
Charlotte, NC

Joseph W. Howe, DC, DACBR
Sylmar, CA

Tracy Hoyt, DC
Placentia, CA

Nancy E. Hudgins, JD
San Francisco, CA

Carl Robert Humphreys, MS, DC
Lombard, IL

Grant C. Iannelli, DC, DAAPM
Lombard, IL

Trevor Ireland, DC, FICA, FPC,
 FPAC, FICC
Anchorage, AK

Paul A. Jaskoviak, DC, DACAN
Bedford, TX

Jerilynn S. Kaibel, DC
San Bernardino, CA

Joseph C. Keating, Jr., PhD
Los Gatos, CA

Ronald G. Kelemen, DC
Little Rock, AR

Charles J. Keller, DC, FICA, FACC
Yonkers, NY

Davis L. Kinney, DC
Albany, GA

J. Todd Knudsen, DC
Whittier, CA

Matthew H. Kowalski, DC
Lombard, IL

Karl Kranz, DC
Schenectady, NY

Donald J. Krippendorf, DC, DABCN
St. Petersburg, FL

Thomas M. LaBrot, DC
Glendale, AZ

Dana J. Lawrence, DC
Lombard, IL

Craig Liebenson, DC
Los Angeles, CA

Vincent P. Lucido, DC, DABCO
Lakeland, FL

Jerome F. McAndrews, DC
Fairfax, VA

Kevin McCarthy, DC, DABCO
Sunnyvale, CA

Lawrence T. Markson, DC
New Hyde Park, NY

Duane J. Marquart, DC, DACBR
Ballwin, MO

Peter Martin, DC
Lancaster, CA

Edward L. Maurer, DC, DACBR
Kalamazoo, MI

Thomas B. Milus, DC, DABCO
Sunnyvale, CA

Robyn Mitchell, DC
Los Angeles, CA

Henry B. Morrison, DC
Toronto, Ontario, Canada

Kenneth S.J. Murkowski, BS, DC
Jackson, MI

William A. Nelson, DC
San Francisco, CA

Bruce Nordstrom, DC
Washington, DC

Michael W. Olff, DC
Hayward, CA

Paul J. Osterbauer, DC
Phoenix, AZ

D. Brent Owens, DC, FACO
Waldorf, MD

John Pammer, DC, DACBR
Catasaugua, PA

Marino R. Passero, DC
Norwalk, CT

Daniel J.M. Proctor, BSc, DC (Hon),
  FCCS(c)
Toronto, Ontario, Canada

Jeffrey B. Prystupa, DC
Longmont, CO

David J. Redding, DC
Dansville, NY

Gary D. Schultz, DC, DACBR
Costa Mesa, CA

Ronald Scott, DC
Perrine, FL

Dennis G. Semlow, DC
Fremont, MI

Ray Sherman, DC
East Aurora, NY

Robert P. Sherman, JD
Columbus, OH

Thomas Souza, DC
San Mateo, CA

Virgil V. Strang, DC
Davenport, IA

Patrick Sullivan, DC
Tequesta, FL

Gary Tarola, DC
Fogelsville, PA

John M. Taylor, DC, DACBR
San Diego, CA

Thomas J. Terenzi, MA, MS, MEd,
  DC, EdD
Rye, NY

A. Grant Thomson, DC
San Lorenzo, CA

Herbert J. Vear, DC, FCCS
Pickering, Ontario, Canada

Richard E. Vincent, DC
Burlington, MA

Frederick W. von Arx, DC
Redlands, CA

Dana Weary, DC
Spokane, WA

David Wickes, DC
Lombard, IL

Michael R. Wiles, BSc, MEd, DC,
  FCCS(c)
Scarborough, Ontario, Canada

Kerwin P. Winkler, DC
Aberdeen, SD

Francis Wisniewski, DC
Pittsburgh, PA

Terry R. Yochum, DC, DACBR
Federal Heights, CO

SUPPORT STAFF

Arlene Basilico
Debra da Silva
Doreen McIntyre
Anne O'Brien
Debi Pugliese

Chairman's Preface

Scott Haldeman, DC, MD, PhD

When the suggestion was made that a national consensus conference should be convened by the chiropractic profession, my first reaction was that this might be impossible. The divisions within the profession seemed to be large, and prior attempts to achieve agreement on how chiropractic should be practiced had often led to bitter argument which often became personal.

Although I agreed that national consensus on practice guidelines was essential for the advancement of chiropractic, initially I felt that the effort would be a waste of time and energy. The first indication that it might be possible was the positive response from leaders of the major associations to questions on the need for such a meeting. It then became evident that a consensus conference would only succeed if convened by a neutral sponsoring agency and governed by a completely independent Steering Committee. The sponsoring of a commission by the Congress of Chiropractic State Associations and the terms of that commission were the factors which allowed for the initial consensus protocol. Without COCSA the process would not have even begun.

COCSA, however, did not have the capacity to finance the conference and did not have the political influence to give the commission the prestige necessary to draw the quality of participants which a national consensus process required. The co-sponsorship of the commission by virtually every major association and agency within the chiropractic profession answered these needs, and removed any doubt that a conference was going to take place. It also greatly increased the importance of the commission as well as its visibility. It was the sponsoring of the commission that ensured the widespread involvement and input of the profession in the consensus process.

The primary decisions dealing with the consensus process and methods were the responsibility of the Steering Committee. The demands of the commission became the priority of each of the committee members for almost two years. The credit or criticism of the consensus process itself can be given to the Steering Committee. These individuals, with their understanding of the profession and of the mechanisms of gaining consensus, were responsible for the organization of the commission.

The hard work, however, was done by the 35 commission members. For over a year they were required to write and repeatedly read and correct the different drafts of the consensus document. They were asked to consult with authorities and prominent individuals in the profession and debate with each other to reach consensus. The captains had the responsibility of ensuring that all points of view were accurately included in the final document. Finally, the commission members had to debate and reach consensus at the Mercy Conference. This entailed four 16-hour days of high pressure concentration. In the final analysis all of the final document, as the consensus process requires, is the agreed views of these 35 chiropractors.

Special thanks must be given to the five wonderful staff members who assisted both before and after the conference but especially during the meeting itself. Their tremendous energy and skill was necessary for the repeated updating of the consensus document. Through their efforts the members of the commission were able to walk away from the conference with a completed text.

The commission has completed its task and has now disbanded. It can be said with confidence that this is the greatest consensus that has ever been achieved by the chiropractic profession. The document represents the best effort possible by a representative cross-section of the profession. Like any consensus process, there will and should be further discussion on many of the specific recommendations. There needs to be additional consensus conferences and meetings in the future. It is unlikely in the near future, however, that the resources and support that this first commission was able to generate will be repeated.

One important point made clear from this commission is that the chiropractic profession, given the right conditions, can reach a high degree of agreement on methods of practice. It has been a privilege to be part of this commission. As chairman, I offer this document to the chiropractic profession and request that the recommendations of this commission be endorsed as reasonable guidelines for chiropractic quality assurance and practice parameters.

Secretary's Report

Donald M. Petersen, Jr., BS, HCD(hc)

Never before in the history of the chiropractic profession has an event enjoyed such widespread support. From the initial commissioning by the Congress of Chiropractic State Associations (representing 42 state associations), to the industry sponsors, almost every branch of the chiropractic profession has supported and participated in the development of these proceedings.

Reviewing the list of organizations which sponsored the conference, it is clear that the academic, clinical, political (on both a national and state level), and regulatory sectors of the profession were well represented. The industry sponsors include some of the most respected companies supplying and supporting the chiropractic profession.

In a profession that hasn't yet accomplished substantial unity in any other way, unity by consensus on practice parameters was an impressive achievement. Even though the 35 members of the conference were from the full spectrum of chiropractic backgrounds they all had one thing in common: they were licensed chiropractic practitioners. This common bond was reflected in every opinion stated or position taken; in every deliberation the chiropractic profession came first.

This undertaking was far more ambitious than most thought wise. But it was driven by a frank understanding of what is being demanded by the political and economic environments that are shaping the future of the profession in the 1990s. The demands placed upon the committee captains, members, consultants, council, chairman, and staff were great, but in all cases the participants were more than equal to the task.

The entire process, from the initial discussion phase through to completion of the proceedings, required more than three years of work. The entire effort was funded for only $50,000. Each sponsor contributed $2,500. With the exception of staff time and very modest honorariums for the committee captains, all participants volunteered their time and talents. A conservative estimate of the market cost for development of such guidelines is at least $500,000. The difference was the dedication of those who gave of themselves to make it happen.

The majority of the funds collected was used to pay for travel and lodging for the conference at the Mercy Center.

This site was chosen because its retreat atmosphere was the most conducive to the long hours and effort required to produce these proceedings. All staff time was donated with the exception of the six days of the conference, for which the staff members were paid on a nominal basis, despite working more than 80 hours in that time.

There are many, many individuals throughout the chiropractic profession who made the event possible. Most of these have already been recognized at the beginning of this text. Obviously, without their commitment and vision, this conference would not have occurred.

In addition, there were five staff members who put forth exceptional effort to facilitate the smooth progress of the conference. Their dedication was exemplary, and shows the commitment many non-chiropractors have to the chiropractic profession. Each of them volunteered for the job and worked long hours at the side of the captains and their committees. The Commission would like to extend its special thanks to them:

Arlene Basilico
Debra da Silva
Doreen McIntyre
Anne O'Brien
Debi Pugliese

There should also be recognition for three observers who provided practical support to the Commission during the conference. Special thanks to:

Dr. Herb Vear
Karl Krantz
Thomas Bergman.

After the conference the editors were greatly assisted by Drs. Silvano Mior and Howard Vernon. The Commission and the editors wish to thank them.

One of the most important tasks involved in the development of practice guidelines is distribution to the field. The distribution of these proceedings is another example of the spirit of selflessness that has surrounded this effort. The industry that serves the chiropractic profession, having recognized the importance of these guidelines to the practitioner, has financed the distribution of the proceedings to every member of the chiropractic profession in the United States.

It is impossible at this point to predict the exact impact that these proceedings will have. The effects will certainly be far reaching; to some extent incalculable. The knowledge that this first effort at establishing national guidelines for practice provides a major step toward addressing the needs of the patient and assuring the quality and acceptance of chiropractic health care services is most reassuring. As the call for explicit standards of practice within health care increases, the public will know that the chiropractic profession respects and will continue to meet that call.

The Agency for Health Care Policy and Research and the Development of Clinical Practice Guidelines:

The Importance of the Consensus Process in the Development of National Health Policy

Hervé Guillain, MD, MPH
Senior Policy Analyst
Agency for Health Care Policy and Research
Washington, D.C.

The Agency for Health Care Policy and Research (AHCPR) was established by Congress in December 1989 as the successor to the National Center for Health Care Technology Assessment. AHCPR is one of eight agencies of the U.S. Public Health Service within the Department of Health and Human Services.

The mission of the Agency is to enhance the quality, appropriateness, and effectiveness of health care services as well as to improve access to these services.

The Agency pursues a variety of activities that fall under the following categories:

1. Developing a broad base of scientific research, methods and databases.
2. Demonstrating and evaluating new ways to organize, finance and direct health care services.
3. Assessing technologies being considered for reimbursement by federally-funded programs.
4. Facilitating the development of clinical practice guidelines and measurements of quality care.
5. Promoting the utilization of research findings and practice guidelines through a systematic effort of information dissemination.

These activities are carried out with the active involvement of health care providers, professional groups, and consumer organizations.

The Congressional legislation creating AHCPR also established within the Agency the Office of the Forum for Quality and Effectiveness in Health Care ('the Forum'). This Forum is responsible for facilitating the development, review and updating of clinically relevant guidelines, as well as standards of quality, performance measures, and medical review criteria. Guidelines are defined as:

Systematically developed statements to assist practitioner and patient decisions about appropriate health care for specific clinical circumstances.

In selecting guideline topics a variety of factors are taken into consideration, including:

1. High risks or potentially large benefits for large numbers of persons.
2. Wide variations among different treatment options and outcomes.
3. Costly services and procedures.
4. Evaluation data that are readily available or that can be readily developed.

As of April 1992, the following topics have been selected by AHCPR for guideline development:

- Management of Functional Impairment Due to Cataract in the Adult
- Diagnosis and Treatment of Benign Prostatic Hyperplasia
- Acute Pain Management: Operative or Medical Procedures and Trauma
- Management of Cancer-Related Pain
- Diagnosis and Treatment of Depressed Outpatients in Primary Care Settings
- Sickle Cell Disease
- Prediction, Prevention and Early Intervention of Pressure Ulcers
- Treatment of Stage Two and Greater Pressure Ulcers

Note: The opinions expressed in this article are solely those of the author and do not necessarily reflect those of the Agency for Health Care Policy and Research or the U.S. Public Health Service.

- Urinary Incontinence in Adults
- HIV Positive Asymptomatic Patients: Evaluation and Early Intervention
- Low Back Problems
- Development of Quality Determinants of Mammography
- Screening for Alzheimer's and Related Dementia
- Diagnosis and Treatment of Otitis Media in Children
- Diagnosis and Treatment of Heart Failure Secondary to Coronary Vascular Disease
- Post Stroke Rehabilitation

ESTABLISHING GUIDELINES

The Congressional legislation describes two mechanisms to promote the establishment of guidelines: (1) by convening panels of experts and health care consumers, and (2) by contracting with public and nonprofit private organizations. After electing to utilize the panel process for the initial set of guidelines, the Forum has issued Requests for Proposals (RFPs) and awarded several contracts on a competitive basis.

For each guideline topic, a panel of private-sector experts is convened, either by the Forum or the contractor. The selection of the panel chairperson and members is an important step in the guideline development process. Through a notice published in the Federal Register, nominations are sought from a broad range of interested individuals and organizations, including medical physicians representing specialty and general practices, nurses, allied health professionals and other health care practitioners as well as consumers with experience or information pertinent to the guideline being developed. At least one consumer representative sits on every guideline panel sponsored by AHCPR.

Whatever the mechanism through which guidelines are established, the foundation of the methodological approach to their development must be explicitness and scientific evidence. In the guideline development process, all available scientific evidence must be considered and the consequences of diagnostic or therapeutic alternatives weighed. This requires an extensive literature search followed by the critical review of all the relevant publications. To the extent possible, recommendations made in the guidelines should be based on the results of well designed studies. Evidence tables and methods such as meta-analysis are used to synthesize scientific information. All significant outcomes (especially those important to patients), benefits and harms are assessed.

In this process, some interventions may turn out to be much less or much more effective than generally recognized and conclusions may fly in the face of conventional medical thinking. But it should be remembered that the purpose of guidelines is to improve the quality and effectiveness of health care, not to codify the current practice of health care providers.

Only when scientific evidence is not available can subjective judgments be applied to make specific recommendations.

In this case, a formal consensus method such as the Delphi technique may be used.

Whether based on science or opinion, each statement included in the guideline must be explicit, i.e., methods, rationale and assumptions must be clearly explained.

ATTRIBUTES OF GUIDELINES

In addition to explicitness, the Institute of Medicine of the National Academy of Science has developed seven other attributes of practice guidelines to provide guidance for their establishment and evaluation:

Validity: Practice guidelines are valid if, when followed, they lead to the expected improvement in health outcomes. Clearly, it is essential to assess the impact a guideline has in order to determine its validity.

Reliability/reproducibility: This attribute refers both to the development and implementation of guidelines. Practice guidelines are reproducible and reliable if (1) given the same evidence and methods for guideline development, another set of experts produces the same statements, and (2) given the same clinical circumstances, the guidelines are interpreted and applied consistently by practitioners or other appropriate health care providers.

The assessment of the reliability/reproducibility of guidelines necessitates additional resources. It can be done by conducting studies in which two or more adequately selected panels establish guidelines on the same topic and two or more health care providers use the same guideline under the same clinical circumstances.

Clinical applicability: Practice guidelines should be as inclusive of appropriately defined patient populations as evidence and expert judgment permit, and they should explicitly state the populations to which statements apply.

Clinical flexibility: Practice guidelines should identify the specifically known or generally expected exceptions to their recommendations. Unless they have both clinical applicability and flexibility guidelines will be criticized for promoting "cookbook medicine."

Clarity: Practice guidelines should use unambiguous language, define terms precisely, and use logical, easy-to-follow modes of presentation.

In many instances graphics, flow charts and algorithms help users better understand the content of a guideline.

Multidisciplinary process: Practice guidelines should be developed by a process that includes the participation by representatives of key affected groups.

This issue is addressed not only through the careful selection of panel members, but also the Open Forum and the peer and pilot review described below.

Scheduled review: Practice guidelines should include statements about when they should be reviewed to determine whether revisions are warranted, given new clinical evidence or changing professional consensus.

As a result, the Forum is implementing a mechanism for updating guidelines after their initial release.

While developing a guideline, each panel holds a hearing session called "Open Forum." This session is announced in the Federal Register and every individual interested in providing oral or written testimony relevant to the guideline is invited to do so.

Once drafted, guidelines undergo peer and pilot review. They are sent to external experts for review and comments. They are also sent to practitioners who are asked to apply the draft guidelines and make suggestions to improve their usability.

DISSEMINATION OF GUIDELINES

When a guideline is completed, it is released in different formats, including:

Guideline report: This is the technical version that contains all the recommendations with complete supporting materials, including background information, methodology, literature review, scientific evidence tables, discussion, and a comprehensive bibliography. It serves as the source document for other guideline versions, and it is of particular interest to researchers, educators, professional organizations, and similar audiences.

Clinical practice guideline: This is the provider version that presents the specific statements and recommendations that constitute the actual guideline with brief supporting documentation and pertinent references for use as a desk reference for clinical decision-making in the care of patients.

Quick reference guide: This is the shortest of the provider versions of the guideline and serves as a companion to and a memory jogger for the Clinical Practice Guideline. It provides summary points of prevention, diagnosis, and treatment/management for ready reference on a day-to-day basis.

Patient's guide: This is the consumer version that features those aspects of the actual guideline that are the necessary knowledge base for the patient to be an active partner in care, especially where patients' preferences are involved, and a self-advocate for quality treatment. This booklet may be distributed directly to consumers or by clinicians to their patients when discussing and evaluating treatment options. In addition to the English version, a Spanish version is produced that reflects the same content but uses language and reading level appropriate to Hispanic populations.

To disseminate guidelines, a multi-pronged approach is used to reach target audiences. Health care providers and consumer organizations are encouraged to send the guidelines to their members and constituents. Print and electronic media are used to announce the formation of panels and the release of new guidelines, and to reinforce messages over time to facilitate adoption by the various users. AHCPR is also working jointly with the National Library of Medicine to make guidelines available through medical libraries and indexing services.

EVALUATION OF GUIDELINES

Finally, assisting health care providers and consumers in making decisions is not the same as evaluating practice. The former is done through practice guidelines, the latter through other instruments defined by the Institute of Medicine as follows:

Medical review criteria: Systematically developed statements that can be used to assess the appropriateness of specific health care decisions, services and outcomes.

Standards of quality: Authoritative statements of: (1) minimum levels of performance or results; or (2) excellent levels of performance or results; or (3) the range of acceptable performance or results.

Performance measures (provisional definition): Methods or instruments to estimate or monitor the extent to which the actions of a health care practitioner or provider conform to practice guidelines, medical review criteria, or standards of quality.

Since principles for translating guidelines into evaluation instruments are needed, the Forum has recently convened a work group to develop methods for deriving practice evaluation tools from recommendations made in the guidelines.

CONCLUSION

In conclusion, the establishment of clinical practice guidelines is a challenging task. It requires the careful selection of panel chairs and members; the involvement of content experts, consumers and methodologists; the participation of academicians and practitioners in the peer and pilot review process; the collaboration of communication specialists to disseminate the final products and make them acceptable and useful to health care providers and patients; and a comprehensive evaluation of the impact of guidelines after their release and implementation. The potential benefits that can be derived from such a major effort are considerable, particularly in terms of quality and effectiveness of health care. Furthermore, the development of guidelines will help identify the areas where scientific evidence is missing and outcomes research is needed.

BIBLIOGRAPHY

Institute of Medicine, Marilyn J. Field and Kathleen L. Lohr, editors. *Clinical Practice Guidelines: Directions for a New Program.* Washington, D.C.: National Academy Press, 1990.

Steven H. Woolf. *Interim Manual for Clinical Practice Development: A Protocol for Expert Panels Convened by the Office of the Forum for Quality and Effectiveness in Health Care.* AHCPR Pub. No. 91-0018. Rockville, MD: Agency for Health Care Policy and Research, Public Health Service, U.S. Department of Health and Human Services. May 1991.

Acute Pain Management Guideline Panel. *Acute Pain Management: Operative or Medical Procedures and Trauma. Clinical Practice Guideline.* AHCPR Pub. No. 92-0032. Rockville, MD: Agency for Health Care Policy and Research, Public Health Service, U.S. Department of Health and Human Services. February 1992.

Urinary Incontinence Guideline Panel. *Urinary Incontinence in Adults: Clinical Practice Guideline.* AHCPR Pub. No. 92-0038. Rockville, MD: Agency for Health Care Policy and Research, Public Health Service, U.S. Department of Health and Human Services. March 1992.

To order guideline products or to obtain further information on their availability, call the AHCPR Clearinghouse toll-free at 1-800-358-9295, or write to:

Center for Research Dissemination and Liaison
AHCPR Clearinghouse
P. O. Box 8547
Silver Spring, MD 20907

The Evolution and Mechanics of a Consensus Process

Paul Shekelle, MD, MPH
Rand Corporation

All of health care is being scrutinized. Providers are being asked to produce evidence that the care they deliver is effective. Variations in the medical care received by similar patients in differing geographic areas, or between the same patient seeing different providers in the same city, or even between the same patient seeing the same provider at two different points in time, have demonstrated that not all the health care delivered is appropriate. Part of the problem is that doctors often times don't know what is effective and what isn't, and are frequently left to make decisions based on anecdotal reports or limited clinical experience. Our task is to improve the capacity for providers to make informed decisions.

Chiropractic is no different from other health care professions in this respect. Large geographic variations in the intensity of chiropractic care delivered to those who seek care have been documented, even between areas only 90 miles apart. When the clinical faculty of one prominent chiropractic college were asked to estimate the effectiveness of a common chiropractic treatment on a representative patient with low-back pain in terms of a particularly important patient outcome, the estimates of the probability of the outcome ranged from 5% to 90%. Leading chiropractic clinicians and researchers from around the country had trouble agreeing on whether spinal manipulation was appropriate for certain types of patients with low-back pain. Clearly, the chiropractic profession is not immune to the questions of appropriateness and cost-effectiveness that face allopathic health care.

We would like to base our decisions about these matters on scientific demonstrations of benefit to patients, preferably in the form of well-conducted randomized controlled trials. "Benefit to patients" means outcomes that matter to patients. For patients with back pain, this means outcomes such as relief of pain and ability to resume usual activities. It does not mean outcomes such as improvement in straight-leg raising, or the appearance of lumbosacral radiographs, or the findings on palpation examination of the spine. For many tests and procedures, these data simply don't exist, either for allopathic care or chiropractic care. In the absence of such data, though, we may still provide some guidance to the clinician about the approach to common clinical conditions. The people assembled for this conference represent leading chiropractic clinicians and researchers, and their studied consideration of the issues in front of them may produce statements that reflect the consensus of chiropractic clinical judgment at this time.

In the deliberations that follow, the panel participants should be guided by the following principles when considering a test or procedure:

1. Is there any scientific data to support a conclusion about the use of this test or procedure, and what is the strength of that data?

2. In the absence of conclusive scientific data, is there a consensus of clinical opinion about the use of this test or procedure, and what is the magnitude of that consensus?

The reader of this document will want to know:

"Where recommendations are different from my current practice, why am I to believe this document is right?"

This gets to the question of validity of the statements made. Statements based on conclusive scientific evidence are more likely to be valid than statements based on weak clinical consensus, and the reader must be able to distinguish between the two. Each clinically important statement should be identified with the information that supports it: conclusive scientific evidence; some scientific evidence and true consensus of clinical judgment; weak or no scientific evidence but still true consensus of clinical judgment; less than true consensus of clinical judgment; disagreement.

Lastly, after the deliberations are through, the participants should be able to prioritize the needs of new clinical research. The first priority will be those areas of clinical importance which have true consensus of clinical judgment but no scientific data to support them, and those areas where there is frank disagreement among groups of clinicians as to the appropriate way to proceed. It is through efforts like these that the quality of health care, and the chiropractic profession, can continually improve.

History of the Commission

INTRODUCTION

Chiropractic is approaching its official centennial in 1995. The past decade has been the most challenging in the short history of this profession. Chiropractic is recognized and licensed in every state and province in North America, as well as many jurisdictions in Europe, Australia, New Zealand, Africa and the Middle East. There is increasing interest in chiropractic in multiple other countries in Europe, Africa, Asia, South and Central America, as well as numerous smaller countries where access to highly sophisticated and expensive medical and surgical treatment is limited.

This acceptance of chiropractic as a legitimate health care profession has occurred in part through an increasing emphasis on research by professional organizations and colleges. Research foundations have been formed in the United States, Canada, and Australia which have collected and spent millions of dollars funding research scholarships and research centers, as well as funding numerous specific proposals over the past two decades.

In the United States and Canada, chiropractic has been included in Medicare, most private insurance programs, workers' compensation, and personal injury reimbursement systems. Increasing numbers of health maintenance organizations (HMOs), preferred provider organizations (PPOs), and other managed health care systems are including chiropractic in their consideration of services and costs. An increasing number of research papers comparing the costs of chiropractic care in well-selected groups of patients have led to the conclusion that chiropractic may well be the most cost effective method of treatment for certain types of conditions. The new level of recognition of chiropractic has led to a search for quality assurance measures and practice parameters to better determine the exact nature of chiropractic practice.

The 1980s saw a growing acknowledgement by the major chiropractic associations that uniform standards would have to be developed within the chiropractic profession. Government agencies were in the process of determining the role of each of the health care professions in such programs as Medicare, workers' compensation, no-fault automobile insurance, and other managed health care delivery systems. At the same time, private insurance companies were increasing their control over the costs of health care. While negotiating with various agencies, chiropractic organizations were repeatedly told that only one standard of chiropractic practice would be tolerated. It became obvious that if the profession did not develop practice parameters itself then rules governing the practice of chiropractic would be imposed by these agencies without chiropractic input.

The acceptance of chiropractic also had the effect of forcing greater responsibility on the profession to improve the overall quality of care given by individual chiropractors. A rapid increase in the number of malpractice suits against chiropractors demanded expert opinion on the basis by which chiropractic standards should be judged. The lack of well-defined practice guidelines has contributed to a proliferation of chiropractic "experts" and texts that, more often than not, are contradictory.

By the end of the 1980s the need for a consensus within the chiropractic profession on guidelines for practice and quality assurance had become critical. The general crisis in health care costs in North America had resulted in an overhaul of Medicare and other health insurance programs. The cost of malpractice was approaching that of the non-surgical medical specialties. Attempts to unify the chiropractic profession under one national association had failed. Each of the chiropractic associations, however, acknowledged the necessity for a forum to discuss and develop standards. Statements supporting a national consensus conference on guidelines for practice were made by the presidents of the four national associations. The following excerpts from letters serve as examples of the support by the professional organizations:

> "The board of the Congress of Chiropractic State Associations enthusiastically endorses your concept of a chiropractic summit meeting." Brad M. Hayes, DC, President COCSA, April 1989.

"I am enthusiastic about the idea of interested parties coming together and discussing, in a constructive fashion, the needs of the profession and our patients." Kenneth L. Luedtke, DC, FICC, President ACA, April 1989.

"We agree that a meeting of the organizational leaders of the profession would be constructive and that professional facilitators should be utilized at such a conference." Fred H. Barge, DC, Ph.C., President ICA, April 1989.

"We are in agreement with a summit conference which encourages communication between the factions in chiropractic." Douglas Gates, DC, President and Joseph Donofrio, DC, Chairman FSCO, April 1989.

PRIOR GUIDELINES CONFERENCES

A number of conferences and workshops were held in 1989 and 1990 in an attempt to define priorities for the chiropractic profession and to develop a consensus on practice parameters. In August 1989, the American Chiropractic Association convened a "Think Tank" in Chicago which brought together a number of prominent academic and politically active individuals within the profession. A professional facilitator was able to help the participants at this workshop develop a consensus on the priorities of the profession. One of the major goals and objectives for the profession was "to identify, adopt, and implement standards of practice maximizing quality of care." At this workshop, it was pointed out that the federal government was requiring that each health profession have established guidelines for practice within two years.

The California Chiropractic Association and the Consortium for Chiropractic Research established a joint committee in 1987 with the view to researching, understanding, and making recommendations on standards of care in chiropractic. A number of other state associations convened conferences or established task forces on quality of care issues. A meeting was held in Seattle on March 2-3, 1990, sponsored by the ACA Council on Technique, the Washington Chiropractic Association and the Consortium for Chiropractic Research to investigate the consensus process, to evaluate techniques, and to set agendas for further investigation.

At the same time standards of practice were developed in a number of states such as California, Georgia and Ohio. The Canadian Chiropractic Association established a committee to develop practice guidelines which would assist in negotiations on new legislation being planned in different provinces. At the same time the Chiropractors Association of Australia had developed a Committee on Chiropractic Clinical Practice and was investigating standards in other countries. It became clear, however, that varying standards in different states or regions was not the ideal situation. A national, or preferably a North American or international, standard was by far the most desirable situation.

In 1989 and early 1990, intensive informal discussions were taking place throughout the country on the various mechanisms which were available to develop national guidelines. The RAND Corporation was commissioned to evaluate the appropriateness of spinal manipulation for low-back pain and to develop specific indications and contraindications for chiropractic care. By using the consensus process and literature review developed by the RAND panel it was demonstrated that, given the right situation, a group of chiropractors could reach a high level of consensus on the indications for spinal manipulation. It was even possible to gain consensus when chiropractors and medical specialists and scientists were placed on the same panel.

Although the RAND project proved valuable in developing a list of categories of low-back pain which are most likely to respond to chiropractic care, it did not address many larger issues of chiropractic practice and quality assurance. It became clear that the only way a wide consensus could be achieved was to bring together varied and representative points of view, clinical practice methods, and philosophies. This could only occur if a neutral forum could be found, one which was not dominated by any association, school of thought or geographical region. It was also of fundamental importance that such a forum represented the practicing chiropractor as strongly as academic and scientific members of the profession.

THE COMMISSION

On February 16, 1990, after considerable discussion, the Congress of Chiropractic State Associations (COCSA) agreed to commission an independent steering committee to convene a workshop on chiropractic quality assurance. The letter of commission provided:

"The Board of Directors and the delegates to the Congress of Chiropractic State Associations unanimously agreed to the following:

1. To commission your committee to convene a workshop on chiropractic quality assurance with the express purpose of developing a consensus of chiropractic opinion and providing a document outlining recommendations on this issue.

2. To permit the committee to independently develop a list of participants in the workshop which should include individuals with academic, scientific, clinical and political knowledge and reputation.

3. Not to directly interfere or attempt to influence the program or the published proceedings of the workshop. However, this recognizes that at least one representative from COCSA will be invited to participate in the workshop.

4. That the published document will list COCSA as a primary sponsor of the workshop.

5. That the committee may approach other professional organizations, academic institutions, and corporations as co-sponsors of the workshop and solicit funds for sponsorship."

The function of the Steering Committee was thus to establish a consensus group of participants and a procedure for them to follow that would lead to a meeting at which guidelines or standards for quality assurance in chiropractic practice throughout North America would be agreed upon and recommended. The Steering Committee included:

Scott Haldeman, DC, MD, PhD, Chairman/Editor
David Chapman-Smith, Esq., Counsel/Editor
Donald Petersen, Jr., BS, Secretary/Editor
Alan Adams, DC, MS
Gerard W. Clum, DC
Daniel T. Hansen, DC
William Meeker, DC, MPH
Reed Phillips, DC, PhD
John J. Triano, DC, MA

Committee members were chosen on the basis of their understanding of the consensus process, their representation of different points of view, and their ability to encourage the most appropriate members of the profession to participate in the Commission—the body that would represent the profession in the actual work of establishing guidelines.

The Steering Committee met on three occasions during 1990 and had a number of conference calls as it developed the process. Discussion was held with professional facilitators. Intense discussion and consultation took place with multiple individuals within chiropractic colleges, state and national organizations, and the practicing profession.

SPONSORSHIP OF THE CONFERENCE

A primary concern of the Steering Committee was that the Commission not be considered under the excessive influence of any one organization or group within the profession. This required that the Commission be sponsored by the widest possible spectrum of organizations and agencies. This, in turn, required that the sponsorship fee be kept low enough to allow smaller organizations to participate. The final fee decided upon was $2,500 per sponsor, with all organizations and agencies to be given an equal level of sponsorship.

Industries which provided products and services to the chiropractic profession were then approached to sponsor the Commission at the same level as the professional organizations and agencies.

Twenty sponsors came forward, 10 from industry and 10 professional organizations and agencies. This gave the Commission a budget of $50,000 to develop a consensus document on chiropractic quality assurance and parameters of practice.

The following is a list of the sponsors:

CHIROPRACTIC ORGANIZATIONS AND AGENCIES
Congress of State Chiropractic Associations
American Chiropractic Association
International Chiropractors Association
Canadian Chiropractic Association
Federation of Chiropractic Licensing Boards
Foundation for Chiropractic Education and Research
Association of Chiropractic Colleges
Southeastern Chiropractic Federation
Texas Chiropractic Association
National Upper Cervical Chiropractic Association

INDUSTRIAL SPONSORS
Activator Methods
The Chiropractic Report
Foot Levelers, Inc.
Leander Technologies
Motion Palpation Institute
National Chiropractic Mutual Insurance Company
Nutri-West
OUM Group, Inc.
Superfeet
Worldwide Chiropractic Placement Service

THE PROCESS OF CONSENSUS DEVELOPMENT

The Steering Committee spent approximately six months developing the list of potential participants for the Commission. Extensive consultation was held with members of different chiropractic organizations throughout North America. The initial 30 invitees were supplemented with five additional members later in the process, when certain areas of the profession were considered to be under-represented. On February 10, 1991, the members of the Commission were formally invited to participate in the consensus development process. All members, as with Steering Committee members, volunteered their time without compensation. The final distribution of the Commission was as follows:

1. **TOTAL NUMBER:** 35 members, all graduate chiropractors.
2. **PRIVATE PRACTICE:** 23 members from 14 states and provinces: Arizona, California, Florida, Illinois, Michigan, New York, North Carolina, Ohio, Ontario, Pennsylvania, Saskatchewan, Texas, Washington, and Wisconsin.
3. **COLLEGES:** 24 members with some college affiliations; 8 full-time, 12 with some research experience. The following colleges were represented: Canadian Memorial Chiropractic College, Life Chiropractic College West, Logan College of Chiropractic, Los Angeles College of Chiropractic, National College of Chiropractic, Northwestern College of Chiropractic, Palmer College

of Chiropractic, Palmer College of Chiropractic West, Southern California College of Chiropractic, and Texas Chiropractic College.

4. **ASSOCIATIONS:** 18 members, either currently or in the past, held senior offices in national, state or other associations. The following associations were represented: American Chiropractic Association, Canadian Chiropractic Association, International Chiropractors' Association, Federation of Chiropractic Licensing Boards, Congress of Chiropractic State Associations, National Chiropractic Mutual Insurance Company, National Institute of Chiropractic Research, American Chiropractic College of Radiology, Straight Chiropractic Academic Standards Association, Association of Chiropractic Colleges, various state associations and licensing examining boards.

PREPARATION OF THE GUIDELINES

The guidelines took over a year to develop and the process was designed to have the greatest amount of professional input that was possible. At the same time no formal input was allowed from any association or special interest group. It was necessary to produce multiple drafts of the guidelines, each of which was to be the subject of debate and discussion at different levels.

1. Initial Literature Review and Topic Development

Development of guidelines was divided into 15 chapters based on the classic patient-doctor contact. Committees were chosen for each chapter, each with a captain or chairman. Captains were instructed to develop consensus statements on their topic and describe how a practicing practitioner should evaluate and/or manage patients. Purposes of guidelines were to: a) Protect patients; b) Provide defined defensible practice parameters which could be followed by practitioners as a general rule; c) Provide guidelines as opposed to imposing rigid standards, by which outside agencies could judge the practice of individual practitioners.

The captains were instructed to conduct a literature search and complete an outline by May 3, 1991. The captains then met with the Steering Committee in Toronto at the World Chiropractic Congress in May 1991, to review and obtain input on their chapters. The final format for the guidelines document was developed and discussed.

2. The First Draft—Input from Consultants

The captains were now given three months to complete the first draft of the guidelines on their topics. They were instructed to seek consultants to assist them in this process. No limit to the number or type of consultants was established. Consultants could be from colleges, state or national associa-

tions, those in general chiropractic practice or from other professions. The deadline for the first draft was August 1, 1991.

3. Expert Review

The captains were then instructed to submit the completed first draft to at least two experts to ensure accuracy of the literature review and the rationale for the various recommendations. Following this they were required to complete a second draft of the guidelines, incorporating the suggestions of the experts where appropriate. The second drafts were supposed to follow similar formats and include specific guideline recommendations. Where specific difficulties were encountered, the Steering Committee was available for consultation. Deadline for the second draft was October 1, 1991.

4. Review by the Topic Committee

Each second draft chapter or topic was referred to seven appointed members of the Commission for critical review. The captain was to begin the consensus process by mail, telephone or direct meetings with members of the committee. An amended literature review, and definitions and an introduction were included in the third draft. Discussion of the assessment criteria for the chapter and specific recommendations on guidelines took place. At this time the first minority opinions were to be written into chapters. The committee had the opportunity to invite input from consultants to ensure full discussion of the topic. A list of all members of the Commission was published in a number of major national chiropractic publications. Any correspondence received at the secretariat was referred to the committee discussing the topic. Deadline for the third draft was December 24, 1991.

5. Review by the Entire Commission

The third draft of all the chapters was sent to all 35 members of the Commission, who reviewed the entire document with special emphasis on the recommendations. This was the final opportunity for input by members of the profession other than the Commission. It was suggested that any serious disagreement with the formal recommendations be drafted as a minority report for consideration at the conference. In this way, before attending the workshop meeting at the Mercy Center, the entire document was reviewed by all participants. The stage was set.

THE MERCY CONSENSUS CONFERENCE

The climax of the consensus process to develop the guidelines was held in a workshop retreat at the Mercy Conference Center in Burlingame, California, on January 25-30, 1992. This center was picked because of its seclusion, facilities and lack of distractions. The participants were supported by an outstanding administrative unit with appropriate computer equipment and a staff of five with superior word processing and editorial skills. They ensured that all proposals were promptly available for debate and that decisions made during the meeting were included in the guidelines. This entailed 16-20 hours of work each day, and allowed the final document to be complete except for final editing by the end of the meeting.

The conference was opened with presentations by Hervé Guillain, MD, from the federal Agency for Health Care Policy and Research (AHCPR) who discussed "the importance of the Consensus Process in the Development of National Health Policy," and Paul Shekelle, MD, MPH, one of the primary investigators of the RAND Study. His presentation was "The Evolution and Mechanics of a Consensus Process." This helped to set the stage for the actual work of reaching a consensus on the multiple recommendations which had been proposed.

1. The Committee Deliberations

On each of the first three days of the conference the Commission members were divided into five committees of seven members under the chairmanship of the captain initially responsible for developing the chapter. After three days, at five chapters a day, all topics had been reviewed.

The committees deliberated for at least three hours each morning, and were directed to reach a consensus on the chapter being discussed. Any two members of the committee could propose a minority opinion. The committee was to vote on each recommendation. A vote of four members or more constituted a majority position. A vote of two or three members constituted a minority opinion. The final recommendations and changes to the chapter were then inserted by the captain assisted by the staff member assigned to that committee.

2. The General Session

The general session each afternoon was conducted in a round table format. The Commission members had reviewed the third draft of each chapter in advance. The committee captains were asked to present only the changes that had been made in the committee session. These were all duplicated on overhead transparencies. Each recommendation was taken in order and voted on by the Commission members. If there was any dissenting vote, the recommendation was opened to amendment. Only formal amendments were accepted and had

to be supported by five members of the Commission for further discussion. Each amendment was then voted on and a majority of the members (18) was necessary for changes to the recommendation to be included as part of the majority opinion. Any amendment which was not accepted by the majority could then be submitted at any time during the conference by 25 percent (nine members) of the Commission.

No chapter was closed until the final discussion on the fourth day when each chapter was summarized and a table of all recommendations was presented to the Commission. The members were then asked to vote that the chapter, with all recommendations as amended and any minority opinions, accurately reflected the consensus of the Commission on that chapter. All chapters were unanimously accepted by the Commission. The final draft recommendations or guidelines in each chapter as accepted had to be signed off by the committee captains as being accurate.

When all debate was complete, all chapters had been closed by unanimous vote, and all captains had signed off on their chapters, the conference was adjourned.

PUBLICATION OF THE CONSENSUS DOCUMENT

Extensive deliberations took place within the Steering Committee and with corporate sponsors and national associations concerning the publication of the consensus document. Inexpensive publication and widespread distribution were known to be essential to the overall impact and success of the venture. Funding was not available to the Steering Committee for publication. At the Mercy Conference it was decided to form an independent publication committee to arrange for publication. It was elected on the last day of the conference. The Steering Committee ceased to exist on the last day of the consensus workshop or conference, having completed its commission.

It was recommended that the Publication Committee submit the final consensus document to the various chiropractic organizations for discussion and possibly endorsement. On April 11th, 1992, the Federation of Chiropractic Licensing Boards expressly endorsed the recommendations of this Commission at its annual meeting, thus making this the first officially sanctioned chiropractic consensus process. The actual wording of the endorsement has been included at the end of this document. The work of this Commission is currently being considered by a number of other official bodies and associations.

Introduction and Guide to Use of These Guidelines

A. INTRODUCTION

The majority of standard treatments provided by all health providers for all disorders, whether these disorders be minor or life-threatening, have not been validated by formal scientific methodology. Only about 15 percent of medical interventions are supported by valid evidence and many have never been assessed at all. [1,2]

These facts, together with the unacceptable variations in practice and cost of health care, explain why the public and governments are now insisting that there be better guidelines for practice. To ensure that improved national guidelines for each health care specialty were developed without delay, the U.S. federal government established the Agency for Health Care Policy and Research in December 1989. At the time the message was clear—either the health professions developed their own guidelines or third parties would impose them.

These guidelines, developed according to established consensus methods, are the initial response of the chiropractic profession.

B. FORMAT

These guidelines appear in topic chapters under the following headings:

History and Physical Examination
Diagnostic Imaging
Instrumentation
Clinical Laboratory
Record Keeping and Patient Consents
Clinical Impression
Modes of Care
Frequency and Duration of Care
Reassessment
Outcome Assessment
Collaborative Care

Contraindications and Complications
Preventive/Maintenance Care and Public Health
Professional Development

Each chapter is organized according to the same outline, namely:

    I. Overview
    II. Definitions
    III. List of Subtopics
    IV. Literature Review
    V. Assessment Criteria
    VI. Recommendations
    VII. Comments, Summary or Conclusion
    VIII. References
    IX. Minority Opinions

The "Recommendations" (Part VI) in each chapter are the guidelines. Subjects covered by guidelines in each chapter are indicated in the "List of Subtopics" (Part III).

For easy reference all recommendations are numbered sequentially, and repeated in summary form in tables at the end of the publication.

C. ASSESSMENT CRITERIA—RATINGS SYSTEMS

Part V of each chapter lists the "Assessment Criteria" or ratings system(s) used to evaluate each recommendation. The key to comprehending the new chiropractic guidelines lies in understanding the ratings systems.

Developing appropriate ratings was a major challenge because the technique of ratings is still evolving and the guidelines cover a broad territory, the whole practice of chiropractic. Ratings for one aspect (e.g., when it is appropriate to use plain film x-rays or a given treatment approach—i.e., technical matters) are not suitable for other aspects of practice (e.g., what records should be kept or when patient consents are required—i.e., procedural matters).

Two basic systems were adopted and appear in Figures 1 and 2. Some chapters use System I, some System II, and others both systems. To identify which system(s) is/are used in a given chapter look at Part V (Assessment Criteria) in that chapter.

Procedure Ratings (System I)

This system is suited to scientific/technical areas of practice.

1. Procedures are judged, in descending order of approval, established, promising, equivocal, investigational, doubtful and inappropriate. See Figure 1 for definitions.
2. The first three ratings (established, promising, and equivocal) are all positive. Procedures with any of these ratings are approved for use and reimbursement in clinical practice.

The remaining three ratings (investigational, doubtful, and inappropriate) are negative. A procedure currently rated "investigational" has the potential to be raised to an acceptable level and a positive rating on the basis of future clinical and scientific evidence.

A specific procedure may have more than one current rating depending upon the circumstances in which it is used—see examples below.

3. As noted in Figure 1, the rating chosen for a procedure is linked to the quality of evidence in support of utilization of that procedure.

The following examples illustrate how the rating should be interpreted.

a. In Chapter 2, on Diagnostic Imaging, Recommendations 2.8.1 and 2.8.2 deal with stress radiographs. The value of their use is rated as *established* in the assessment of degenerative, traumatic or post-surgical instabilities, but *equivocal* for other conditions and circumstances.

Both are positive recommendations. In the first case there is Class I evidence in support (i.e., controlled clinical trials—for full definition of Class I evidence see Figure 1). This quality of evidence justifies the rating *established*. The strength of this rating is Type A.

In the second case there can only be a rating of *equivocal* because, as Recommendation 2.8.2 indicates, there is no Class I evidence. Most evidence is Class III. This has led to a Type C positive recommendation—which is *equivocal*.

Figure 1 Procedure Ratings (System I)

Established: Accepted as appropriate by the practicing chiropractic community for the given indication in the specified patient population.

Promising: Given current knowledge, this appears to be appropriate for the given indication in the specified patient population. As more experience and long-term follow-up are accumulated, this interim rating will change. This connotes provisional acceptance, but permits a greater role for the current level of clinical use.

Equivocal: Current knowledge exists to support a given indication in a specified patient population, though value can neither be confirmed nor denied. As more evidence and experience accumulates this rating will change. Expert opinion recognizes a need for caution in general application.

Investigational: Evidence is insufficient to determine appropriateness. Further study is warranted. Use for a given indication in a specified patient population should be confined to research protocols. As more experience and evidence accumulates, this rating will change.

Doubtful: Given current knowledge, this appears to be inappropriate for the given indication in the specified patient population. As more experience and long-term follow-up are accumulated, this interim rating will change.

Inappropriate: Regarded by the practicing chiropractic community as unacceptable for the given indication in the specified patient population.

Quality of Evidence

Class I: Evidence provided by one or more well-designed controlled clinical trials; or well-designed experimental studies that address reliability, validity, positive predictive value, discriminability, sensitivity, and specificity.

Class II: Evidence provided by one or more well-designed controlled observational clinical studies, such as case-control, cohort studies, etc.; or clinically relevant basic science studies that address reliability, validity, positive predictive value, discriminability, sensitivity, and specificity; and published in refereed journals.

Class III: Evidence provided by expert opinion, descriptive studies or case reports.

Strength of Recommendation Ratings

Type A: Strong positive recommendation. Based on Class I evidence or overwhelming Class II evidence when circumstances preclude randomized clinical trials.

Type B: Positive recommendation based on Class II evidence.

Type C: Positive recommendation based on strong consensus of Class III evidence.

Type D: Negative recommendation based on inconclusive or conflicting Class II evidence.

Type E: Negative recommendation based on evidence of ineffectiveness or lack of efficacy based on Class I or Class II evidence.

b. There must be one or more controlled trials (Class I evidence) for a Type A rating of *established*. Other forms of studies (Class II evidence) or clinical experience, expert opinion and case reports (Class III) may be a perfectly adequate basis for a positive recommendation, but the strength of that recommendation can only be Type B (*promising*) or Type C (*equivocal*).

c. For completeness every recommendation or guideline should have both a rating (e.g., *equivocal*) and a strength (e.g., Type C).

Strength of rating is included in two chapters only, Instrumentation (Chapter 3) and Frequency and Duration of Care (Chapter 8). In the latter, for example, Recommendation 8.4.1. includes guidelines for adjustive procedures for acute, uncomplicated, low-back disorders. Here the rating is *established*, but it is not presented in the same manner as the other example given above. There is reference to the rating of *established* and the class of evidence in support, but the fact ultimately highlighted is strength of recommendation—which is Type A.

Procedure Ratings (System II)

This system is suited to procedural/administrative aspects of practice. Accordingly it is used in chapters such as History and Physical Examination (Chapter 1), Record Keeping and Patient Consents (Chapter 5) and Collaborative Care (Chapter 11). Again, one can discover which rating system is being used by looking at Part V (Assessment Criteria) of each chapter.

1. Rating levels are necessary, recommended, discretionary and unnecessary.

2. Rating is once again linked to quality of evidence—see Figure 2 for details.

Special Rating System for Complications

A special third rating system has been developed for the unique area of potential complications of high-velocity thrust procedures. See Part V (Assessment Criteria), Chapter 12. The basic rating is the level of contraindication, which may be:

- No contraindication
- Relative contraindication: "high-velocity thrust procedures may be used with appropriate care and/or modification"
- Relative to absolute contraindication: "careful clinical judgment dictates whether contraindication is relative or absolute with each specific patient"
- Absolute contraindication

The recommended level of contraindication appears as a short paragraph in each recommendation and is supported by specific evidence. For example Recommendation 12.1.2, which relates to high-velocity thrusts in the presence of subacute or chronic ankylosing spondylitis, reads:

12.1.2 Sub-acute and/or chronic ankylosing spondylitis and other chronic arthropathies in which there are no signs of ligamentous laxity, anatomic subluxation or ankylosis are *not contraindications* to high-velocity thrust procedures applied to the area of pathology.
Risk-of-Complication Rating:
Severity: Minimal
Condition Rating: Type I, II
Quality of Evidence: Class II, III

Figure 2 Procedure Ratings (System II)

Necessary: Strong positive recommendation based on Class I evidence, or overwhelming Class II evidence when circumstances reflect compromise of patient safety.

Recommended: Positive recommendation based on consensus of Class II and/or strong Class III evidence.

Discretionary: Positive recommendation based on strong consensus of Class III evidence.

Unnecessary: Negative recommendation based on inconclusive or conflicting Class II, III evidence.

Quality of Evidence

The following categories of evidence are used to support the ratings:

Class I: A. Evidence of clinical utility from controlled studies published in refereed journals.
B. Binding or strongly persuasive legal authority such as legislation or case law.

Class II: A. Evidence of clinical utility from the significant results of uncontrolled studies in refereed journals.
B. Evidence provided by recommendations from published expert legal opinion or persuasive case law.

Class III: A. Evidence of clinical utility provided by opinions of experts, anecdote and/or by convention.
B. Expert legal opinion.

What this means is:

1. The conditions mentioned are not contraindications to high-velocity thrust procedures.
2. The severity of potential complications is not high—for definitions of minimal, moderate, and high-level severity of complication see Part V, Assessment Criteria, paragraph B.
3. On the basis of the severity rating just given and probability or likelihood of harm, there is now a "condition rating" of Type I—for definitions of Type I, Type II and Type III conditions ratings see Part V, paragraph A.
4. Finally, there is a rating for quality of evidence—for definitions of Class I, Class II and Class III evidence see Part V, paragraph D.

Chapter 12 lists the various potential complications of high-thrust procedures under categories of:

Articular Derangements
Bone Weakening and Destructive Disorders
Circulatory and Cardiovascular Disorders
Neurological Disorders

D. THE RECOMMENDATIONS IN CONTEXT

Individual recommendations or guidelines must be read in context. Thus:

1. Each chapter has a section entitled "Definitions" (Part II). It is often important to consult this section to understand the recommendations.

For example under Modes of Care (Chapter 7) high-velocity thrust procedures are rated *established* for neuromusculoskeletal disorders (Recommendation 7.1.2). The question might be raised whether this includes respiratory or digestive dysfunctions assessed as having a somatovisceral component. In chiropractic practice the basis for management is the presence of subluxation or spinal dysfunction, and such disorders can be seen as neuromusculoskeletal.

In this context the answer is no—see the definition (Part II —end). For the purposes of this chapter the term "neuro-musculoskeletal" excludes internal organ dysfunctions.

2. The rest of the chapter may modify a particular recommendation. The overview (Part I in each chapter) often does. In addition, other recommendations often qualify a given recommendation.

Under Chapter 8 on Frequency and Duration of Care, for example:

a. Recommendation 8.4.1 suggests a guideline for management of patients with acute, uncomplicated disor-
ders—four weeks of manual procedures, two weeks of two different approaches, with continuing care only if there is "significant" documented improvement.
b. The determination whether this recommendation applies to patients with neck pain and headache as well as low-back pain may only become apparent on reading comments in the overview (Part I, paragraph 3). It does.
c. The number of treatments recommended per week appears in Recommendations 8.2.1 and 8.5.1, i.e., 3-5 per week during the first two weeks, depending upon the individual patient, then decreasing in frequency.
d. The answer to whether four weeks of treatment is an absolute time within which there must be significant documented improvement is found in the Overview (Part I), and Recommendation 8.1.1. which provides for some of the factors that modify the guideline and treatment plan—e.g., severe pain, previous episodes, or pre-existing conditions.
e. In summary, Recommendation 8.4.1 can only be understood when read in context, and together with other recommendations.

Properly understood, these recommendations do not give a "cookbook" approach to duration of care or number of treatments. The guidelines on these matters may be modified by multiple factors, including pre-existing conditions, re-injury or failure to comply with other aspects of management. The facts may explain why the guideline is exceeded and the care still considered appropriate in an individual case.

Individual chiropractic practice should conform with the guidelines in general, and document reasons for continuing with manual procedures in the absence of anticipated improvement in specific cases. A problem arises only when the management of a specific case is outside the guidelines with no apparent reason.

E. CONSENSUS LEVELS

Next to each recommendation or guideline there appears a level of consensus on a scale of 1-5. This defines the level of agreement for that recommendation as voted by the 35 members of the consensus panel at the Mercy Center meeting. Consensus levels adopted were:

Level 1 (Full agreement)—over 85% (more than 30 votes out of 35)

Level 2 (Consensus)—70-85% (25-29 votes)

Level 3 (Majority/Minority Opinions)—51-69% (i.e. a majority)

Level 4 (Multiple Minority Opinions)—26-50%

Level 5 (No Consensus)—no agreement by more than 25%

The great majority of recommendations received Level 1 consensus or full agreement. In the few cases where there was Level 3 consensus a minority opinion is noted in the recommendations and there is a cross-reference to the minority opinion which appears at the end of the chapter (Part IX).

The meeting produced an extremely high level of consensus. Most recommendations received Level 1 consensus, a few received Level 2 and Level 3, none received Level 4 or Level 5.

F. PROFESSIONAL TITLE

The use of professional title is governed by law and individual preference, and varies according to jurisdiction. Common titles used for the general practice of chiropractic include "chiropractor," "chiropractic physician," and "doctor of chiropractic."

Throughout this document, for reasons of uniformity and clarity, the word "practitioner" is used. This has the additional benefit of being inclusive, and denoting chiropractic and medical practitioners where the context requires.

Specialties exist in chiropractic, in areas such as orthopedics, radiology, and sports chiropractic. Specialist practitioners are given their common and usual titles (e.g., chiropractic radiologist).

G. CONCLUSION—HOW TO FIND A GUIDELINE

It is suggested that the following process be followed:

1. Consider which chapter will cover the guideline topic in question. (e.g., adequate patient identification in office records will be found in Chapter 5 on Recordkeeping and Patient Consents).

2. Consult Part III (List of Subtopics) of the relevant chapter. This gives a breakdown of the guideline topics in that chapter. (In Chapter 5, patient identification appears under Part III, paragraph A).

3. Turn to Part VI of the chapter, which lists the recommendations or guidelines, and consult the relevant guidelines. (Paragraph 3, which includes Guidelines 5.1.4 to 5.1.6., deals with patient identification).

4. Read the guidelines carefully. Guideline 5.4.1 rates the clear identification of the patient as *necessary,* but does not mean or say that every element listed is necessary. Identifying information "may" include all of the elements listed.

5. Check other recommendations in case they modify the guidelines. (Here Recommendation 5.1.5 is that it is *necessary* to include both sex and occupation, and Recommendation 5.1.6 lists other elements that might be recorded but that are rated *discretionary*).

6. Refer to other parts of the chapter, especially the overview (Part I) and the Definitions (Part II). (In the example being considered, patient identification, there are no introductory statements which modify the recommendation. However, a disclaimer at the beginning of Part VI is relevant and notes that all guidelines on patient records and consents "may necessarily be superseded by statutory law" in a specific jurisdiction.)

REFERENCES

1. Smith R (1991) *Where is the Wisdom: The Poverty of Medical Evidence*, BMJ 303:798-799. Quoting David Eddy MD, Professor of Health Policy and Management, Duke University, NC.

2. Rachlis N and Kuschner C (1989) *Second Opinion: What's Wrong with Canada's Health Care System and How to Fix It,* Collins, Toronto.

1

History and Physical Examination

Chapter Outline

I. OVERVIEW

The main objective in practice is to find a solution to the patient's problem. To accomplish this goal the nature and cause of the problem must be known before appropriate management can be instituted.

Initially, this requires data collection and interpretation. The patient interview represents an important opportunity to obtain the information necessary to make a correct diagnosis. A careful examination is then necessary to verify that diagnosis. Responses to pertinent historical queries suggest how the examination should be planned, what course it should take, and what areas may require special consideration. Several methods of examination are known to exist. From the choices made during the examination a management plan is finally formulated.

It is the initial patient contact that establishes the nature of the doctor/patient relationship and determines the degree of confidence and trust involved in case management.

II. DEFINITIONS

Consultation: Any combination of history taking, physical examination, and explanation and discussion of the clinical findings and prognosis. A consultation can also be the service provided by a practitioner whose opinion or advice regarding evaluation and/or management of a specific problem is requested by another practitioner or other appropriate source.

Diagnosis: A decision regarding the nature of the patient's complaint; the art or act of identifying a disease or condition from its signs and symptoms.

Examination: Those varied procedures performed by the practitioner necessary to determine a working diagnosis. The goal of the examination is not to attain diagnostic certainty but rather to reduce the level of uncertainty sufficient to make optimal recommendations for care.

Gold Standard Test: An accepted reference test or procedure used to define the true state of the patient's health.

History: The patient's account of the clinical problem(s) given in response to the practitioner's questions.

Neurologic Examination: Most commonly refers to evaluating deep tendon reflexes, sensation and muscle strength.

Provocative Testing: Those tests or procedures that are performed to elicit physical or physiological expressions of a given disorder.

Sensitivity: The likelihood of a positive test result in a person with a disorder (also true-positive rate or TPR).

Specificity: The ability to correctly identify negative test results among subjects who truly do not have a specific disorder.

Vascular Examination: Most commonly refers to auscultation and palpation of appropriate blood vessels.

III. LIST OF SUBTOPICS

A. History
   1. General considerations
   2. Components

B. Examination Procedures
   1. Generally
   2. In presence of head complaints
   3. Neck and adjacent structures
   4. Thoracic complaints and/or chest complaints
   5. Lower back and adjacent structures
   6. Extremity complaints
   7. Independent chiropractic examinations

IV. LITERATURE REVIEW

Specific literature on the appropriate history and examination techniques for the chiropractic practitioner can be found in numerous texts. The reader is directed to those texts listed in the bibliography for detailed description of such techniques. The intent of this chapter is not to serve as a teaching tool. Rather, the purpose is to assist in establishing guidelines related to acceptable history techniques to be used by the practitioner.

Many journals published for the chiropractic profession, including the *Journal of Manipulative and Physiological Therapeutics, Chiropractic Technique,* and *Chiropractic Sports Medicine*, provide articles on the appropriateness of various examination procedures, but there is little information on history taking procedures. The articles range from describing the measurement of lumbar range of motion to objectively measuring the strength of the biceps muscle. These articles often reflect only one individual's perspective, and in some instances have associated economic ramifications. These considerations increase our need for objective information gained from well-designed research projects.

The history-taking procedure has been considered the most clinically sophisticated and complex task used by health care providers. [21] Its purpose is to provide the clinician with one or more diagnostic impressions. These are then confirmed or altered following the judicious selection of additional tests — and it can be noted in the literature that this process does indeed occur. [43] One study determined that a sample group of practitioners determined their first hypothesis regarding the diagnosis of a random sample of patients an average of 28 seconds after hearing the chief complaint. The correct hypothesis (which was identified in 75% of these cases) was found on average within the first six minutes of a half-hour work-up.[2] Much of the information that will lead a clinician to a management plan, then, is gained very early in the doctor/patient interaction.[44]

Sandler[44] also emphasized the importance of the history. He found that the percentage of diagnostic completion was as high as 73% after the history and physical examination alone. He suggested that further tests were often unnecessary and costly. Cutler[16] stated that 70%-90% of diagnoses are derived from the history alone. The art and skill of the doctor in the history-taking process includes the ability 1) to obtain an appropriate description of the patient's complaints; 2) to elicit data vital to the case that may not have been volunteered; and 3) to know that the patient does not have clinically relevant factors that are left unmentioned.[21]

These skills can be diminished in a number of ways. Previous experience, while of great value, may result in the clinician prejudging a patient's condition, coming to a conclusion too quickly. This may result in unnecessary testing procedures in order to determine that the hypothesis made during the history is incorrect, or may result in an appropriate confirmatory test not being used and the patient being treated inappropriately. Further, the meaning of words used by the patient may not be the same as that of the practitioner. "Night pain," for example, may signify a pain when resting in bed which has high sensitivity (greater than 0.90) for the detection of malignancy;[1] or it might mean that the patient wakes up whenever he/she rolls over and that the movement irritates an inflamed facet. A practitioner's arbitrary use of professional jargon, and the assumption that the patient understands it, can lead to further confusion. All of the above are further complicated when the first language of the clinician is not the same as that of the patient. It is perhaps for these reasons that the accuracy of patient histories has been questioned,[14, 35] and significant variability noted.[19]

Mishler et al.[39] state that there are three parameters involved in the interview process: attentiveness, facilitation and collaboration. Attentiveness is defined as the degree to which the practitioner takes the patient's concerns seriously. Facilitation is the encouragement given by the clinician to allow patients to tell their own stories in their own words, and collaboration is the degree to which patients are considered partners in the process by which they receive care.

The biologic/diagnostic sciences, then, are aids to the decision-making process. This process, however, must take place within the social context of our society. As a result a social interactive component must be recognized and taken into account in order to make appropriate choices during the physical examination and any additional testing procedures.

There are several examination styles that are currently recognized. Not all of them are practical in a clinical setting. One is the exhaustive approach, with the completion of a comprehensive series of all tests that may significantly contribute to determining the diagnosis. A study by Durbridge,[18] performed in a hospital setting, showed that exhaustive testing produced no improvement in mortality rate, morbidity, duration of monitoring, disability, medical opinions of the patient's progress or length of stay.

Another style, the one generally used to obtain the history and perform the physical examination, is the hypothetic-deductive approach.[16, 43] This consists of generating one hypothesis after hearing the patient's chief complaint(s), or several possible working hypotheses. The practitioner then attempts to gather historical and physical information to either support or refute the potential working hypotheses. The goal is to narrow the number of working hypotheses to one.

The physical examination, while apparently objective, is no less riddled with social issues than the history. It has been noted that the assessment of the observer,[21] instructions given to the patient, and sincerity of response are important. When, for example, an almost 30% difference is found in the sensitivity of a test such as sensory loss used to help diagnose a herniated lumbar nucleus pulposis for two different samples,[1] it is difficult to know if the difference lies in the test itself or in the doctor-patient relationship. The more motivated patients are, the more likely they are to fairly represent their maximum capacity on a physical performance test.[26, 40, 46] The less anxious patients are, the more likely they are to reach forward despite their pain.

The literature is sorely lacking with respect to controlled randomized clinical trials directed at measuring reliability and validity of specific history taking procedures. A thorough review of practitioner reliability studies performed by Koran[30] did not include any studies relating to history taking. Earlier studies, in which practitioners interviewed different samples of patients drawn from one population, found considerable disagreement in symptom prevalence rates.[19]

Although there are many studies of examination techniques, high quality randomized trials do not exist. Koran's review[30] revealed very poor reliability amongst medical physicians regarding agreement greater than chance in the examination of many components of the cardiovascular, gastrointestinal and respiratory systems. Chiropractic studies of examination techniques often omit an accurate description of the inherent properties of a test including reliability and validity, or fail to comment on the utility of the diagnostic procedure in relation to the therapeutic impact and patient outcome. Further, a gold standard of diagnosis is not often available for many of the conditions treated by the chiropractic profession. Thus tests of sensitivity and specificity may be open to bias.

Cooperman et al.[13] attempted to assess intertester and intratester reliability and validity of Lachman's test in determining the integrity of the anterior cruciate ligament (ACL). They found the test judgments had limited reliability. They were more reliable for predicting absence of ACL injury than the presence of ACL injury.

Another study analyzing a sample of patients with objectively determined anterior cruciate ligament tear or chondral damage found patients were not correctly diagnosed using a battery of usual orthopedic tests. Under anesthesia, however, Lachman's test proved to be highly sensitive and specific. This suggests that even in the face of well-performed maneuvers, compensatory defense reactions from soft tissue may prevent stressing the targeted tissues in the manner necessary for adequate diagnosis.[25]

Mierau et al.[37] determined that the correlation between straight leg raising (SLR) and low-back pain may be poor when evaluating children and adolescents, with the exception of male adolescents with a history of low-back pain. When evaluating various populations it has been observed that ipsilateral SLR is a highly sensitive indicator (72%-97%) of lumbar disc herniation, and contralateral SLR is highly specific for the same condition (88%-100%).[1]

A study performed by physical therapists attempting to measure lumbar lordosis with a flexible ruler showed poor intertester reliability with slightly increased intratester reliability. [38] Similar studies done within the chiropractic profession to measure intersegmental range of motion show similar poor intertester reliability.[29] Furthermore, out of eight conservative evaluations of lumbar segmental abnormality (including palpating for pain, assessing temperature differentials, active and passive motion palpation, muscle tension and misalignment palpation), the subjective finding (of pain) was found to be the most reliable.

Brunarski[8] evaluated two physical measurements, plumbline analysis and lateral bending dynamic roentgenograms. These two measures demonstrated greater predictive value and accuracy in differentiating patients with myofascial pain from asymptomatic patients than sacroiliac motion palpation and straight leg raising. This information is of limited clinical use because myofascial pain is poorly defined.

The Quebec Task Force on Spinal Disorders[41] concluded that, with few exceptions, there were currently no objective procedures which usefully diagnosed any type of spinal pain of less than seven weeks duration. It is noted that there were no chiropractic representatives on this Task Force, and that palpation findings and other subtle forms of evaluation may not have been considered.

LeBoeuf [32] evaluated eight different orthopedic tests and found that only one (heel to buttock test) had predictive value for low-back pain. Orthopedic tests that appeared to strain several adjacent anatomical structures were commonly positive. This may indicate that these tests have poor discriminative ability.

Three common cervical orthopedic tests used to determine the presence of cervical disc disease were evaluated as they related to radicular, neurologic and radiologic signs. Neck compression, axial manual traction and shoulder abduction tests were found to be highly specific for radicular pain, neurologic and radiologic signs. Despite their low sensitivity, these tests were deemed valuable in the clinical examination of a patient with neck and arm pain.[51] In the presence of a negative finding from an accepted test, a practitioner needs to recognize that many tests have low sensitivity.

In conclusion, much of the basis of history taking and performing a physical examination stems from clinical experience rather than scientific data. As clinicians we must remain flexible in our approach to the patient, and recognize consultative procedures that may assist in establishing an effective working diagnosis.

V. ASSESSMENT CRITERIA

Note: Two rating systems are employed in this chapter because of the diverse subject matter.

Procedure Ratings (System I)

Established: Accepted as appropriate by the practicing chiropractic community for the given indication in the specified patient population.

Promising: Given current knowledge, this appears to be appropriate for the given indication in the specified patient population. As more evidence and experience accumulates this interim rating will change. This connotes provisional acceptance, but permits a greater role for the current level of clinical use.

Equivocal: Current knowledge exists to support a given indication in a specified patient population, though value can neither be confirmed nor denied. As more evidence and experience accumulates this interim rating will change. Expert opinion recognizes a need for caution in general application.

Investigational: Evidence is insufficient to determine appropriateness. Further study is warranted. Use for a given indication in a specified patient population should be confined to research protocols. As more evidence and experience accumulates this interim rating will change.

Doubtful: Given current knowledge, this appears to be inappropriate for the given indication in the specified patient population. As more evidence and experience accumulates this interim rating will change.

Inappropriate: Regarded by the practicing chiropractic community as unacceptable for the given indication in the specified patient population.

Quality of Evidence

The following categories of evidence are used to support the ratings.

Class I:
Evidence provided by one or more well-designed controlled clinical trials; or well designed experimental studies that address reliability, validity, positive predictive value, discriminability, sensitivity, or specificity.

Class II:
Evidence provided by one or more well-designed uncontrolled, observational clinical studies, such as case control, cohort studies, etc.; or clinically relevant basic science studies that address reliability, validity, positive predictive value, discriminability, sensitivity, specificity; and published in refereed journals.

Class III:

Evidence provided by expert opinion, descriptive studies or case reports.

Suggested Strength of Recommendations Ratings

Type A. Strong positive recommendation. Based on Class I evidence or overwhelming Class II evidence when circumstances preclude randomized clinical trials.

Type B. Positive recommendation based on Class II evidence.

Type C. Positive recommendation based on strong consensus of Class III evidence.

Type D. Negative recommendation based on inconclusive or conflicting Class II evidence.

Type E. Negative recommendation based on evidence of ineffectiveness or lack of efficacy based on Class I or Class II evidence.

Procedure Ratings (System II)

Necessary: Strong positive recommendation based on Class I evidence, or overwhelming Class II evidence when circumstances reflect compromise of patient safety.

Recommended: Positive recommendation based on consensus of Class II and/or strong Class III evidence.

Discretionary: Positive recommendation based on strong consensus of Class III evidence.

Unnecessary: Negative recommendation based on inconclusive or conflicting Class II, III evidence.

Quality of Evidence

The following categories of evidence are used to support the ratings.

Class I:
A. Evidence of clinical utility from controlled studies published in refereed journals.
B. Binding or strongly persuasive legal authority such as legislation or case law.

Class II:
A. Evidence of clinical utility from the significant results of uncontrolled studies in refereed journals.
B. Evidence provided by recommendation from published expert legal opinion or persuasive case law.

Class III:
A. Evidence of clinical utility provided by opinions of experts, anecdote and/or by convention.
B. Expert legal opinion.

VI. RECOMMENDATIONS

A. History

1. The process by which one determines the diagnosis should be adequately recorded and interpretable.

   1.1.1 **Rating:** Necessary
   Evidence: Class II, III
   Consensus Level: 1
   (For detailed recommendations see Chapter 5)

2. The history plays a critical role in the diagnostic process. A well performed history will appropriately identify the region to be examined and the extent of the condition.

   1.1.2 **Rating:** Established
   Evidence: Class I, II, III
   Consensus Level: 1

3. The components of the history may include any or all of the following, dependent on the presentation of the patient and the judgment of the practitioner.
   a. Data on identity, including age and sex
   b. Chief complaint (problem list)
   c. History of present complaint
      history of trauma
      description of chief complaint(s)
      quality/character
      intensity
      frequency
      location and radiation
      onset
      duration
      palliative and provocative factors
   d. Family history
   e. Past health history
      general state of health
      prior illness
      surgical history
      previous injuries, i.e., MVA, workers' comp.
      past hospitalizations
      previous treatment and diagnostic tests
      medications
      allergies
   f. Psycho-social history
      occupation
      activities
      recreational activities
      exercise
   g. Social history
      marital status
      level of education
      social habits
   h. Review of systems
      musculoskeletal
      cardiovascular

respiratory
gastrointestinal
genitourinal
central nervous system
eye, ear, nose and throat
endocrine
peripheral vascular disease
psychiatric

1.1.3 **Rating:** Necessary
Evidence: Class I, II, III
Consensus Level: 1

B. Examination

1. Practitioners may use any or all diagnostic procedures pertinent to the physical examination, however sophisticated, dependent on individual training and the legal statutory framework within which they work.

1.2.1 **Rating:** Necessary
Evidence: Class II, III
Consensus Level: 1

2. Examination procedures regardless of chief complaint(s) may include:
    a. Evaluation of blood pressure and pulse rate
    b. Recording of height and weight
    c. Record of temperature in the presence of pertinent subjective complaints

1.2.2 **Rating:** Recommended
Evidence: Class III
Consensus Level: 1

3. In the presence of head complaints evaluation may include examination of the neck and adjacent structures as well as appropriate vascular and cranial nerve testing.

1.2.3 **Rating:** Established
Evidence: Class II, III
Consensus Level: 1

4. In the presence of reported or observed changes in cognition, coordination, special sensory function or recent head trauma, it is necessary to perform a neurologic evaluation or obtain a more extensive neurologic/vascular workup in a timely fashion.

1.2.4 **Rating:** Established
Evidence: Class II, III
Consensus Level: 1

5. Examination of the neck and adjacent structures may include:
    a. Inspection and observation to include postural presentation of the region
    b. Regional palpation

c. Range of motion including active and/or passive movement
d. Muscle strength
e. Provocative maneuvers which might include compression and stretching
f. Neurologic examination
g. Vascular examination

as is safe and effective in diagnosing the patient.

1.2.5 **Rating:** Established
Evidence: Class II, III
Consensus Level: 1

6. Examination procedures for thoracic and/or chest complaints may include:
    a. Inspection and observation to include postural presentation of the region
    b. Regional palpation
    c. Auscultation of the chest in the presence of pertinent subjective complaints to be performed by the practitioner or appropriate specialist
    d. Auscultation of heart sounds in the presence of pertinent subjective complaints to be performed by the practitioner or appropriate specialist
    e. Auscultation and palpation of the abdomen
    f. Range of motion including passive and/or active movements
    g. Muscle strength
    h. Provocative maneuvers which may include compression and stretching
    i. Neurologic examination

as is safe and effective in diagnosing the patient.

1.2.6 **Rating:** Established
Evidence: Class II, III
Consensus Level: 1

7. Examination procedures for lower back and adjacent structures may include:
    a. Inspection and observation to include postural presentation of the region
    b. Regional palpation
    c. Evaluation of the abdominal aorta to include palpation and auscultation in the presence of pertinent subjective and objective findings
    d. Evaluation of the abdominal/pelvic viscera to include palpation and/or auscultation in the presence of pertinent subjective complaints
    e. Range of motion including passive and/or active movements
    f. Muscle strength
    g. Provocative maneuvers which may include compression and stretching
    h. Neurologic examination
    i. Vascular examination
    j. Recording the circumference of the involved extremity in the presence of pertinent subjective complaints

as is safe and effective in diagnosing the patient.

1.2.7 **Rating:** Established
Evidence: Class I, II, III
Consensus Level: 1

8. Examination procedures for extremity complaints may include:
   a. Vascular examination
   b. Neurologic examination
   c. Regional palpation
   d. Range of motion including passive and/or active movements
   e. Provocative maneuvers which may include compression and stretching.
   f. Recording the circumference measurements of the involved extremity in the presence of pertinent subjective complaints.

as is safe and effective in diagnosing the patient.

1.2.8 **Rating:** Established
Evidence: Class I, II, III
Consensus Level: 1

9. Independent chiropractic examinations (ICE) should be performed in accordance with the recommendations put forth in this chapter.

1.2.9 **Rating:** Recommended
Evidence: Class II
Consensus Level: 1

VII. COMMENTS, SUMMARY OR CONCLUSION

None.

VIII. REFERENCES

1. Andersson G: Sensitivity, Specificity and Predictive Value. *The Adult Spine: Principles and Practice.* New York, Raven Press, 1991.

2. Barrows HS, Norman GR, Neufeld VR, Feightner JW: The clinical reasoning of randomly selected physicians in general medical practice. *Clin Invest Med* 1982; 5:49.

3. Bates B: *A guide to physical examination.* Philadelphia, Lippincott, 1982.

4. Beede, Scott et al: Positive predictive value of clinical suspicion of abdominal aortic aneurysm. *Arch Intern Med* 1990; 150: 549-41.

5. Biering-Sorenson F: Physical measurements as risk indicators for low-back trouble over a one year period. *Spine* 1984;9:106-119.

6. Boachie-Adjei O: Evaluation of the patient with low-back pain. *Post Grad Med* 1988; 84:110-119.

7. Bolton PS, Stick PE, Lord RSA: Failure of clinical tests to predict cerebral ischemia before neck pain. *J Manip Physiol Ther* 1989; 12:304-7.

8. Brunarski D: Chiropractic biomechanical evaluations: validity in myofascial low-back pain. *J Manip Physiol Ther* 1982; 5:155-61.

9. Cailliet R: *Low Back Pain Syndrome.* Philadelphia, FA Davis Co, 1968.

10. Cailliet R: *Soft Tissue Pain and Disability*, Philadelphia, FA Davis Co, 1977.

11. Cailliet R: *Scoliosis: Diagnosis and Management.* Philadelphia, FA Davis Co, 1977.

12. Cipriano J: *Regional Orthopedic Tests.* Maryland, William and Wilkins, Fourth Ed. 1985.

13. Cooperman JM: Reliability and validity of judgements of the integrity of the anterior cruciate ligament of the knee using the Lachman's test. *Phys Ther* 1990; 70:(4) 225-232.

14. Corwin R, Krober M, Roth H: Patients' accuracy in reporting their past medical history: a study of 90 patients with peptic ulcer. *J Chron Dis* 1971; 23: 875-879.

15. Cox JM: *Low-back pain: mechanism, diagnosis and management. 4th ed.* Baltimore, Williams and Wilkins, 1985.

16. Cutler P: *Problem Solving in Clinical Medicine: from Data to Diagnosis. 2nd ed.* Baltimore, Williams and Wilkins, 1985 p.13.

17. Cyriax J: *Textbook of Orthopaedic Medicine.* Great Britain, Spottiswoode Ballantyne Ltd, 1978.

18. Durbridge TC, Edwards F, Edwards RG, Atkinson M: An evaluation of multiphasic screening on admission to hospital. Precis of a report to the National Health and Medical Research Council. *Med J Aust* 1976. 1:703.

19. Fairbairn AS, Wood CH, Fletcher CM: Variability in answers to a questionnaire on respiratory symptoms. 1959 *Br J. Prev Soc Med* 13: 175-93.

20. Fields K, Delaney M: Focusing the pre-participation sports examination. *J Fam Pract,* 1990 30 (3):304-12.

21. Feinstein AR: Scientific methodology in clinical medicine-Acquisition of clinical data. *Clinical Methodology* 1964 Dec.61 (6): 1162-1193.

22. *Guides to the Evaluation of Permanent Impairment, 3rd ed,* AMA, 1988.

23. Haldeman S: *Modern Developments in the Principles and Practice of Chiropractic.* New York, Appleton-Century-Crofts, 1980.

24. Halzeman B, Bulgen D: Low-back pain. *Med Inter* 1982; 11: 932-6.

25. Hardaker WT, Garrett WE, Bassett FH: Evaluation of acute traumatic hemarthrosis of the knee joint. *South Med J.* 1990 Jun. 83 (6): 640-4.

26. Hazaerd FG, Reid S, Fenwich J, Reeves J: Isokinetic trunk and lifting strength measurements: variability as an indicator of effort. *Spine* 1988; 13:(1) 54-57.

27. Hoppenfield S: *Orthopaedic Neurology.* Philadelphia, JB Lippincott Co, 1977.

28. Hoppenfield S: *Physical Examination of the Spine and Extremities.* New York, Appleton-Century-Crofts, 1976.

29. Keating J, Bergman T, Jacobs G, Finer B, Larson K: Interexaminer reliability of eight evaluative dimensions of lumbar segmental abnormality. *J Manip Physiol Ther* 13 (8): 463-70.

30. Koran L: The reliability of clinical methods, data and judgements. *New Eng J of Med* 1975; 293 (13): 1642-46.

31. Kirkaldy-Willis WH: *Managing Low-back Pain.* New York, Churchill Livingstone, 1983.

32. LeBoeuf C: The sensitivity and specificity of seven lumbo-pelvic orthopedic tests and the arm-fossa test. *J Manip Physiol Ther* 1990; 13(3): 138-143.

33. Lovell FW, Rothstein JM, Personius WJ: Reliability of clinical measurements of the lumbar lordosis taken with a flexible rule. *Phys Ther* 1989 Feb, 69 (2): 96-105.

34. Magee DJ: *Orthopedic Physical Assessment.* Philadelphia, WB Saunders Co, 1987.

35. Manning A, Wyman JB, Heaton JW: How trustworthy are bowel histories: Comparison of recalled and recorded information. *BMJ* 1976: July: 213-214.

36. Mazion JM: *Illustrated Manual of Orthopedic Signs/Tests/Maneuvers for Office Procedure.* Orlando, Daniels Publishing Co, 1980.

37. Mierau D, Cassidy JD, Yong-Hing K: Low-back pain and straight leg raising in children and adolescents. *Spine* 1989; 14 (no 5): 526-28.

38. Million R, Hall W, Haavik-Nilson K, Baker RD, Jason MIV: Assessment of the progress of the back pain patient. *Spine* 1982; 7:204-212.

39. Mishler E, Clark J, et. al: The language of attentive patient care. *J Gen Int Med* 1989; 4: 325-335.

40. Niebuhr BR, Marion R: Detecting sincerity of effort when measuring grip strength. *Spine* 1985; 8: 765-772.

41. Quebec Task Force: Scientific approach to the assessment and managment of activity related spinal disorders. *Spine* 1987 12 (7):5-59.

42. Rube N, Secher NH: Paradoxical influence of encouragement on muscle fatigue. *Eur J Appl Physiol* 1981; 46: 1-7.

43. Sackett DL, Haynes RB, Tugwell JP: *Clinical Epidemiology: a basic science for clinical medicine. 1st ed.* Toronto, Little, Brown and Company, 1985.

44. Sandler G: The importance of the history in the medical clinic and the cost of unnecessary tests. *Am Heart J.* 1980; 100: 928.

45. Shiging X, Quanzhi A, Dehao F: Significance of the straight leg raising test in the diagnosis and clinical evaluation of lower lumbar IVD protrusion. *J Bone and Jt. Surg,* 1987; 69: 517-521.

46. Smith GA, Nelson RC, Sadoff SJ, Sadoff AM: Assessing sincerity of effort in maximal grip strength tests. *Am J Phys Med 1989*;2: 73-80.

47. Sweetman BJ, Anderson JAD, Dalton ER: The relationship between little finger mobility, straight leg raising and low-back pain. *Rheumat Rehabil,* 1974; 13: 161-66.

48. Triano J, Baker J, McGregor M, Torres B: Optimizing measures of maximum voluntary contraction: verbal instructions vs. instruction plus visual feedback. Provisionally accepted for publication, *Spinal Rehabilitation,* 1992.

49. Van Allen MW, Rodnitzky RL: *Pictorial Manual of Neurologic Tests. 2nd ed.* Chicago, Year Book Medical Publishers, Inc, 1981.

50. Vernon H: Chiropractic manipulation in the treatment of headache: a retrospective and prospective study. *J Manip Physiol Ther* 1982; 5: 109-112.

51. Viikari-Juntura E, Porras M, Laasonen EM: Validity of clinical tests in the diagnosis of root compression in the diagnosis of cervical disc disease. *Spine* 1989; 14 (3): 253-7.

52. White AA, Panjabi MM: *Clinical biomechanics of the spine.* Philadelphia, JB Lippincott Co, 1978.

IX. MINORITY OPINIONS

None.

2

Diagnostic Imaging

Chapter Outline

I. OVERVIEW

The fundamental purpose of diagnostic imaging is to gain information to aid diagnosis, prognosis and therapy. Studies are performed to confirm or contribute to the clinical picture. Each study requires the informed consent of the patient and appropriate documentation.

Diagnostic imaging is a field which has undergone revolutionary changes because of the explosion of advanced imaging technology. The rapid advancement of technology and information means that it is not possible to write static guidelines regarding diagnostic imaging.

Diagnostic imaging, especially plain film radiography, continues to be a mainstay in the assessment of chiropractic patients. This document presents current knowledge regarding the proper utilization of diagnostic imaging in the assessment of chiropractic patients. An overview of diagnostic imaging in regards to education, services, patient selection, imaging modalities and recommendations is presented. It is beyond the scope of this paper to discuss all available radiology services.

II. DEFINITIONS

A. Personnel

Radiologic Technologist or Radiographer: A person educated and trained to perform appropriate diagnostic studies under published guidelines in a safe and reasonable manner. The technologist or radiographer does not practice independently but performs studies by referral under the direction of a licensed practitioner.

General Chiropractic Practitioner: A practitioner licensed to practice diagnostic radiology and educated in radiation protection, standards of quality, clinical indications for radiography and interpretation.

Radiologist: A licensed practitioner certified by a recognized national certification board in the specialty of diagnostic imaging. Trained chiropractic radiologists typically have over 6,000 hours of education during their post-professional training.

B. Services

Technical Component: That portion of radiology services that includes providing the facilities, equipment, resources, personnel, supplies and support needed to perform and produce the diagnostic study.

Professional Component: Represents the services performed by a licensed practitioner to interpret each study and to document the diagnostic conclusions of the study in a formal written radiology report. The practitioner may assign any right or claim to the professional component service if, upon prior agreement, all duties of interpretation, diagnosis and reporting are relegated to a radiologist. When the primary professional component is performed by a radiologist it is not considered as a second opinion.

Second Opinion or Consultation: Is requested in circumstances when a practitioner or radiologist feels more input in the case is in the best interest of the patient.

C. Other

Diagnostic Significance: Information has diagnostic significance if it results in a change of diagnosis. (This does not necessarily imply a change in therapy.)

Spinal Instability: Interruption of the anatomic elements resulting in abnormal or excessive motion which may or may not carry the risk of neurologic injury.

Therapeutic Significance: Information has therapeutic significance if it indicates a need for a change in therapy.

III. LIST OF SUBTOPICS

    A. Sequence of Services
    B. Patient Selection Procedures
    C. Radiographic Interpretation and Reporting
    D. Legal Issues in Radiography
    E. Radiation Technology and Protection
    F. Plain Film Radiographs
    G. Full Spine Radiography
    H. Stress Radiography
    I. Videofluoroscopy
    J. Plain Film Contrast Studies
    K. Computed Tomography
    L. Magnetic Resonance Imaging
    M. Radionuclide Bone Scanning
    N. Diagnostic Ultrasound

IV. LITERATURE REVIEW

A. Selection Procedures

Diagnostic imaging procedures are diverse and span a wide spectrum ranging from traditional plain film radiographs to complex computer generated images. Plain film x-rays should not be acquired unless the results could reasonably affect treatment (Seelentag,1989; Wyatt, 1987). Overutilization may be the result of inexperience, habit, peer pressure, patient education or reassurance, and fear of litigation (Deyo, 1987).

1. **Diagnostic efficacy.** Effectiveness can be measured and varies with each type of imaging (Baddley, 1984). Efficacy can be assessed at three levels: diagnostic, therapeutic and prognostic (Lusted, 1977). Imaging studies are useful when

they reduce diagnostic uncertainty. Imaging also contributes to management decisions for prognosis and plan of therapy. (Baddley, 1984).

2. **Accuracy and clinical certainty.** An important feature in selection of diagnostic studies is accuracy. A test must be selected on the basis of its ability to discriminate between those patients who have the disease in question and those who do not.

3. **Decision making for patient selection.** The selection of patients for radiographic examination is based on the following guidelines:
   a. Need for radiographic examination should be based on history and physical examination findings.
   b. Potential diagnostic benefits must be weighed against the risks of ionizing radiation.
   c. The purposes of radiographic examination are to assist the practitioner in diagnosis of pathology, identify contraindications to chiropractic care, identify bone and joint morphology, and acquire postural, kinematic and biomechanical information.
   d. Routine radiography of patients as a screening procedure is inappropriate.
   (Sinclair, 1988; Maurer, 1988; Ontario Gvt. Publ., 1987; Mootz; Kovach, 1983; Vernon, 1982; Aspegren, 1987)

4. **Additional selection considerations**
   a. Non-responsive patient. It is not appropriate to image patients simply because of clinical uncertainty or prior negative results (Kemp, 1984; Mjoen, 1990). The entire clinical picture needs to be re-evaluated.
   b. Progressive pathology. In cases of progressive pathology re-examination may be important to evaluate progression and the effect of treatment. Frequency of re-examination depends on the nature of the disease.
   c. Discharge examination. There is little documented need to image patients prior to release from care. Exceptions are the utilization of a diagnostic imaging test to establish disability or permanency of an abnormality where this is helpful in determining the disposition of a claim.
   d. Frequent re-examination. The need for frequent diagnostic images for purely biomechanical analysis is not well documented.
   e. Health policy. Medicare requirements mandate that radiographs be obtained in every case regardless of clinical opinion. This is contrary to appropriate imaging selection and practice. Routine radiographs acquired as a pre-employment screen have been thought to be of diagnostic or prognostic value with respect to the potential for development of occupational back pain (Diveley, 1956). More recently this belief has come under severe criticism due to the extremely low diagnostic yield, unproven predictive value and pro-

hibitive cost (Wyatt, 1987; Joseph et al., 1986; Eisenberg et al., 1979).
   f. Therapeutic indications. In some circumstances, although the clinical picture may not indicate a need for diagnostic imaging, it is required because of the therapy being considered by the practitioner. This may be contraindicated with certain clinically silent conditions that may be apparent on radiographic examination (Yochum, 1987).

B. Interpretation and Reporting of Diagnostic Studies

1. **Components.** The professional component of an imaging study may be performed by the general chiropractic practitioner or a specialist chiropractic practitioner with advanced training in radiology. This decision is based upon practitioner preference, liability considerations, availability of services and other issues. An interpretation of the imaging study must be included as part of the patient's permanent record. Performing the professional component of an imaging study by the practitioner is not mandated, and may be relegated to the radiologist. It must be performed by one or the other in each case. This decision is based on preference of practice, liability consideratons, availability of services and other issues.

2. **Content of report.** The necessary components of a formal written radiology report include patient identification, location where studies were performed, study dates, types of studies, radiographic findings, diagnostic impressions, and signature with professional qualifications. Other components may include recommendations for follow-up studies and comments on further clinical patient evaluation (Taylor, 1990). Unique radiology reports are generated for each study. The use of check-list forms is not supported.

3. **Function.** The main function of the radiological report, an important part of the patient record, is to document the findings of the imaging study. It forms only part of the clinical picture however and is not the sole determinant of management. Comment in reports suggesting or directing patient management is generally inappropriate. The treating practitioner integrates other information from clinical history, physical examination, and the other diagnostic procedures to form a complete clinical impression.

Yochum (1987) lists five other functions and reasons for recording radiographic findings in a written report: 1) medicolegal circumstances; 2) allowing comparison with prior or subsequent exams; 3) providing a reference if radiographs are lost or not available for review; 4) communication with other health practitioners; 5) expediting care by providing a resume of important indications and contraindications for therapy.

4. **Timing.** A radiology report should convey the findings of the diagnostic study to the treating practitioner in a timely manner and the radiologist has a duty to ensure such commu-

nication. In appropriate circumstances the general chiropractic practitioner may institute the initial treatment plan based on patient history and physical findings prior to obtaining the formal written radiology report.

C. Regulations and Professional Responsibilities

Legislation governing chiropractic practice provides that radiography is to be used solely for diagnostic purposes. The laws and regulations governing the use of diagnostic radiology are established by individual state radiation protection authorities. The U.S. National Council on Radiation Protection (1975, 1987) has established recommendations for the safe and effective use of diagnostic radiology. Those who operate chiropractic radiographic facilities should implement the NCRP recommendations.

1. **Diagnostic procedures and instruments.** Those typically allowed for use in chiropractic practice include plain films, fluoroscopy, tomography, thermography, ultrasound, nuclear medicine imaging, computed tomography, digital radiography, and magnetic resonance imaging.

2. **Legal and ethical issues**. Practitioners should be aware that it is not only unethical but also illegal in most states for any health professional to receive financial compensation (kick-back payments) for ordering studies. Ownership, limited partnerships, and stock purchase are ethical ways to have financial investment in imaging facilities or centers. Any offer or advertising of free x-rays to actual or potential patients shall be accompanied by the statement "if necessary". Any facility utilizing two or more fee schedules for their services is engaging in unethical and potentially illegal activity. Services should be billed at the same rate whether payment is direct or by a third party. No out-of-pocket expense (NOOPE) billing schemes are unethical and generally illegal.

3. **Clinical responsibility.** Individuals or institutions are responsible to the level of service provided. Adequate technology is the responsibility of the facility and personnel providing the technical services. Radiologic diagnosis is the responsibility of the general chiropractic practitioner or the specialist chiropractic practitioner with advanced training in radiology. Chiropractic practitioners performing duties in general practice may not be held responsible at the level of the specialist in radiology.

4. **Patient consent**. Each patient should be informed in advance of the need and nature of radiographic examinations to be performed, and any significant potential risks or contraindications. Consent should be obtained in the case of minors. This should be from a parent or legal guardian.

D. Standards of Billing

Standard Current Procedural Terminology codes for reimbursement of radiology services are technical fee, professional fee, global fee (combined technical and professional), and level of office service for practitioner involvement. Radiology procedures, or groups of procedures are billed in an available single, comprehensive CPT-4 code. Body areas are billed as a series or study. Billing of individual views when more than one view is obtained is considered unbundling. Manipulation of reimbursement codes to gain higher reimbursement (e.g., performing partial studies on various office visits to allow code gaming) by any professional providing radiology services is inappropriate.

E. Plain Film Radiography

1. **Radiation technology and radiation protection**
    a. **Technique factor selection** (Maurer, 1989; Mootz, 1989; Sherman, 1982; Curry et al., 1990; Bushong, 1984; Yochum, 1987; Moilanen et al., 1983; Jaeger, 1988). Practitioners should have the following goals for each radiographic examination:
      - Patient exposure to radiation on the ALARA ("As Low as Reasonably Achievable") principle;
      - Images with quality "As High as Reasonably Achievable" (AHARA);
      - Proper procedures to ensure minimum need for repeat studies.
      i) Technique Charts. Chiropractic radiographic installations make use of accurate technique charts or other reliable methods of calculating exposure factors. These charts vary for each installation because of variances in tube current and voltage output in each location.
      ii) kV Selection (Yochum, 1987; Jaeger, 1988). Technique selection is based on a fixed optimum kV basis. This procedure is best suited for use with rare-earth intensifying screens. These are sensitive to a specific kV range and requirements for specific degrees of penetration based on body part thickness and density. Selection of optimum kV is based on the body part being radiographed. Tube current and/or time (mAs) is altered according to body part thickness. Table 1 provides optimum kV values as a range—rather than a fixed value to accommodate voltage output variances from one installation to another.
      iii) mAs Selection. The mAs signifies the quantity of x-ray photons emitted from the x-ray tube and affects radiographic density. The mAs is calculated as the product of tube current (milli-amperage [mA]) and time (seconds-[s]) according to the formula $mAs = mA \times s$. The amount of mAs required is calculated for each exposure and is easily determined by referring to a standardized technique chart or calculating device. Thicker and denser body regions typically re-

quire more mAs than thinner and less dense body regions. Selection of minimum exposure times with adequate milli-amperage helps avoid patient motion. In certain cases the heat capacity of the tube may be exceeded using the maximum milli-amperage available. In these cases lower mA values and longer exposure times are more appropriate to protect the tube.

iv) Focal-Film Distance Selection. Most radiograph procedures use a 40" (Yochum, 1987; Jaeger, 1988) or 48" (Gray et al., 1981) focal-film distance (FFD). The main exceptions are chest, full-spine, and some cervical spine radiographs which typically use a 72" FFD. There is growing interest in the use of FFDs at 72" or 80" to reduce patient skin exposure (Sherman, 1982). 84" provides similar advantages for full spine radiography (Aikenhead, 1989). Increased FFD requires a corresponding increase in mAs according to the Inverse Square Law. Use of long FFD is encouraged in facilities with adequate capacity of x-ray generator, x-ray tube and control and the appropriate grid focal range.

b. **Radiographic quality assurance** (Sherman, 1981; Gray, 1983). Proper maintenance and use of all radiographic equipment significantly contributes to image quality. A prescribed diagnostic and maintenance schedule helps achieve this goal. Table 2 outlines appropriate procedures and intervals of performance.

c. **Radiographic equipment specifications** (Sherman, 1981; Gray, 1983, Samuel, 1985). Many chiropractic radiographic installations are equipped with single-phase, fully rectified x-ray units. Three-phase x-ray units provide superior results with less patient radiation exposure. The cost of three-phase equipment however is often prohibitive for a low-volume radiographic installation.

The relatively new technology of medium-frequency x-ray generators holds promise as a more affordable alternative to three phase technology. Most medium-frequency units (Siemens, Gendex, Bennett) have the dual advantage of reducing patient exposure as well as the capacity to "plug-in" to standard 120V electrical outlets without any special electrical modifications. Some authors (Hildebrandt, 1981) have recommended a minimum x-ray generator-control capacity of 300 mA/125kV. There is no scientific evidence to support this recommendation. Some radiographic generators of less capacity, such as 200 mA/100 kV, are capable of producing excellent quality radiographs. The major concern about lower capacity x-ray units is the possibility of long exposure time leading to excessive patient motion. This may cause a frequency of repeat studies which is unacceptable. The use of patient immobilization devices, such as compression bands, is recommended in these cases.

i) Gonad shields (NCRP#39, 1974; Mootz, 1989; Sherman, 1981; Bushong, 1984; Curry et al., 1990; Moilanen et al., 1983; Jaeger, 1988; Aikenhead et al., 1989; Hildenbrandt, 1981; Gyll, 1988). Male and female reproductive organs are especially sensitive to ionizing radiation. Lead shields covering the ovaries and testicles should be used in most examinations of the pelvic region in patients with reproductive potential. The only exception is where shields will obscure an area of diagnostic interest. (See Table 5).

ii) Intensifying screen/film combinations (Sherman, 1981; Curry et al., 1990; Bushong, 1984; Aikenhead et al., 1989; Picus et al., 1984; Skukas, 1980; Cohen et al., 1984). The most significant recent advance in reducing ionizing radiation is the rare earth intensifying screen. All practitioners with radiographic installations should consider the use of rare-earth screens. Suggested film-screen speed combinations are provided in Table 3. It is essential that the spectral sensitivity of the radiographic film matches that of the intensifying screens used (e.g., orthochromatic screens must be used with orthochromatic [green sensitive] film while blue-emitting screens must be used with blue-sensitive film). Very fast film-screen combinations may reduce patient radiation exposure. The direct increase of film graininess and quantum mottle with increasing speeds results in a drastic loss of radiographic definition. The use of film-screen speeds of 800-1200 is insufficient for identifying subtle changes in bone and joint architecture. Use of 800-1200 film-screen combinations is acceptable in full spine radiography for assessing biomechanical relationships (such as Cobb's angle and Risser's sign). Slower speed systems are used in cases where subtle changes are suspected and higher detail is necessary. Extremity radiography uses screens and films that demonstrate high detail.

iii) Collimator (Sherman, 1981; Curry et al., 1990; Bushong, 1984; Yochum, 1987). Chiropractic practice generally employs adequate vertical and horizontal beam limitation (collimation) on all radiographs. Certain jurisdictions require the use of semi-automatic or automatic collimation devices.

iv) Cassettes (Sherman, 1981; Gray, 1983; Herman et al., 1987; Hufton et al., 1987; Russell, 1985). Adequate film-screen contact and film protection from white light are dependent on good quality cassettes. Routine testing of cassettes for light leaks is advisable. Defective cassettes should be repaired or replaced. Conventional cassette fronts are made of aluminum. Newer materials such as carbon-fiber and Kevlar are now in use. These materials attenuate less x-ray, are lighter, and result in reduction of patient radiation, especially at lower (50-70) kV levels. Improvements should be considered when purchasing new cassettes.

v) Grids (Sherman, 1981; Curry et al., 1990; Bushong, 1984). The radiographic grid absorbs scattered radiation after it leaves the patient and before it reaches the image receptor. A grid ratio of 12:1 is ideal for spine radiography up to 100 kV. Grid ratios of 8:1 and 10:1, while resulting in less radiation exposure than 12:1, do not provide adequate scatter radiation absorption in radiography using kV of greater than 100. A moving bucky is usually not necessary for the newer grids which are manufactured with greater than 100 lines per inch. Chiropractic facilities employ focal film distances which reflect the focal length of the grid. Non-grid techniques are preferable for the thinner extremities.

vi) Patient immobilization (Sherman, 1981). Many practitioners take weight-bearing (standing) radiographs which have the dual advantage of providing diagnostic as well as postural or biomechanical information. When radiographing thicker body parts such as the lumbar spine it is sometimes impossible to reduce exposure times sufficiently to avoid patient motion. Recumbent radiography and compression devices are two methods of patient immobilization. The disadvantage of placing the patient in the recumbent position on a radiographic table is decreased accuracy in assessing posture or biomechanical relationships. Compression devices made of a wide band of radiolucent, flexible, naugahyde material are effective in immobilizing patients. These bands, fitted with a ratchet-type tightening device, can be used with upright or recumbent radiography. The compression device not only immobilizes patients during the exposure but also compresses the soft tissues, reducing patient thickness which allows less radiation exposure. Use of such bands may affect patient posture.

vii) Processing and darkroom (Ontario Ministry of Health, 1987; Sherman, 1981; Curry et al., 1990; Bushong, 1984; Gray, 1983). The darkroom and processing equipment, manual or automatic, are monitored and serviced on a regular basis. Modern automatic processors are de-signed to process large numbers of films (over 50 films daily). Oxidation of the developer chemistry solution occurs over time. Excessive oxidation of the developer solution results in a visible decrease in film optical density. In these circumstances increased patient exposure to compensate for underdevelopment and maintain optimum density is not acceptable. The useful life of automatic developer solution is typically a maximum of one month. Solutions should be disposed of in accordance with environmental protection recommendations, not poured down the drain.

viii) Filtration (NCRP #33,1975;39,1987; Sherman, 1981; Shrimpton et al., 1988; Merkin, 1982; Buehler, 1985; Kohn et al., 1988; Gatterman, 1985; Johnson, 1981; Burgess, 1981; Gray and Stears, 1983). Minimum total filtration represents the sum of inherent filtration within the tube and added filtration outside the tube port. Chiropractic radiographic installations must comply with the NCRP#33 recommendations for total filtration. Minimum requirements are listed in Table 4. Additional filtration is often used to further decrease patient exposure. Acceptable filtration materials for this purpose include aluminum, copper, gadolinium, erbium, yttrium, and niobi.

Density-equalizing filtration (DEF) is used when radiographing body parts with unequal densities. Such filtration is typically used with thoracic spine or full-spine projections. DEF is typically composed of aluminum, copper, and/or lead. The filters are positioned in the primary beam between the collimator and patient. DEF, easily attached to most collimators, provides the dual advantage of reducing radiation and enhancing radiographic quality.

ix) Full-spine radiography patient protection (Ontario Ministry of Health, 1987; Aikenhead et al., 1989; Hildebrandt, 1980; Merkin, 1982; Gatterman, 1985; Gray, 1983; Field, 1981; Gonstead, 1977; Drummond et al., 1983; Manninen et al., 1988; Kling et al., 1992; Butler et al., 1986; Daniel et al., 1985; Frank et al., 1983; De Smet et al., 1981; Hellstrom et al., 1983; Boice et al., 1979; Adran et al., 1980; Fearon et al., 1988 Nykolation et al., 1986). The chiropractic profession has established procedures to ensure reduction of patient exposure and optimal film quality in full-spine radiography. These procedures are listed in Table 5.

d. **Other issues.**

i) Radiography and pregnancy (Howe, 1985; Mossman, 1982). Genetic and somatic damage to the embryo following radiation exposure during the first trimester of pregnancy is well documented. The following precautions should be taken:

- Appropriate patient selection, determination of the most appropriate examinations, and the proper number of films consistent with diagnostic objectives.
- Explanation of the degree of risk if the person is or may be pregnant.
- Completion and signature of standard forms by every pre-menopausal patient prior to radiographic examination of the pelvic region. Forms must include an express inquiry about the patient's pregnancy status.

ii) Office staff (NCRP #39, 1975; NCPR #91,1987; Maurer, 1989). All chiropractic radiographic facilities should comply with recommendations for protection of radiation workers and occasional radiation workers from ionizing radiation as outlined in NCRP report #91. Precautions must also be taken to ensure that non-radiation workers are fully protected at all times. Practitioners may use thermo-luminescent dosimeters (TLD) to monitor radiation exposure levels.

2. **Plain film studies**
   a. **Availability.** Most chiropractic facilities have in-house radiographic equipment which allows quick and efficient acquisition of needed studies. A wide variety of technology is available to the field practitioner.
   b. **Indications and advantages.** The plain film radiograph is considered an adequate first step in the evaluation of degenerative and inflammatory joint disease, fracture, infection and neoplasm. Deyo and Diehl (1986) found plain film radiography to be 90% sensitive to these conditions when therapeutically significant. Certain other conditions, evident on plain films, particularly transitional segment and tropism, have a role in the development of back complaints (Cox, 1989; Miller, 1982; Giles, 1981; Giles, 1981). Evaluation of biomechanical relationships continues to be an important reason to acquire radiographs. Prediction of developing pain, the duration, location and severity of symptoms, and presence of complicating factors cannot be reliably ascertained from the radiograph alone. The decision to use plain film radiography must follow history and clinical examination, and be justified by clinical findings.
   c. **Radiographic series.** Sufficient radiographic evaluation of an area requires (1) clear views of relevant anatomy, (2) special views of special structures and (3) at least two films at right angles to appreciate three dimensions. (Wyatt, 1987; Gehwhiler, 1983; Hall F, 1983; Scavone, 1981). Some consider oblique views important in the evaluation of low- back pain (Howe,

1976). However the majority of published research is to the contrary, and finds the diagnostic utility of this view to be low for therapeutically significant conditions (Hall et al., 1990; Rhea et al., 1980; Schultz et al., 1990). The routine use of the lateral lumbosacral spot view has been criticized for poor diagnostic yield (Scavone, 1981; Eisenberg et al., 1979).

   d. **Disadvantages.** Plain film radiography has some inherent limitations. Soft tissue disorders, central nervous disease and abnormalities of the pelvis and abdomen are frequently not apparent on plain film until late in their course. Neither are abnormalities of the bone marrow, reproductive organs and other tissues. There is no completely safe level of radiation exposure. Mensuration and other geometric assessments have been criticized for their lack of intra- and inter-examiner reliability, and lack of association to patient complaints (Phillips, 1986; Phillips, 1975; Rozeboom, 1983; Sigler, 1985: Meeker, 1985; Wyatt, 1987). This low reliability and validity is ascribed to inherent variability in structure, geometric distortion and positional error (Davis, 1983; Rupert, 1980; Schram, 1981 & 1982; Meeker, 1985; Howe, 1972; Nash, 1969; Saraste et al., 1985; Zengle; Cypress, 1983).

   Correlation of patient complaints of mechanical pain and objective findings on the plain film radiograph remains unreliable. (Hanssen et al., 1985; Frymoyer, 1984; Fullenlove, 1957; Saraste et al., 1985; LaRocca, 1970; Rockey et al., 1978; Wyatt, 1987; Meeker, 1985; Deyo, 1986; Kelen et al., 1986; Gehwiler, 1983). Despite this, mensuration and postural analysis continue to be a significant part of the overall assessment of chiropractic patients (Jackson et al., 1989).

3. **Full spine radiography**
   a. **Availability.** Standing radiographs of the full spine, exposed on a 14" x 36" film, remain an important diagnostic tool in chiropractic practice. With proper patient selection and technical detail, full-spine radiography is safe and effective. Criticism for excessive radiation exposure and overuse is warranted when factual. Various technical improvements have resulted from continuing research.
   b. **Indications and advantages.** Patient selection for full-spine radiography is based upon similar criteria to other imaging procedures. Particular indications for frontal (A-P and P-A) full-spine radiographs are:
- Scoliosis evaluation where appropriate following clinical assessment.
- Evaluation of complex biomechanical or postural disorders.
- Evaluation of multi-level spinal complaints as a result of biomechanical compensations.

c. **Disadvantages.** Full-spine imaging procedures that are promising, but have yet to gain widespread use because of practical considerations including prohibitive cost, are:
- Large-screen image intensifier photofluorography (Manninen, 1988);
- Digital radiography (Kling, 1990) and digitizing procedures;
- Segmented-field radiography (Daniel, 1985);
- Ultra long focal film distance (10 feet or more) with air-gap, non-grid technique.

d. **Contraindications and complications.** The following are not acceptable reasons for using full-spine radiography:
- Routine evaluation or screening of patients;
- Routine re-evaluation of biomechanical or postural disorders other than scoliosis;
- Replacement for sectional radiography.

The use of split-screen or gradient screen cassettes is unacceptable because of unnecessary radiation exposure and/or inferior film quality.

4. **Stress studies**

a. **Availability.** Stress views are frequently used in chiropractic practice for the purpose of evaluating spinal instability and joint dysfunction. They are films acquired as the patient holds a posture at end-range of a motion, and the purpose is to view joint structures in that position. This gives information regarding the integrity of soft tissues surrounding the bones.

b. **Indications and advantages.** Dupuis et al. (1985) commented on the need of a quick and readily available method to evaluate spinal motion. Consistency of positioning, accuracy in measurement and satisfactory technique in performing stress views were listed as obstacles which have not been overcome outside the laboratory. Stress radiographs of the cervical spine in the initial evaluation of the post-traumatic neck allow adequate detection of integrity of the retaining fibers and to rule out late post-traumatic instability. Lateral bending and flexion/extension views of the lumbar spine are reported by some to be reliable for the detection of motion segment laxity (Dupuis et al., 1985). This study admitted that the sensitivity, specificity and validity of stress views was unproven. Some descriptive articles suggest significant clinical utility of stress films in the assessment of spinal pain syndromes (Grice, 1979; Begg, 1949; Weitz, 1981; Farfan, 1984). Speiser et al. (1989, 1990) advocated multiple stress radiographs to determine the direction and duration of lateral bending and flexion/extension exercise to improve spinal posture. The therapeutic significance of using radiography in this instance is not documented appropriately.

c. **Disadvantages.** Haas et al. (1990), in a controlled study utilizing three examiners (radiology residents), felt that the use of stress radiographs in clinical practice should be questioned. Phillips et al. (1990) concluded that there was poor correlation between the radiographs and clinical findings, rendering this a questionable technique in the evaluation of low-back pain patients. Dvorak et al. (1991) determined stress views of the low-back served only to reliably demonstrate reduction in motion, which added little to the clinical management or diagnostic picture. They concluded that stress views for mechanical back pain patients were not warranted. They further concluded that stress views were of limited diagnostic value and of no therapeutic significance. Currently the weight of published opinion supports this view (Weisel, 1991; Roberts et al., 1978; Haas et al., 1990; Nachemson, 1985; Phillips et al., 1990).

d. **Contraindications and complications.** Judicious use of stress radiography will avoid iatrogenic injury. Where obvious osseous or ligamentous abnormalities exist (e.g., dislocation and/or fracture on non-stress studies) stress studies are inappropriate.

e. **Patient outcome and therapeutic significance.** The literature clearly states that clinically significant information cannot be obtained from these studies alone. Stress radiographs are safe and can be effective in obtaining therapeutically significant information in defined circumstances.

F. Videofluoroscopy

1. **Availability.** Equipment. For clinical utility, exposure to the patient must be kept as low as reasonably achievable (ALARA) (NCRP #91, 1987). Breen et al. (1989) were able to reduce dosage in each plane (sagittal and coronal) to less than the same assessment with plain films. This is not universally achieved, however, as patient exposure levels vary from system to system.

2. **Effectiveness.** Videofluoroscopy may be valuable for evaluating the quality of spinal motion. It is unique in this respect since, unlike stress views, it not only provides a view of total excursion, but also how the segments arrived there. Unfortunately, quantification of motion is only possible with digitization. Digitization is not considered possible outside the laboratory at this time (Breen,1991).

3. **Disadvantages.** Quantification can only be done with real time fluoroscopy using a digitizer (Breen et al., 1988; Cholewicki et al., 1991). Quantification of normal has not been adequately defined. Breen et al. (1989) in a study with digital VF on a single asymptomatic subject noted that "intersegmental coronal plane rotation was not always regular, and if this phenomenon is common, similar degrees of irregularity

in symptomatic subjects cannot be regarded as pathological." Bell (1990) purports that VF is an established reliable method of evaluating spinal mechanics. While joint motion can be observed, drawing conclusions about the normalcy or abnormality of that motion appears to be unreliable and has not been evaluated for clinical correlation. Antos et al. (1990) evaluated the inter-examiner reliability of videofluoroscopy in the detection of cervical "fixations" and achieved substantial agreement, but this requires confirmation in future studies. Jones (1967) concluded that the total degree of instability or the combination of instability and restricted motion are no better depicted by cineradiography than by plain roentgenogram if adequate flexion/extension views are obtained. It would appear that for the purpose of visualizing real-time spinal motion, VF is excellent but as one attempts to quantify that motion, issues of reliability become problematical (Howe, 1976; Breen, 1989). In addition, standardized training and protocols in the use of VF are still lacking.

4. **Contraindications and complications.** Radiation dosage and unreliability are two major factors of concern.

5. **Patient outcome and therapeutic significance.** Following an extensive literature review, the Quebec Task Force on Spinal Disorders (1987) asserted that the usefulness of VF as a diagnostic procedure to evaluate presumed radicular compression, confirmed spinal stenosis, and symptomatic patients at six months or more post-surgery has been demonstrated by non-randomized controlled trials. The same Task Force concluded that there was no scientific validity to the use of VF for chronic pain syndromes, localized spinal pain, pain radiating into the extremities with or without neurologic signs, or post surgery up to six months. In addition, the role of VF remains undisputed in interventional radiology and in the evaluation of gastrointestinal, myelographic and other studies requiring the injection of contrast material. The literature does not speak strongly for spinal videofluoroscopy as a technique for clinical use at this time.

G. Plain Film Contrast Exams

1. **Myelography**
   a. **Availability and cost effectiveness.** Myelography is effectively used for demonstrating the subarachnoid space, spinal cord and nerve roots sheaths. However it is more costly and more invasive than CT or MRI, which can be performed on an out-patient basis. (Resnick,1988; Boulay et al., 1990).
   b. **Indications and advantages.** Conventional myelography has few indications today. It is used on a very limited basis in the evaluation of cervical spine radiculopathy when the CT and/or the MRI findings are ambiguous (Resnick,1988). In most instances lack of availability of CT or MRI is the only rationale for ordering myelography rather than CT or MRI. Myelography

still has usefulness in the evaluation of torn meningeal coverings of the nerve roots, or frank nerve root avulsion injuries in the post-traumatic circumstance. Some surgeons prefer myelography over MRI. Metallic surgical implants, patient size, and claustrophobia sometimes preclude the use of MRI or CT as well.
   c. **Disadvantages.** MRI has more diagnostic accuracy than myelography and is better able to visualize the internal matrix of the disc, the bone marrow, the spinal cord and the surrounding soft tissues. CT also clearly outlines soft-tissue/fat planes allowing for gross visualization of the thecal sac. It also provides superior detail of the bony elements and articulations (Boulay et al., 1990; Hesselink, 1988).
   d. **Contraindications and complications.** Many complications are possible as a result of insertion of a needle into the subarachnoid space. In addition, hypersensitivity reaction to the contrast media is well documented. "Spinal headache" following the procedure is infamous and experienced by most patients.
   e. **Patient outcome and therapeutic significance.** Acceptable diagnostic accuracy with reasonable cost are reasons that myelography has survived the imaging technology explosion. Real-time visualization of the anatomy is another reason that this modality remains viable in diagnostic imaging.

2. **Conventional arthrography**
   a. **Availability.** This modality is widely available on an outpatient basis at most imaging centers and hospitals with fluoroscopy.
   b. **Costs and effectiveness.** Arthrography is an adequately sensitive and specific modality for the assessment of intra-articular derangements. Arthrography is less expensive than sectional imaging techniques, but is considerably more invasive.
   c. **Indications and advantages.** Current literature regards arthrography and digital subtraction arthrography as the procedures of choice for the assessment of ligamentous disruption or instability in the wrist (Gundry et al., 1990; Koenig et al., 1986; Weiss et al., 1986; Belsole et al., 1990; Wilson et al., 1991). MRI appears to be useful for evaluating the ligaments of the wrist but it is difficult to interpret because of the small size of the ligaments and the varied signal intensities within them. A thorough knowledge of the anatomy and various tissue signal intensities is required (Gundry et al., 1991; Barry et al., 1991). Intra-articular loose bodies and osteochondral fractures are sometimes best demonstrated by arthrography, particularly in the ankle and elbow. Arthrography of the temporomandibular joint is reportedly very accurate for disc perforations and internal derangements. However, less invasive imaging modalities such as tomography and/or MRI are generally considered prior to

arthrography. All three studies have their strengths and weaknesses in assessing the TMJ (Rao et al., 1990; Schellhas, 1989; Nance, 1990).

d. **Disadvantages.** The diagnostic accuracy and the non-invasive pain-free nature of MRI outweighs the cost-effectiveness and invasiveness of arthrography of the knee and shoulder. MRI is now considered the study of choice for the evaluation of internal derangements and general assessments of the knee and shoulder (Dalinka et al., 1989; Habibian et al., 1989; Morrison, 1990).

e. **Contraindications and complications.** The same generic complications for this invasive technique exist as for myelography.

f. **Patient outcome and therapeutic significance.** Conventional arthrography remains a valuable study for the assessment of articular defects, loose bodies, ligamentous (or joint capsules) and/or tendinous integrity of most extra-axial joints. Less invasive imaging modalities have replaced arthrography as a routine procedure except in the wrist where it is still considered the procedure of choice for assessing ligamentous integrity (Dalinka,1990). Consultation with a radiologist is crucial in deciding upon the correct imaging modality for each given circumstance.

3. **Barium contrast examinations of the gastrointestinal tract**

a. **Availability.** Barium contrast examinations are still considered the initial imaging modality of choice for the evaluation of the gastrointestinal tract and are conducted in most radiologic centers.

b. **Cost and effectiveness.** These examinations are an inexpensive method of evaluating the morphology and course of the viscera. In addition, they are an adequately sensitive modality for the assessment of mucosal disease of the GI tract and have the advantage of real-time visualization of the functional anatomy.

c. **Indications and advantages.** Barium contrast examinations are the cornerstone for assessment of the gastrointestinal tract (Putman, 1988). Controversy exists concerning single versus double contrast studies, but the prevailing opinion is that smaller lesions of the colon such as aphthous ulcers and small polyps can be detected better with the double contrast method (Juhl, 1987). Radioisotope and CT scans, endoscopy, sigmoidoscopy and colonoscopy are secondary imaging modalities used to complement contrast studies. All of these modalities are more costly than contrast examinations, the latter three yielding a higher risk of complication (Gelfand, 1991).

d. **Disadvantages.** Ionizing radiation dosage to the organs and gonads is comparatively high.

e. **Contraindications and complications.** Reactions to the contrast media are extremely rare. However, recent publications report that anaphylactic reactions can occur from the latex bulbs used to hold enema tubes in place. Perforations as a result of overzealous per rectum introductions of contrast or air are a recognized, albeit rare, complication.

f. **Patient outcome and therapeutic significance.** As an initial evaluation, barium studies are adequately sensitive and specific. They can provide unique and important information.

H. Computed Tomography

1. **Availability.** CT is an important modality utilized in the imaging of various systems within the body, including the neuromusculoskeletal system and the abdomen. It is a proven non-invasive method of evaluating the spine and spinal cord and is widely available.

2. **Costs and effectiveness.** CT is one of the best modalities available for the assessment of spinal, musculoskeletal, central nervous, visceral and thoracic pathologies. It is an established part of any sectional imaging protocol, and has replaced conventional tomography as the sectional imaging modality of choice for musculoskeletal abnormalities. It is more expensive than most plain film techniques, but provides enhanced tissue contrast, better detail, and less radiation dose in most instances.

3. **Indications and advantages.** CT is an excellent imaging modality for the spine (Sartoris, 1989; Dalinka et al., 1990; Genant, 1981; Mirvis et al., 1989), particularly in patients with low-back pain or sciatica to demonstrate facet joint abnormalities, infection or suspected infection, radiculopathy and/or signs of nerve root irritation, chronic mechanical and neurogenic back pain, severe bony hypertrophy, neoplasm, various rheumatologic diseases, complex congenital anomalies and dysplasia including spinal stenosis, recurrent disc disease, and metabolic disease. Indications for use of CT following spinal trauma include: suggestion of vertebral fracture on plain film x-rays, further evaluation of an evident fracture or dislocation, disparity between the plain film x-rays and neurological symptoms, and inadequate imaging of the lower cervical spine vertebrae with plain film radiography. There is a higher percentage of positive findings on CT scans when there are signs and symptoms indicating possible cervical spine or cord injury.

CT is also a good adjunctive imaging modality for appendicular trauma. It is particularly valuable in the diagnosis and evaluation of hip and sternoclavicular trauma (Sartoris, 1989; Dalinka et al., 1990; Sartoris, 1988,1987). It has been suggested that CT is the modality of choice for evaluating occult fractures of the acetabulum and femoral head and to identify any intra-articular fragments. CT is an excellent modality to image sacral and sacroiliac joint fractures, and surpasses plain film radiography in this regard. It is useful in assessing the intra-articular extension of fractures in and about joints, fractures in complex anatomical areas such as the foot/ankle and hand/wrist, and is the modality of choice for evaluation of acute post-traumatic intracranial hemorrhage (Taveras, 1990).

Imaging of the spinal cord and thecal sac can be done with CT, often with a contrast agent introduced into the subarachnoid space. CT myelography can differentiate epidural from intradural lesions. Most intramedullary lesions can be distinguished from intradural extramedullary lesions as well.

Computed tomography has a secondary role in the evaluation of both osseous and soft tissue neoplasms. The major indications for CT in patients with neoplasms of bone or soft tissue include defining the extent of the neoplasm, aiding in selection of biopsy sites, surgical planning, and evaluating response to therapy. CT is most useful when the plain films do not adequately characterize the lesion or when there is uncertainty after magnetic resonance imaging. CT is best for evaluation of fine periosteal reaction, tumor mineralization, and cortical integrity. It is recommended that CT or MRI imaging of solitary neoplasms be obtained before biopsy (Sundaram et al., 1990). CT is also valuable in the diagnosis of arthritis (Kaye, 1990; Sartoris, 1987; Sartoris Part II, 1988; Resnick, 1988; Moss, 1983).

While CT is not a screening modality, some have suggested that CT is the most widely available and most effective non-invasive technique for demonstrating discogenic and bone-related pain (Pelz, 1989). In comparative studies, CT and MRI compare favorably; however, most describe the superiority of CT in the evaluation of osseous detail.

4. **Disadvantages.** CT plays a small role in the imaging of primary joint diseases and should be considered a complementary approach to rheumatologic disease as compared to other imaging modalities. It is most useful in areas of complex anatomy or areas which are difficult to evaluate with plain film x-ray such as the spine.

5. **Contraindications and complications.** CT should be used in conjunction with plain film in the spine and other areas of the body (Dalinka et al., 1990; Sartoris, 1989). In general, regardless of what system of the body is being imaged, the plain film exam or other screening type procedures such as scintigraphy should precede computed tomography.

6. **Patient outcome and therapeutic significance.** CT is relatively non-invasive (unless used with contrast medium), has excellent spatial and contrast resolution, and the ability to evaluate both osseous and soft tissue structures during a single examination.

I. Magnetic Resonance Imaging (MRI)

1. **Availability.** MRI systems have not proliferated as rapidly as CT in the same time period for technical and financial reasons. To date there are about 2,000 MRI units operating worldwide, 1,200 of these located within the United States.

Except for Japan, most countries have very limited access to MRI scanners (Hillman, 1986; Rothschild et al., 1990).

2. **Costs and effectiveness.** Estimating the cost of performing a scan is very complicated, and ranges widely depending on financing and patient volume. The average technical cost is around $250, but cost can be much higher (Milliren, 1989). The full cost of a scan depends on technical costs, the type of scan, location, professional fees and profit margins. An MRI scan without contrast can cost between $500 and $1,500. Use of contrast can increase this charge significantly (Benness, 1991; Milliren, 1989). Comparison studies with MRI and plain film myelography indicate that MRI is less expensive to perform. The most important element of the increased cost of myelography is the need to admit the patient to the hospital overnight (du Boulay et al.,1990). Boden et al. (1990) estimate that with knee trauma patients MRI would not be a cost-effective procedure compared to arthroscopy if more than 78% of the patients referred for MRI proceeded to have an arthroscopy.

3. **Indications and advantages.** MRI is best suited for stable, cooperative patients. It also lacks significant streak or beam hardening artifacts from thick bone or metallic surgical implants, structures that can severely degrade the CT image (Council on Scientific Affairs, 1989; Dalinka et al., 1990; Hillman, 1986; Hinshaw, 1989). In the head and brain, MRI is considered superior to CT in evaluating the temporal lobes, posterior fossa, cranio-cervical junction, paranasal sinuses, and nasopharynx. It is considered superior or equal to CT with contrast in evaluating many inflammatory or demyelinating disorders, cases in which detailed anatomic assessment is necessary, most vascular disorders, the extent and distribution of disease, and in locating pathology (Benness,1991; Deck et al., 1989; Hinshaw, 1989; Levy et al., 1990; Milliren, 1989; Wallace, 1991).

In the spine, there is still considerable controversy over whether CT or MRI is the better initial imaging modality. While MRI and CT (with or without myelography) are of relatively equal sensitivity in evaluating herniated disc, many authors consider MRI the modality of choice because it is less expensive and invasive and does not expose the patient to ionizing radiation. Other advantages of MRI over CT in general include direct multiplanar imaging, easily obtainable images of the entire spine, excellent tissue contrast, and the ability to detect myelopathies of the cord (Carmody et al., 1989; Jackson et al., 1989; Kormano, 1989; Lee, 1990). MRI has been found to be as sensitive and specific as plain film myelography in evaluating cord compression, but with increased sensitivity in finding bony changes. It is usually better tolerated by the patient and is non-invasive (Carmody et al., 1989). MRI with intravenous contrast (GD-DPTA) is very helpful at differentiating epidural scar from recurrent or residual disc material in the post-operative patient. Scar will enhance diffusely within 15 minutes, while disc may show minimal enhancement after 30 minutes (Kormano, 1989; Lee, 1990).

With regard to the musculoskeletal system, MRI has been found to be of value in staging bone and soft tissue tumors, evaluation of normal and diseased menisci and ligaments of the knee, early detection of articular cartilage damage, determining a specific arthritic diagnosis, evaluating for tendinitis, differentiating septic joints from cellulitis from osteomyelitis, demonstrating the soft tissue and marrow effects of trauma, and evaluating most conditions of the TMJ (Council on Scientific Affairs, 1989; Dalinka et al., 1990; Hinshaw, 1989; Kaye, 1990). MRI is considered more sensitive than scintigraphy for detecting stress fractures, and gives better anatomic detail. It is also considered the most sensitive imaging modality for diagnosing avascular necrosis (Council on Scientific Affairs, 1989). Visceral evaluation is limited. Some authors suggest that MRI is an excellent means for evaluating pelvic mass lesions (Hinshaw, 1989), but the cost and availability of the procedure won't allow MRI to be competitive with other established procedures.

4. **Disadvantages.** MRI is not considered cost-effective for routine use in many body areas. It cannot compete with scintigraphy in whole body evaluation for suspected bone metastasis. The high cost of MRI contrast exams and limited availability will limit the role it will play in determining disease activity in arthritis.

It is not competitive with mammography in evaluation of the breast, nor ultrasound in evaluation of the prostate (Council on Scientific Affairs, 1989; Frank et al., 1990; Jackson et al., 1990; Kaye, 1990; Milliren, 1989). In general, MRI is nonspecific in differentiating benign from malignant lesions in most body areas, and in distinguishing between specific disease processes in the brain (Council on Scientific Affairs, 1989; Dalinka et al., 1990; Levy et al., 1990; Rothschild et al., 1990). MRI is not considered as sensitive as CT in the evaluation of osteoarthritis of the TMJ, acute cranial trauma (fractures and acute hemorrhage), and the skull base and temporal bones (if bone windows are used). It is also considered inferior to CT in assessing acute strokes, calcification in brain lesions, meningiomas, and most forms of epilepsy (Benness, 1991; Council on Scientific Affairs, 1989; Milliren, 1989; Wallace, 1991).

Many insurance carriers won't cover MRI of the lumbar spine for suspected disc herniation. There is more difficulty differentiating herniated disc from posterior osteophyte in the cervical spine with MRI. Evaluation of facet joint disease is less efficient with MRI than CT. For the trauma patient CT and plain film radiography are the mainstay, especially in the acute phase (Kormano, 1989; Lee, 1990).

5. **Contraindications and complications.** Because of the magnetic fields generated by this procedure, there are contraindications for having an MRI scan. These include cochlear implants, metallic foreign bodies in the eye, ferromagnetic heart valves, intracranial aneurysm clips, IUDs with metallic loops, permanent TENS units, and some pacemakers. Additionally, because of the confined space in the scanner, patients with claustrophobia are not good candidates for this exam

(Council on Scientific Affairs, 1989; DeLuca, 1990). It is still recommended that pregnant women forgo this procedure unless absolutely necessary, not because of any known complications, but because of the uncertainty of its effects. There has been no evidence to suggest that significant heating of metallic implants occurs during this procedure, and accordingly most orthopedic implants (joint replacements, etc.) are not a contraindication. These implants do cause focal image degradation (Dalinka et al., 1990; Deluca, 1990). While most authors indicate that there are no known detrimental side effects to this procedure, it is still relatively new. One suggested complication is the potential for hearing loss after an exam performed on a high field strength scanner, secondary to the excessive noise of the machine during the exam (Rothschild et al., 1990).

6. **Patient outcome and therapeutic significance.** Boden et al. (1990) in their study of 63 asymptomatic cervical spine patients emphasized the danger of predicting therapeutic decisions on diagnostic tests without precisely matching those findings with clinical signs and symptoms. The increased sensitivity of MRI does not alone justify the addition of an expensive diagnostic test. The availability of the modality will also greatly affect its usage. To insist on an MRI because it is the best modality when it is not readily available is unrealistic. Additionally, if diagnostic imaging is to be performed, conventional radiography is almost invariably the initial procedure of choice.

J. Radionuclide Scanning

1. **Availability.** Nuclear medicine scanning (e.g., bone scanning) is a highly effective imaging modality in the assessment of structure and function of many organ systems. The technique is based upon biochemistry or, more accurately, organ metabolism. The increased or decreased uptake of the radiopharmaceutical allows the doctor to visualize areas of abnormal metabolism. Technetium-99m phosphate is the primary radiopharmaceutical used in skeletal radionuclide scanning (SRC). (Many other radionuclides, such as radioisotopes of thallium and indium, are used to image non-skeletal organs.) SRC is available at most imaging centers.

2. **Costs and effectiveness.** SRC is highly sensitive but often non-specific (Kognon et al., 1983). The radionuclide scan allows the doctor to evaluate large areas of the body with relatively low radiation dose to the patient. In fact, radionuclide scanning is the most useful screening test for evaluating the entire skeleton for pathology (Frank et al.,1983).

3. **Indications and advantages.** SRC is actually a measure of the metabolic activity of bone and may detect lesions when plain film radiographic studies are negative. Technetium's short half-life makes it useful for diagnostic radiology. Gallium-67 is the preferred radiopharmaceutical for imaging suspected infection or lymphoma. Gallium-67 is unsatisfactory for almost all other bone disorders (Alazraki et al., 1985;

Kognon et al., 1984). SRC is the most commonly used imaging technique for the staging and evaluation of bone metastasis. Magnetic resonance imaging has greater sensitivity in detecting focal disease, but SRC is the most useful screening test for the entire skeleton (Frank et al., 1983). Degenerative joint disease, fractures, and infection can all produce an abnormal bone scan. Scintigraphic studies permit the early detection of stress injuries to bone when plain film radiographs are negative, and SRC is therefore the study of choice if clinical findings suggest a stress fracture (Pennell et al., 1985). Osteomyelitis and septic arthritis may be diagnosed only by scintigraphic studies in their early stages. In cases where infection is clinically suspected and a technetium-99m scan is equivocal or negative, a gallium-67 scan should be performed.

Radionuclide scanning is also commonly used for extra-skeletal organ systems. The most common organ and organ systems imaged are the cardiopulmonary system, the gastrointestinal system, and the genitourinary system. This imaging modality has many advantages over other modalities. These include 1) function of the organ or organ systems can be evaluated; 2) contrast material is not needed; 3) low radiation dose to the patient; 4) fairly low cost; 5) prior patient preparation is not required; and 6) sequential studies of other organ systems can be performed easily (Stine, 1988). Indications for extra-skeletal radionuclide scanning include but are not limited to the following: 1) assessment of organ function; 2) evaluation of organs in trauma; 3) diagnosis of infection within organs; 4) evaluation for congenital anomalies; and 5) evaluation for malignancy (Velchik, 1985).

4. **Disadvantages.** Radionuclide scanning is a sensitive but not a specific imaging technique for detection of malignant tumors because other conditions, some benign in nature, can result in positive tests (Frank et al., 1983).

5. **Contraindications and complications.** The most important contraindication is that radionuclide scanning should not be performed on the pregnant patient.

6. **Patient outcome and therapeutic significance.** Skeletal radionuclide scanning is a very sensitive, cost effective method of evaluating the metabolic activity of a single region of the skeleton, or in evaluating the activity of a known lesion. It also serves as a screening modality for the detection of skeletal metastasis.

K. Diagnostic Ultrasound (Ultrasonography)

1. **Availability.** Ultrasonography is a widely used diagnostic imaging procedure which employs the use of sound waves transmitted into the body, and then received back as echoes to a receiver. It is the most commonly used imaging procedure in the female genitourinary tract. More recently ultrasonography has been used to evaluate the musculoskeletal system.

2. **Costs and effectiveness.** This non-invasive modality is a highly effective and inexpensive tool to evaluate the soft tissues of the body. Real-time visualization of the anatomy allows even more accurate evaluation of an area.

3. **Indications and advantages.** Primary use is for the gastrointestinal and genitourinary tracts. Diagnostic ultrasound is also an established modality in the assessment of obstetric and gynecologic conditions. The advantages of ultrasonography include: 1) it is non-invasive; 2) absence of ionizing radiation; 3) relatively low cost; 4) it is a fast procedure; 5) as it is non-destructive to tissues, frequent examinations of the same region can be performed without tissue damage; 6) it does not require contrast material; and 7) it does not depend on the function of an organ to visualize the anatomy (Terenzi, 1990; Stine et al., 1988).

   a. **Ultrasound of the abdomen.** Ultrasonography is the most commonly employed diagnostic procedure of the abdomen. In the abdomen it is primarily used to evaluate solid organs, to differentiate masses from cysts, and to evaluate the patient for intra-abdominal calcification. Ultrasound is the imaging method of choice in the investigation of gallbladder disease, and the method of choice in the assessment of bile duct obstruction or dilatation (Lindsell, 1990). Ultrasound can help to correctly identify the origin of a focal mass which allows expeditious acquisition of additional diagnostic studies (Carroll, 1989). In the genitourinary system ultrasound plays a key role in the diagnosis of tumors and cysts of the kidneys, bladder, prostate, and intrascrotal structures (Stine, 1988). In patients with palpable pelvic masses, ultrasonography has demonstrated superiority to retroperitoneal pneumography, barium enemas, and intravenous pyelography (O'Brien et al., 1984). Ultrasonography is very useful for evaluation of a patient for genitourinary infections and intraluminal calcification. Ultrasonography is an extremely sensitive modality for diagnosing hydronephrosis (Coleman, 1985). If renal failure is suspected clinically, ultrasonography should be the initial exam because it shows the anatomy better than an intravenous pyelogram given the poor function of the kidney (Coleman, 1985). It is a commonly used modality for patients with ureteral calculi who have renal failure or are allergic to the intravenous pyelogram contrast media (Stine et al., 1988). It may be useful in the early diagnosis of bladder carcinoma and it is sometimes helpful in determining benign versus malignant nodules in the prostate (Rifkin, 1985).

   b. **Musculoskeletal ultrasound.** Ultrasonography of the musculoskeletal system is a relatively new and controversial technique. The consensus of opinion is that it is best used to evaluate muscles, tendons, ligaments, and bursae. It is a reliable means for diagnosing intramuscular and muscular boundary lesions (Van Holsbeeck, 1991). It is a very useful diagnostic tool to evaluate soft tissue trauma of the shoulder (Lind et al., 1989). It is a commonly used procedure to evaluate for tears of the rotator cuff. Real-time ultrasonography with static ultrasonography is diagnostically as sensitive and specific as arthrography in the diagnosis of rotator cuff tears (Drakeford et al., 1990). It is, however, more accurate in detecting full thickness tears than in detecting thin, incomplete tears. Ultrasound is also now being used to detect osteomyelitis. It is used to visualize the inflammatory fluid underneath the periosteum (Kaplan et al., 1990).

4. **Disadvantages.** The main disadvantage of ultrasonography is that it is a difficult modality to perform and requires highly qualified doctors to interpret (Kaplan). Other disadvantages are that it requires the patient to have a full bladder and that bowel gas may interfere with the image (Stine et al., 1988).

5. **Contraindications and complications.** Because ultrasound employs only sonic waves, there are no direct complications or contraindications to the study. However, since skin contact is mandatory for the study, patients with severe skin conditions or burns may not be able to receive this study.

6. **Patient outcome and therapeutic significance.** Diagnostic ultrasound currently has definite utility only in the evaluation of intra-abdominal and pelvic abnormalities. However, recently developed musculoskeletal applications show promise, especially in evaluation of musculoligamentous abnormalities.

L. Utilization Review

Decisions on appropriateness of imaging services remain the prerogative of the primary practitioner. A radiologist who provides a service at the request of the primary practitioner is responsible and subject to review, for the service quality and cost but not the decision to utilize these services.

Any requirement for demonstrated radiological abnormality or clinical proof of diagnosis to substantiate claims for radiological services is inappropriate. It would be inconsistent with the proven and proper uses of diagnostic imaging for the detection of suspected disease or injury and evaluation of treatment. Denial of claims because the exam findings prove to be "negative" is a marked disservice to the provision of good patient care. Such exams are expressly obtained for the purposes of excluding or confirming a variety of abnormalities.

Incomplete and/or suboptimal plain film studies may occur for a variety of reasons, including poor patient cooperation, the habitus of the patient, and technical factors.

Careful patient selection by the practitioner and open consultation with specialists will prevent inappropriate examinations. A variety of advanced imaging modalities are available,

and consultation with experts is bound to have a positive impact on the overall patient management.

V. ASSESSMENT CRITERIA

Procedure Ratings (System I)

Established: Accepted as appropriate by the practicing chiropractic community for the given indication in the specified patient population.

Promising: Given current knowledge, this technology appears to be appropriate for the given indication in the specified patient population. As more evidence and experience accumulate this interim rating will change. This connotes provisional acceptance, but permits a greater role for the level of current clinical use.

Equivocal: Current knowledge exists to support a given indication in a specified patient population, though value can neither be confirmed nor denied. As more evidence and experience accumulates this interim rating will change. Expert opinion recognizes a need for caution in general application.

Investigational: Evidence is insufficient to determine appropriateness. Further study is warranted. Use for a given indication in a specified patient population should be confined largely to research protocols. As more evidence and experience accumulates this interim rating will change.

Doubtful: Given current knowledge, this appears to be inappropriate for the given indication in the specified patient population. As more evidence and experience accumulate this interim rating will change.

Inappropriate: Regarded by the practicing chiropractic community as unacceptable for the given indication in the specified patient population.

Quality of Evidence:

The following categories of evidence are used to support the rating.

Class I:
Evidence provided by one or more well designed controlled clinical trials; or well designed experimental studies that address reliability, validity, positive predictive value, discriminability, sensitivity, and specificity.

Class II:
Evidence provided by one or more well designed uncontrolled, observational clinical studies such as case control, cohort studies, etc.; or clinically relevant basic science studies that address reliability, validity, positive predictive value, discriminability, sensitivity, and specificity; and published in refereed journals.

Class III:

Evidence provided by expert opinion, descriptive studies or case reports.

Suggested Strength of Recommendations Ratings

Type A. Strong positive recommendation. Based on Class I evidence or overwhelming Class II evidence when circumstances preclude randomized clinical trials.

Type B. Positive recommendation based on Class II evidence.

Type C. Positive recommendation based on strong consensus of Class III evidence.

Type D. Negative recommendation based on inconclusive or conflicting Class II evidence.

Type E. Negative recommendation based on evidence of ineffectiveness or lack of efficacy based on Class I or Class II evidence.

VI. RECOMMENDATIONS

A. Sequence of Services

The practitioner, in most instances, is the person that initiates a radiographic study. The study is performed by the technologist or qualified person in a safe environment in a manner consistent with published guidelines regarding quality and performance. It is the standard of care that all studies are viewed for interpretation by the practitioner or radiologist to obtain the maximum level of diagnosis which is achievable based on the type of study performed. Standard and customary billing procedures are followed.

2.1.1 **Rating:** Established
Evidence: Class III
Consensus Level: 1

B. Patient Selection Procedures

The decision on whether or not to use diagnostic imaging studies is made following a carefully performed history, physical and regional evaluation, and consideration of cost/benefit/radiation exposure ratios. It is based on sound clinical reasoning and the likelihood that significant information can be obtained from the study in regards to diagnosis, prognosis and therapy. The decision remains solely the domain of the examining (primary) practitioner.

2.2.1 **Rating:** Established
Evidence: Class I, II, III
Consensus Level: 1

Comment: It is difficult to weigh the impact of the political, litigious, and social climate on the perceived need of many practitioners to have prior radiographic evidence of the area to be manipulated. This issue needs further study before firm conclusions about the prophylactic acquisition of radiographs can be made.

C. Radiographic Interpretation and Reporting

Imaging studies are performed primarily to contribute to a diagnostic impression. Interpretation of each imaging study should be documented in the patient's permanent record.

2.3.1 **Rating:** Established
Evidence: Class II, III
Consensus Level: 1

D. Legal Issues in Radiography

Federal regulations (Public Law 97-35 sec. 978) state that radiography, as applied to chiropractic practice, is used for diagnostic purposes only, and not for radio-therapeutic purposes. The National Council on Radiation Protection has established recommendations for the safe and effective use of radiography. It is the responsibility of every practitioner to be informed of and abide by all relevant legal requirements.

2.4.1 **Rating:** Established
Evidence: Class III
Consensus Level: 1

E. Radiation Technology and Protection

Practitioners should keep the radiation exposure of patients as low as reasonably achievable. This includes use of modern equipment and techniques as outlined in the literature review section of this document. A suboptimal radiograph should be repeated. The decision on whether or not to expose a patient to radiation is only valid before the series is ordered. Once committed to the acquisition of a series, the practitioner is obligated to produce high quality radiographs.

2.5.1 **Rating:** Established
Evidence: Class I, II, III
Consensus Level: 1

F. Plain Film Radiographs

The plain film radiograph is considered an adequate first step in the evaluation of degenerative and inflammatory joint disease, fracture, infection and neoplasm. Not every patient with these conditions will require radiography for diagnosis. Orthogonal views are a necessary minimum for visualizing any body area. Additional views are used as appropriate to demonstrate conditions which could exist given the findings of the clinical diagnosis.

2.6.1 **Rating:** Established
Evidence: Class I, II, III
Consensus Level: 1

For postural and biomechanical assessment.

2.6.2 **Rating:** Promising
Evidence: Class II, III
Consensus Level: 1

G. Full Spine Radiography

For scoliosis evaluation where indicated by clinical examination.

2.7.1 **Rating:** Established
Evidence: Class I, II, III
Consensus Level: 1

For evaluation of complex biomechanical or postural disorders and the evaluation of multi-level spinal complaints as a result of biomechanical compensation.

2.7.2 **Rating:** Promising
Evidence: Class II, III
Consensus Level: 1

H. Stress Radiography

Stress views are often of value in the assessment of degenerative, traumatic or post-surgical instabilities with the exception of those that carry the risk of neurologic injury. They provide unique diagnostic information.

2.8.1 **Rating:** Established
Evidence: Class I, II, III
Consensus Level: 1

For other conditions and circumstances.

2.8.2 **Rating:** Equivocal
Evidence: Class II, III
Consensus Level: 1

I. Videofluoroscopy (cinefluoroscopy)

For kinematic and other biomechanical purposes.

2.9.1 **Rating:** Promising
Evidence: Class II, III
Consensus Level: 1

Comment: The authors of the Quebec Task Force (1987) have outlined the limited use criteria which currently appear valid.

For instability of the wrist and contrast studies.

2.9.2 **Rating:** Established
Evidence: Class I, II, III
Consensus Level: 1

J. Plain Film Contrast Studies

Provide valuable unique information in special circumstances. These studies should only be performed by a radiologist.

2.10.1 **Rating:** Established
Evidence: Class I, II, III
Consensus Level: 1

K. Computed Tomography

Valuable in the assessment of most musculoskeletal conditions requiring sectional imaging. Of particular utility in the evaluation of complex fractures in flat bones or the posterior arch of any spinal level. Adequately sensitive and specific for the evaluation of complicated degenerative conditions and herniated nucleus pulposus of the lumbar spine. Ordered only in the presence of specific clinical indications.

2.11.1 **Rating:** Established
Evidence: Class I, II, III
Consensus Level: 1

L. Magnetic Resonance Imaging

The study of choice in the pre-operative evaluation of many internal derangements of articulations, and the evaluation of many central nervous system disorders. Comparisons between CT and MRI have shown similar sensitivity. Limited spatial resolution capabilities and cost are drawbacks. Ordered only in the presence of specific clinical indications.

2.12.1 **Rating:** Established
Evidence: Class I, II, III
Consensus Level: 1

M. Radionuclide Bone Scanning

Has an established role in the evaluation of bone disease. Adequately sensitive, put poorly specific. Ordered only in the presence of specific historical and diagnostic information.

2.13.1 **Rating:** Established
Evidence: Class I, II, III
Consensus Level: 1

N. Diagnostic Ultrasound

Utility and accuracy in the evaluation of musculoskeletal conditions remains limited, but diagnostic ultrasound has promise as a non-invasive, inexpensive alternative to MRI and arthrography. An established modality for evaluation of many intra-abdominal and pelvic organs.

2.14.1 **Rating:** Established
Evidence: Class I, II, III
Consensus Level: 1

VII. COMMENTS, SUMMARY OR CONCLUSION

Imaging has been and continues to be essential in the evaluation of chiropractic patients. It is important to consider the deleterious effects and cost of imaging prior to acquiring a study. The critical issue is *need* for the study. The practitioner considering imaging, from plain film to MRI, must consider this question: "Will the results of this study have an impact on the treatment I propose to deliver?" If this question is asked and answered objectively in every case, there will be proper acquisition of imaging studies. This is particularly true of plain films.

There are many components to each diagnostic study. There is the potential of a variety of individuals to be involved in performing radiology studies. Each individual is responsible for the services they provide in terms of appropriateness, quality and billing for services. It is prudent for the practitioner to consider the value of second opinions and other specialist services as the field of imaging has become increasingly complex.

VIII. REFERENCES

ACBR Candidates Guide; published by the American Chiropractic College of Radiology, 1989.

Adran GM, Coates R, Dickson RA, Dixon-Brown A, Harding FM: Assessment of scoliosis in children: low dose radiographic techniques. *Br J Radiol* 1980, 53:146-7.

Aikenhead J, Triano J, Baker J: Relative efficacy for radiation reducing methods in scoliotic patients. *J Manip Physiol Ther* 1989, 12:259-64.

Alazraki N, Fierer J, Resnick D: Chronic osteomyelitis-monitoring by Techneitium-99m phosphate and Galium-67 citrate imaging. *American Journal of Radiology*. October 1985, 145:767-771.

Albeck MJ, Kjaer L, Praestholm J, Vestergaard A, Hinriksen O, Gjerris F: Magnetic resonance imaging, computed tomography, and myelography in the diagnosis of recurrent lumbar disc herniation. *Acta Neurochir* (Wien) 1990, 102:122-126.

Annertz M, Holtas S, Cronqvist S, Jonsson B, Stromqvist B: Isthmic lumbar spondylolisthesis with sciatica. MR imaging vs myelography. *Acta Radiologica* 1990, 31(5):449-453.

Antos JC, Robinson GK, Keating JC, Jacobs GE: Interrater reliability of fluoroscopic detection of fixation in the mid-cervical spine. *Chiro Technique* 1990, 2:53-55.

Aspegren DD, Cox JM, Trier KK: Short leg correction: a clinical trial of radiographic vs. non-radiographic procedures. *J Manip Physiol Ther* 1987, 10:232-8.

Baddely H: *Radiologic Investigation*. New York, John Wiley and Sons, 1984.

Bailey DN: Plain film vs videofluoroscopy comparison of clinical value in the cervical spine: a retrospective study. *ACA J Chiro* : July, 1991:59-62.

Barry MS, Kettner NW, Pierre-Jerome C: Carpal instability: pathomechanics and contemporary imaging. *Chiropractic Sports Medicine* 1991, 5:(2):38-44.

Lumbar intervertebral disks: a correlation with operative findings. *Br J Surg*. Jan 1949, 26(143):225-239.

Bell GD: Skeletal applications of videofluoroscopy. *J Manip Physiol Ther* 1990, 13(7):396-405.

Belsole RJ, Quinn SF, Greene TL, Beatty ME, Rayhack JM: Digital subtraction angiography of the wrist. *Bone Joint Surg* 1990, 72A(6):846-851.

Benness GT: MRI assessment programme: A clearer picture: *Med J Aust* Feb 1991, 154:229-230.

Boden SD, Labropoulos PA, Vailas JC: MR scanning of the acutely injured knee: sensitive, but is it cost effective: *Arthroscopy* 1990, 6(4):306-310.

Boden SD, McCowin PR, Davis DO, Dina TS, Mark AD, Wiesel S: Abnormal magnetic resonance scans of the cervical spine in symptomatic subjects. *J Bone Joint Surg* Sept 1990, 72-A(8): 1178-1183.

Boice JD, Land CE, Shore RE, Norman JE, Tokunaga M: Risk of breast cancer following low-dose radiation exposure. *Radiology* 1979, 131:589-97.

Boulay GH, Hawks S, Lee CC, Teather BA, Teather D: Comparing the cost of spinal MR with conventional myelography and radiculography. *Neuroradiology* 1990, 32:124-136.

Breen A, Allen R, Morris A: An image processing method for spine kinematics-preliminary studies. *Clinical Biomechanics* 1988, 3:5-10.

Breen AC, Allen R, Morris A: Spine Kinematics: A digital videofluoroscopic technique. *J Biomed Eng* 1989, 11:224-228.

Breen A, Allen R, Morris A: A digital videofluoroscopic technique for spine kinematics. *J Med Eng Technol* 1989, 13:109-113.

Breen A: The digital videofluoroscopic assessment of spine kinematics. *Proceedings 1990 ICSM* Washington D.C. May 1990:86-92.

Breen A: The reliability of palpation and other diagnostic methods. World Chiropractic Congress, *Proceedings of the Scientific Symposium*: May 1991:1-7.11.

Buehler MT, Hrejsa AF: Application of lead-acrylic compensating filters in chiropractic full spine radiography: a technical report. *J Manip Physiol Ther* 1985, 8:175-80.

Buonocare E. Hartman JT, Nelson CL: Cineradiograms of cervical spine in diagnosis of soft-tissue injuries. *JAMA* 1966, 198:25-29.

Burgess AE. Contrast effects of a gadolinium filter. *Med Phys* 1981, 8:203-9.

Buschong SC: *Radiologic science for technologists: physics, biology, and protection. 3rd ed.* St. Louis, Mosby 1984:1-621.

Butler PF, Thomas AW, Thompson WE, Wollerton MA, Rachlin JA: Simple methods to reduce radiation exposure during scoliosis radiography. *Radiologic Technology* 1986, 57:411-17.

Carmody RF, Yang PJ, Seeley GW, Seeger JF, Unger EC, Johnson JE: Spinal cord compression due to metastatic disease: diagnosis with MR imaging versus myelography. *Radiology* 1989, 173:225-229.

Carrera G, Haughton V, Syvertsen A, Williams A: Computed tomography of the lumbar facet joints. *Radiology* 1980, 134:145-148.

Carroll, BA: US of the gastrointestinal tract: *Radiology* 1989, 172:605-608.

Cholewicki J, McGill SM, Wells RP, Vernon H: Method for measuring vertebral kinematics from videofluoroscopy. *Clinical Biomechanics* 1991, 6:73-78.

Cohen G, Wagner LK, McDaniel DL, Robinson LH: Dose efficiency of screen-film systems used in pediatric radiography. *Radiology* 1984, 187-193.

Coleman BG: Ultrasonography of the upper genitourinary tract. *Urologic Clinics of North America*. 1985, 12(4):633-44.

Cooley J, Schultz G, Phillips R: What do chiropractors see on x-rays? in *Proceedings of International Conference on Spinal Manipulation FCER*, May 1990: 24-26.

Council on Scientific Affairs: Musculoskeletal applications of magnetic resonance imaging. *JAMA* 1989, 262(17):2420-2427.

Cox J: *Low-Back Pain.* 4th Ed. Baltimore, Williams and Wilkins, 1989.

Curry TS, Dowdey JE, Murry RC: *Christensen's Physics of Diagnostic Radiology. 4th ed.* Philadelphia, Lea & Febiger, 1990:1-522.

Cypress B: Characteristics of physician visits for back symptoms: a national perspective. *AM J Public Health* 1983, 73(4):389-395.

Dalinka MK, Kricun ME, Zlatin MB, Hibbard CA: Modern diagnostic imaging in joint disease. *AJR* 1989, 152:229-240.

Dalinka MK: Radiographic imaging in orthopedics. *Orthopedic Clinics of North America* 1990, 21:423-559.

Dalinka MK, Zlatkin MB, Chao P, Kricun ME, Kressel HY: The use of magnetic resonance imaging in the evaluation of bone and soft tissue tumors. *Radiologic Clinics of North America* 1990, 28:461-469.

Daniel WW, Barnes GT, Nasca RJ, Annegan DC: Segmented-field radiography in scoliosis. *AJR* 1985, 144:325-329.

Davis B, Roozeboom D: A model to test the radiographically determined pelvic subluxation. *Proceedings from the Advances in Conservative Health Sciences.* National College of Chiropractic Academic Press, Lombard, IL. 1983.

Deck MD, Henschke C, Lee BC, Zimmerman RD, Hyman RA, Edwards J, Saint Louis LA, Cahill PT, Stein H, Whalen JP: Computed tomography versus magnetic resonance imaging of the brain. A collaborative interinstitutional study. *Clin Imaging* 1989, 13(1):2-15.

DeLuca SA, Castronova FP: Hazards of magnetic resonance imaging. *AFP* 1990, 41:145-146.

De Smet AA, Fritz SL, Asher MA: A method for minimizing the radiation exposure from scoliosis radiographs. *J Bone Joint Surg* 1981, 63-A:156-8.

Deyo R, McNiesh L, Cone R: Observer variability in the interpretation of lumbar spine radiographs. *Arth And Theum* 1985, l28(9):1066-1070.

Deyo R, Diehl A: Lumbar spine films in primary care: Current use and effects of selective ordering criteria. *J Gen Int Med* 1986, 1:20-25.

Deyo R, Diehl A: Patient satisfaction with medical care for low-back pain. *Spine* 1986, 11(1):28-30.

Deyo R, Diehl A, Rosenthal M: Reducing roentgenography use: Can patient expectations be altered? *Arch Intern Med* 1987, 147:141-145.

Deyo RA, Bigos SJ, Maravilla KR: Diagnostic imaging procedures for the lumbar spine. *Annals Intern Med* 1989, 111:865-867.

Dimnet J, Pasquet A, Krag MH, Panjabi MM: Cervical spine motion in the sagittal plane: kinematic and geometric parameters. *J Biomechanics* 1982, 15:959-969.

Dively R, Oglevie R: Preemployment examinations of the low-back. *JAMA* 1956, 188:856-858.

Drakeford M, Quinn M, Simpson S, Pettine K: A comparative study of ultrasonography and arthrography in evaluation of the rotator cuff. *Clinical Orthopedics and Related Research* 1990, 253:118-122.

Drummond D, Ranallo F, Lonstein J, Brooks L, Cameron J: Radiation hazards in scoliosis management. *Spine* 1983, 8:741-8.

du Boulay GH, Hawkes S, Lee CC, Teather BA, Teather D: Comparing the costs of spinal MR with conventional myelography and radiculography. *Neuroradiology* 1990, 32:124-136.

Dupuis P, Yong-Hing K, Cassidy D, Kirkaldy-Willis W: Radiologic diagnosis of degenerative lumbar instability. *Spine* 1985, 10(3): 262-276.

During J, Goudfroors H, Keesen W, Beeker ThW: Towards standards of posture: postural characteristics of the lower back system in normal and pathological conditions. *Spine* 1985, 10(1):83-87.

Dvorak M, Panjabi M, Novotny J, Chang D, Grob D: Clinical validation of functional flexion-extension roentgenograms of the lumbar spine. *Spine* 1991, 16(8):943-950.

Edeiken J, Karasick D: Use of radiography for screening employees for risk of low-back disability. *J Occ Med* 1986, 28(10):995-997.

Eisenberg R, Akin J, Hedgecock M: Single well centered lateral view of the lumbosacral spine: is coned view necessary? *AJR* 1979, 133: 711-713.

Farfan H, Gracovetsky S: The nature of instability. *Spine* 1984, 9(7):714-719.

Fearon T, Vucich J, Butler P, et al.: Scoliosis examinations: organ dose and image quality with rare-earth screen-film systems. *AJR* 1988: 359-62.

Field TJ, Buehler MT: Improvements in chiropractic full spine radiography. *J Manip Physiol Ther* 1981, 4:21-25.

Fielding JW: Cineradiography of the normal cervical spine. *NY State J of Med*, 1956:2984-2986.

Frank ED, Stears JG, Gray JE, Winkler NT, Hoffman AD: Use of the posteroanterior projection: a method of reducing x-ray exposure to specific radiosensitive organs. *Radiologic Technology* 1983, 54:343-7.

Frank JA, Ling A, Patronas N, Carrasquillo JA, Horvath K, Hickey AM, Dwyer AJ: Detection of malignant bone tumors: MR imaging vs. scintigraphy. *Am J Radiology* 1990, 155:1043-48.

Frymoyer J: Spine radiographs in patients with low-back pain. *JBJS* 1984, 66A(7):1048-1055.

Fullenlove T, Williams AJ: Comparative roentgen findings in symptomatic and asymptomatic backs. *Radiology* 1957, 68:572-574.

Gatterman B: Filtration in chiropractic. *ICA Int Rev Chiropractic* 1985:62-3.

Gehweiler J, Daffner R: Low-back pain: The controversy of radiologic evaluation. *AJR* 1983, 140:109-112.

Gelfand DW, Ott DJ: The economic implications of radiologic screening for colonic cancer. *AJR* 1991, 156:939-943.

Genant HK: Computed tomography. *Orth Clinics of North America* 1985, 16:359-511.

Giles L: Low-back pain associated with leg length inequality. *Spine* 1981, 6(5):510-521.

Giles L: Lumbosacral facet joint angles associated with leg length inequality. *Rheum and Rehab* 1981, 20:233-238.

Gonstead C: Full spine radiography. In: *Gonstead Chiropractic Science and Healing Art.* U.S.: Sci-Chi Publications, 1977:145-156.

Gratton MC, Salomone JA (III), Watson WA: Clinically significant radiograph misinterpretations at an emergency medicine residency program. *Annals Emergency Med* 1990:497-502.

Gray JE, Raggozzino MW, Van Lysell MS, Burke TM: Normalized organ doses for various diagnostic radiologic procedures. *Am J Roentgenol* 1981, 137:463-70.

Gray JE, Hoffman AD, Peterson HA: Reduction of radiation exposure during radiography for scoliosis. *J Bone Joint Surg* 1983, 65-A:5-12.

Gray JE, Stears JG, Frank ED: Shaped, lead-loaded acrylic filters for patient exposure reduction and image-quality improvement. *Radiology* 1983, 146:825-8.

Gray JE, Winkler NT, Stears J, Frank ED: *Quality control in diagnostic imaging.* Ist ed. Rockville, Aspen. 1983:1-245.

Grice A: Radiographic, biomechanical and clinical factors in lumbar lateral flexion: Part I. *J Manip Physiol Ther* 1979, 2(1):26-34.

Gundry CR, Kurunoglu-Brahme S, Schwaraighofer B, Kang SH, Sartoris DJ, Resnick D: Is MR better than arthrography for evaluating the ligaments of the wrist? In vitro study. *AJR* 1990, 154:337-341.

Gyll C: Gonad protection for the pediatric patient. *Radiography* 1988, 54:9-11.

Haas M, Nyiendo J, Peterson C, Thiel H, Sellars T, Cassidy D, Yong-Hing K: Interrater reliability of roentgenological evaluation of the lumbar spine in lateral bending. *J Manip Physiol Ther* 1990, 13(4):179-189.

Habibian A, Stauffer A, Resnick D, Reicher MA, Rafii M, Kellerhouse LJ, Zlatkin MB, Newman C, Sartoris DJ: Comparison of conventional and computed arthrotomography with MR imaging in the evaluation of the shoulder. *J Computer Assisted Tomography* 1989, 13(6):968-975.

Hall F: Routine oblique projections of the lumbosacral spine in evaluation of chronic low-back pain (letter). *Radiology* 1980, 137: 209-210.

Hall FM: Back pain and the radiologist. *Radiology* 1980, 137:861-863.

Hall F: Back pain and the radiologist. *AJR* 1983, 141:861-863.

Hall T, Schultz G, Phillips R: Why do chiropractors order x-rays? in *Proceedings of international conference on spinal manipulation,* FCER, 1990:21-23.

Halvorsen JG, Kunian A: Radiology in family practice: Experience in community practice. *Family Medicine* 1988, 20(2):112-7.

Halvorsen JG, Dunian A, et al.: The interpretation of office radiographs by family physicians. *J Family Practice* 1989, 28(4):426-432.

Hanssen T, Bigos S, Beecher P, Wortley M: The lumbar lordosis in acute and chronic low-back pain. *Spine* 1985, 10:154-155.

Hashimoto K, Akahori O, Kitano K, Nakajima K, Hitashihara T, Kumasaka Y: Magnetic resonance imaging of lumbar disc herniation, comparison with myelography. *Spine* 1990, 5:1166-69.

Health and Policy Committee, American College of Physicians: How to study the gallbladder. *Annals Internal Med* 1988, 109:752-754.

Hellstrom G, Irstam L, Nachemson A: Reduction of radiation dose in radiologic examination of patients with scoliosis. *Spine* 1983, 8:28-30.

Herman MW, Mak HK, Lachman RS: Radiation exposure reduction by use of kevlar cassettes in the neonatal nursery. *AJR* 1987, 148:969-72.

Hesselink JR: Spine imaging: history, achievements, remaining frontiers. *AJR* 1988, 150:1223-1229.

Hildebrandt RW: Chiropractic spinography and postural roentgenology—part I: history of development. *J Manip Physiol Ther* 1980, 3:87-92.

Hildebrandt RW: Chiropractic spinography and postural roentgenology—part II: clinical basis. *J Manip Physiol Ther* 1981, 4:191-201.

Hillman AL, Schwartz JS: The diffusion of MRI: patterns of siting and ownership in an era of changing incentives. *AJR* 1986, 146: 963-969.

Hinshaw DB: Magnetic resonance imaging versus x-ray computed tomography - which is the appropriate first imaging examination? *West J Med* 1989, 151:569-570.

Howe J: Facts, Fallacies and misconceptions in spinography. *J Clin Chiropractic* 1972, 34:34-45.

Howe JW: Radiological investigation of spinal biomechanics. *JCCA* 1976, 20:16-21.

Howe JW, Yochum TR: X-ray, pregnancy, and therapeutic abortion: a current perspective. *ACA J Chirop* 1985, 19:76-80.

Hufton AP, Crosthwaite CM, Davies JM, Robinson LA: Low attenuation material for table tops, cassettes and grids: a review. *Radiography* 1987, 53:17-18.

Humphreys K, Breen A, Saxton D: Incremental lumbar spine motion in the coronal plane: an observer variation study using digital videofluoroscopy. *Euro J Chiro* 1990, 38:56-62.

Hunter TB, Boyle RR Jr: The value of reading the previous radiology report. *AJR* 1988, 150:697-698.

Jackson RP, Cain JE, Jacobs RR, Cooper BR, McManus GE: The neuroradiographic diagnosis of lumbar herniated nucleus populsuis: II. A comparison of computed tomography (ct), myelography, ct-myelography, and magnetic resonance imaging. *Spine* 1989, 14(12): 1362-1367.

Jaeger SA: *Atlas of radiographic positioning: normal anatomy and developmental variants. 1st ed.* Norwalk, Appleton & Lange, 1988:1-241.

Johnson MA, Burgess AE. Clinical use of a gadolinium filter in pediatric radiography. *Pediatr Radiol* 1981, 10:229-32.

Jones MD: Cineradiographic studies of abnormalities of the high cervical spine. *Arch Surg* 1967, 94:206-213.

Joseph L, Rachlin J: Use and effectiveness of chest radiography and low-back radiography in screening. *J Occupational Med* 1986, 28(10):998-1003.

Juhl J, Crummy A: *Paul and Juhl's Essentials of Radiologic Imaging.* 5th ed. Philadelphia, J.B. Lippincott Co, 1987:393-397.

Ibid:550.

Ibid:566-572.

Kaplan P, Matamoros A, Anderson J: Sonography of the musculoskeletal system. *Am J Radiology.* 1990, 155:237-245.

Kaye JJ: Imaging of joints. *Radiologic Clinics of North America* 1990, 28:905-1072.

Kaye JJ. Arthritis: Roles of radiography and other imaging techniques in evaluation. *Radiology* 1990, 177:601-608.

Kelen G, Noji E, Doris P: Guidelines of the use of lumbar spine radiography. *Annals Emerg Med* 1986, 15(3):245-251.

Kemp S: Low-back pain; a cost effective approach. *Diagnosis* 1984: 47-61.

Kling TF, Cohen MJ, Lindseth RE, DeRosa GP: Digital radiography can reduce scoliosis x-ray exposure. *Spine* 1990, 15:880-5.

Koenig H, Lucas D, Meissner R: The wrist: a preliminary report on high resolution MR imaging. *Radiology* 1986, 160:463-467.

Kognon PL, Buna MP, deGruchy M: An overview of radioisotope scanning—a valuable diagnostic procedure. *Journal of the Canadian Chiropractic Association.* 1984, 28(3):323-326.

Kohn ML, Gooch AW, Keller WS: Filters for radiation reduction: a comparison. *Radiology* 1988, 167:255-7.

Kormano M: Imaging methods in examining the anatomy and function of the lumbar spine. *Ann Med* 1989, 21(5):335-340.

Kottke FJ, Lester RG: Use of cinefluorography for evaluation of normal and abnormal motion in the neck. *Arch Physical Med Rehab*: 1958:228-231.

Kovach SG, Huslig EL: Prevalence of diagnoses on the basis of radiographic evaluation of chiropractic cases. *J Manip Physiol Ther* 1983, 6:197-201.

LACC Curriculum Bulletin, Los Angeles College of Chiropractic, 1991-1992.

LACC Radiology Residency Syllabus; Los Angeles College of Chiropractic.

LaRocca H, McNab I: Value of pre-employment radiographic assessment of the lumbar spine. *Industrial Med* 1970, 30(6):253-258.

Lee KS: The role of magnetic resonance imaging in the evaluation of spinal disorders. *Comprehensive Therapy* 1990, 16(2):43-53.

Leung ST: The value of cineradiographic motion studies in diagnosis of dysfunctions of the cervical spine. *Bulletin Euro Chiro Union* 1977, 25:28-43.

Levy RM, Mills CM, Posin JP, Moore SG, Rosenblum ML, Bredesen DE: The efficacy and clinical impact of brain imaging in neurologically symptomatic AIDS patients: A prospective CT/MRI study. *J Acquired Immune Deficiency Syndromes* 1990, 3(5):461-471.

Liang M, Kamaroff A: Roentgenograms in primary care patients with low-back pain. *Arch Int Med* 1982, 142:1108-1112.

Lind T, Reimann I, Larsen J, Karstrup S: Sonography in soft tissue trauma of the shoulder. *Acta Orthopedica Scandanavia* 1989, 60(1): 49-53.

Lindsell DR: Ultrasound imaging of pancreas and biliary tract. *Lancet* 1990, 335:390-393.

Litt AW, Eidelman EM, Pinto RS, Riles TS, McLachlan SJ, Schwartzenberg S, Weinreb JC, Kricheff II: Diagnosis of carotid artery stenosis: comparison of 2DFT Time-of-flight MR angiography in 50 patients. *AJR* 1991, 156:611-616.

Lusted L: A study of the efficacy of diagnostic radiologic procedures. Chicago, *American College of Radiology*, 1977.

Maglinte DD, Torres WE, Laufor I: Oral cholecystography in contemporary gallstone imaging: a review. *Radiology* 1991, 178:49-58.

Manninen H, Kiekara O, Soimakallio S, Vainio J: Reduction of radiation dose and imaging costs in scoliosis radiography: application of large-screen image intensifier photofluorography. *Spine* 1988, 13:409-12.

Marton KI, Doubilet P: How to image the gallbladder in suspected cholecystitis. *Annals Internal Medicine* 1988, 109:722-729.

Maurer EL: Biological effects of diagnostic x-ray exposure: an update of principles, revised maximum permissible dose recommendations and new patient protection legislation. *Am J Chir Med* 1988, 1:115-118.

Maurer EL: ACCRT: A review. *ACA J Chirop* 1989, 26:54-9.

Mayhue FE, Rust DD, et al.: Accuracy of interpretations of emergency department radiographs: effect of confidence levels. *Annals of Emergency Medicine* 1989:826-830.

Meeker W, Mootz R: Evaluating the validity, reliability and clinical role of spinal radiography. in Coyl B (Ed): *Current Topics in Chiropractic*, Palmer College of Chiropractic-West, Sunnyvale, CA. 1985.

Merkin JJ, Sportelli L: The effects of two new compensating filters on patient exposure in chiropractic full spine radiography: a technical report. *J Manip Physiol Ther* 1982, 5:25-29.

Miller S: Biomechanical and clinical implications of congenital lumbosacral anomalies. *Proceedings of the Palmer College of Chiropractic-West Consortium on Biomechanics of the Spine*. Sunnyvale, CA. 1982.

Milliren JW: Health Policy Analysis and Magnetic Resonance Imaging: The Case of the New York State Demonstration Project. *Clin Imaging* 1989, 13:16-28.

Mirvis SE, Diaconis JN, Chirico PA, Reiner BE, Jolyn JN, Militello P. Protocol-driven radiologic evaluation of suspected cervical spine injury: efficacy study. *Radiology* 1989, 170:831-834.

Moilanen A, Kokko M, Pitkanen M. Gonadal dose in lumbar spine radiography. *Skeletal Radiol* 1983, 9:153-6.

Mjoen D, Zachman Z: Radiographic Re-evaluation in the Non-Responsive Patient. *ACA J Chiro* 1990, 27(5):69-71.

Mootz R, Meeker W: Minimizing Radiation Exposure to Patients in Chiropractic Practice. *ACA J Chiro* 1989, 23(4):65-70.

Morrison DS, Ofstein R: The Use of Magnetic Resonance Imaging In The Diagnosis of Rotator Cuff Tears. *Orthopedics* 1990, 13(6):634-637.

Mortzsohn De Castro J: Fundamental Principles in the Application of Cineroentgenography as an Auxilliary Method to Roentgen Diagnosis. *Am J Roentgen* 1947, 57:103-114.

Moss AA, Gamsu G, Genant HK. *Computed Tomography of the Body*. Philadelphia, W.B. Saunders Co., 1983.

Mossman KL, Hill LT. Radiation risks in pregnancy. *Obst Gyn* 1982, 60:237-42.

Mulligan SA, Matsuda T, Lanzer P, Gross GM, Routh WD, Keller FS, et.al.: Peripheral Arterial Occlussive Disease: Prospective Comparison of MR Angiography and Color Duplex US with Conventional Angiography. *Radiology* 1991, 178:695-700.

Nachemson A: Lumbar Spine Instability: A Critical Update and Symposium Summary. *Spine* 1985, 10(3):290-291.

Nance EP, Powers TA: Imaging of the Temporomandibular Joint. *Radiologic Clinics North America* 1990, 28(5):1019-1031.

Nash C, Moe R: A Study of Vertebral Rotation. *JBJS* 1969, 51-A(2): 223-229.

National Council on Radiation Protection. Basic radiation protection criteria. *NCRP Report* 1974, #39:1-117.

National Council on Radiation Protection. Medical x-ray and gamma-ray protection for energies up to 10 MeV: Equipment design and use. *NCRP Report* 1975, #33:1-66.

National Council on Radiation Protection. Recommendations on limits for ionizing radiation exposure. *NCRP Report* 1987, #91.

Nykolation JW, Cassidy JD, Arthur BE, Wedge JH. An algorithm for the management of scoliosis. *J Manip Physiol Ther* 1986, 9:1-14.

O'Brien WF, Buck DR, Nash JD: Evaluation of Sonography in the Initial Assessment of the Gynecologic Patient. *American Journal of Obstetrics and Gynecology*. 1984, 149(6):598-602.

Ontario Ministry of Health. *The healing arts radiation protection guidelines*, Ontario Government Publication, 1987.

Pammer JC: Videofluoroscopy position statement approved. *J Chiro* 1989, 26:46.

Pelz DM, Haddad RG. Radiologic investigation of low-back pain. *CMA Journal* 1989, 140:289-295.

Pennell RG, Maurer AH, Bonakdarpour A: Stress injuries of the pars

interarticularis: radiologic classification and indications for scintigraphy. *Am J Radiology* 1985, 145:763-766.

Phillips R: An evaluation of the graphic analysis of the pelvis on the A-P full-spine radiograph. *J Am Chiropractic Assn* 1975, 9: 139-148.

Phillips R, Frymoyer J, MacPherson B, Newburg A: Low-Back Pain: A radiographic enigma. *J Manip Physiol Ther* 1986, 9:(3):183-187.

Phillips R, Howe J, Bustin G, Mick T, Rosenfeld I, Mills T: Stress x-rays and the low-back pain patient. *J Manip Physiol Ther* 1990, 13(2):1127-1133.

Phillips R: Plain Film Radiography in Chiropractic: *Proceedings of WFC Symposium*, World Federation of Chiropractic, Toronto, Canada: 1991:5-1—5-12.

Picus D, McAlister WH, Smith E, et al.: Plain radiography with a rare-earth screen: comparison with calcium tungstate screen. *AJR* 1984, 143:1335-1338.

Putman CE, Ravin CE: *Textbook of Diagnostic Imaging*. Philadelphia, W.B. Saunders, 1988, 1:289-293.

Putman CE, Ravin CE: *Textbook of Diagnostic Imaging*. Philadelphia, W.B. Saunders, 1988, 3:695.

Putman CE, Ravin CE: *Textbook of Diagnostic Imaging*. Philadelphia, W.B. Saunders. 1988, 1:1128.

Quebec Task Force on Spinal Disorders: Scientific approach to the assessment and management of activity related spinal disorders: a monograph for clinicians. *Spine* 1987, 12(s-7):s3-59.

Rao VM, Farole A, Karasick D: Temporomandibular joint dysfunction: correlation of MR imaging, arthrography, and arthroscopy. *Radiology* 1990, 174:663-667.

Resnick D, Niwayama G: Conventional tomography. In: *Diagnosis of Bone and Joint Disorders, 2nd ed*. Philadelphia, W.B. Saunders Co., 1988:130-142.

Ibid: 143-202.

Ibid: 188.

Ibid: 270.

Reynolds R: Cineradiography by the indirect method. *Radiology* 1938, 31:177-182.

Rhea J, Delucca S, Llewallyn H, Boyd R: The oblique view: an unnecessary component of the initial adult lumbar spine examination. *Radiology* 1980, 134:45-47.

Rifkin MD: Ultrasonography of the lower genitourinary tract. *Urologic Clinics North America*. 1985, 12(4):645-656.

Roberts G, Roberts E, Lloyd K, Burke M, Evans D: Lumbar spinal manipulation on trial part II: radiological assessment. *Rheum Rehabilitation* 1978, 17:54-59.

Robinson GK, Lantz C: Dynamic Spinal Visualization: Guidelines for the use of videofluoroscopy in chiropractic. *ICA Review*: 1989:24-28.

Robinson GK, Lantz C: Videofluoroscopy in chiropractic management of cervical syndromes. *J Chiro Research & Clinical Investigation* 1991, 6:93-97.

Rockey P, Thompkins R, Wood R, Wolcott B: The usefullness of x-ray examinations in the evaluation of patients with back pain. *J Family Practice* 1978, 7(3):455-465.

Ross JS, Masaryk TJ, Modic MT, Ruggieri PM, Haacke EM, Selman WR: Intracranial aneurysms: evaluation by MR angiography. *AJNR* 1990, 11:449-456.

Rothschild PA, Crooks LE, Margulis AR: Direction of MR imaging. *Invest Radiol* 1990, 25(1):275-281.

Rowe M: Low-back pain in industry. *J Occ Med* 1969, 476-478.

Rozeboom D: Reliability of full spine x-ray analysis. *Proceedings of Advances in Conservative Health Sciences*, National College of Chiropractic, Lombard, IL. 1983.

Rupert R: Anatomical measures of standard chiropractic skeletal references (a preliminary report). *Proceedings of the Biomechanical Conference of the Spine*, University of Colorado, Boulder, CO. 1980.

Russell JGB: Cost and effectiveness of methods of radiation protection in x-ray diagnosis. *Clin Rad* 1985, 36:37-40.

Samuel E, Palmer PES. X-ray equipment for routine investigations—the WHO basic radiological system. *S Afr Med J* 1985, 67:248-51.

Saraste H, Brostrom L-A, Aparisi T, Axdorph G: Radiographic measurement of the lumbar spine: a clinical and experimental study in man. *Spine* 1985, 10(3):236-241.

Sartoris DJ, Resnick D: CT, MRI offer new view of rheumatological disease. *Diagnostic Imaging* 1987:120-126.

Sartoris DJ, Resnick D: Computed tomography of rheumatologic disorders, part I. *Ortho Review* 1988, 17:675-683.

Sartoris DJ, Resnick D: Computed tomography of rheumatologic disorders, part II. *Ortho Review* 1988, 17:757-766.

Sartoris DJ: Musculoskeletal trauma. *Radiological Clinics North America* 1989, 27:855-944.

Scavone J: Use of Lumbar Spine Films. *JAMA* 1982, 246(10):1105-1108.

Scavone J, Latshaw R, Weidner W: Anteroposterior and lateral radiographs: an adequate lumbar spine examination. *AJR* 1981, 136:715-717.

Schellhas KP: Internal derangement of the temporomandibular joint: Radiologic staging with clinical, surgical, and pathological correlation. *Magnetic Resonance Imaging* 1989, 7(5):495-515.

Schram S, Hosek R, Silverman H: Spinographic positioning errors in Gonstead pelvic x-ray analysis. *J Manip Physiol Ther* 1981, 4(4):179-181.

Schram S, Hosek R: Error limitations in x-ray kinematics of the spine. *J Manip Physiol Ther* 1982, 5:5-10.

Schultz G, Phillips R, Howe J, Cherachanko D: Oblique views: useful or useless? *Proceedings of International Conference on Spinal Manipulation*, May 1990:27-30.

Schwerdtner HP: Lumbosakrale ubergangsanomalein als rezidivursach bei chirotherapeutischen behandlungstechniken. *Manuelle Medizin* 1986, 24:11-15.

Seelentag W: Evaluating the role of x-ray diagnosis in public health. *J Manip Physiol Ther* 1989, 12(4):235-237.

Sherman R, Bauer F: *X-ray X-pertise—from A-X.* 1st ed. Fort Worth, PCRF 1982:1-153.

Shippel AH, Robinson GK: Radiological and magnetic resonance imaging of cervical spine instability: a case report. *J Manip Physiol Ther* 1987, 10:316-322.

Shrimpton PC, Jones DG, Wall BF: The influence of tube filtration and potential on patient dose during x-ray examinations. *Phys Med Biol* 1988, 33:1205-12.

Sigler D, Howe J: Intra and interexaminer reliability of the upper cervical x-ray marking system. *J Manip Physiol Ther* 1985, 8(2):75-80.

Sinclair WK: Trends in radiation protection—a view from the NCRP. *Health Physics* 1988, 55:149-57.

Skukas J, Gorski J. Application of modern intensifying screens in diagnostic radiology. *Med Radiography Photog* 1980, 56:25-36.

Speiser R, Aragona R, Heffernan J: The application of therapeutic exercises based on lateral flexion roentgenography to restore biomechanical function. *Chiro Res J* 1990, 1:7-17.

Speiser R, Aragona R, Heffernan J: Applied spinal biomechanical engineering (ASBE): restoration of dynamic function of the lumbar spine. *ICA International Review of Chiropractic* 1989:59-65.

Splitthoff C: Lumbosacral Junction: Roentgenographic comparison of patients with and without backaches. *JAMA* 1953, 152(17):1610-1613.

Stine R, Avila J, Lemons M, Sickorez G: Diagnostic and therapeutic urologic procedures. *Emerg Med Clinics North America* 1988, 6(3):564-566.

Sundaram M, McLeod RA. MR imaging of tumor and tumorlike lesions of bone and soft tissue. *Am J Radiology* 1990, 155:817-824.

Tanagho EA, McAninch JW: *Smith's General Urology.* Norwalk, Connecticut/San Mateo, California, Appleton & Lange 12th ed., 1988:62.

Tasharski CC, Heinze WJ, Pugh JL: Dynamic atlanto-axial aberration: a case study and cinefluorographic approach to diagnosis. *J Manip Physiol Ther* 1981, 4:65-68.

Taveras J, Ferrucci J: GI. *General Abdomen and Pelvic and Genitourinary Radiology.* revised ed. Philadelphia: J.B. Lippincott Co. 1990, 4:13-14.

Taylor JAM: Writing radiology reports in chiropractic. *JCCA* 1990, 34(1):30-34.

Taylor M, Skippings R: Paradoxical motion of atlas in flexion: a fluoroscopic study of chiropractic patients. *Euro J Chiro* 1987, 35: 116-134.

Templeton PA, Caskey CI, Zerhouni EA: Current uses of CT and MR imaging in the staging of lung cancer. *Radiologic Clinics North America* 1990, 28(3):631-644.

Terenzi TJ: The role of the doppler in the differential diagnosis of lower extremity claudication syndromes. *J Manip Physiol Ther* 1990, 13(4):215-220.

Thrall JH, Wittenberg J: Radiology Summit 1990: Specialization in eadiology: trends, implications, recommendations. *AJR* 1991, 156: 1273-1276.

Triano J, Marinelli C: Radiographic reliability of facet orientation. *Proceedings of Conservative Health Sciences Res. Conf.*, Palmer College of Chiropractic-West, Sunnyvale, CA. 1985.

Trout ED, Kelley JP, Cathey GA: The use of filters to control radiation exposure to the patient in diagnostic roentgenology. *AJR* 1952, 62:943-946.

Van Holsbeeck M, Introcaso J: *Musculoskeletal ultrasound.* Mosby Year Book, 1991.

Velchik MG: Radionuclide imaging of the urinary tract. *Urologic Clinics North America* 1985, 12(4):603-631.

Vernon H: Static and dynamic roentgenography in the diagnosis of degenerative disc disease: a review and comparative assessment. *J Manip Physiol Ther* 1982, 5:163-169.

Wallace CJ: Magnetic resonance imaging of the brain. *J Can Assoc Radiol* 1991, 42(1):13-20.

Weitz E: The lateral bending sign. *Spine* 1981, 6(4): 388-397.

Weiss, Beltran, Shamam, Stilla, Levy: High field MR surface-coil imaging of the hand and wrist. *Radiology* 1986, 160:143-152.

White AJ, Panjabi MM: The basic kinematics of the human spine: A review of past and current knowledge. *Spine* 1978, 3:12-29.

Wiesel S: The reliability of imaging (CT, MRI, Myelography) in documenting the cause of spinal pain. *Proceedings WFC Symposium*, World Federation of Chiropractic 1991: 6/1—6/10.

Willson, Gilula, Mann: Undirectional joint communications in wrist arthrography: an evaluation of 250 cases. *AJR* 1991, 157: 105-109.

Witt I, Vestergaard A, Rosenklint A: A comparative analysis of x-ray findings of the lumbar spine in patients with and without lumbar pain. *Spine* 1984, 9(3):289-300.

Wyatt L, Schultz G: The diagnostic efficacy of lumbar spine radiography: a review of the literature. In Hodgsen M (Ed), *Current Topics in Chiropractic.* Palmer College of Chiropractic-West, Sunnyvale, CA. 1987.

Yochum TR, Rowe LJ: Radiographic Positioning and Normal Anatomy. In: *Essentials of Skeletal Radiology.* Baltimore, Williams & Wilkins 1984:1-94.

Ibid: 1067.

Zengle F, Davis B, Rozeboom D: Lack of effect of projectional distortion on Gonstead vertebral endplate lines. *Proceedings of advances in conservative health sciences*, Logan College of Chiropractic, Academic Press, St. Louis, MO. 1982.

Zengle F: Lack of effect of projectional distortion on Gonstead vertebral endplate lines. *Proceedings of the Symposium on Advances in Conservative Health Sciences*, National College of Chiropractic Academic Press, Lombard, IL. 1982:129.

IX. MINORITY OPINIONS

None.

X. TABLES

Table 1

Projection/Area	Optimum kV Range	
	Single-Phase	Three-Phase
Cervical Spine	70-80	60-70
Thoracic Spine	75-85	65-75
Lumbar Spine		
A-P/P-A	80-90	75-85
Oblique	80-90	75-85
Lateral	90-100	85-95
Chest		
Grid	110-125	100-120
Air Gap	90-110	85-100
Ribs	50-70	50-60
Hips	75-85	70-80
Knee	55-65	50-60
Ankle	55-65	50-60
Foot	55-65	50-60
Shoulder	65-75	60-65
Elbow	50-60	50-60
Wrist/Hand	50-60	50-60
Skull	80-90	70-80
Full-Spine (PA)	90-100	80-90

Table 2

Daily:
> Clean processor rollers and crossover racks
> Check processor chemical levels
> Check processor replenisher levels
> Compare sensitometer strips with master

Weekly:
> Check developer temperature
> Compare exposure step-wedge with master
> Inspect processor for leaks, noises, broken parts
> Check darkroom for light leaks

Monthly:
> Check processor replenishment rates
> Replace fresh water filter (if present)
> Replace fixer and developer in processor
> Thorough processor cleaning
> Detailed examination of processor components
> Examine intensifying screens
> Lubricate processor
> Check darkroom for light leaks
> Retake film analysis

Every Six Months:
> *Processor:*
>   Major cleaning and lubrication
>   Drain cleaning solution
>   Major sensitometry: film speed and contrast
> *Image Receptors:*
>   Check film/screen combination speeds
>   Clean all screens (replace if necessary)
>   Check film/screen contact
> *Generating Apparatus:*
>   Grid alignment and servicing
>   mA/mAs linearity
>   kV reproducibility
>   Timer accuracy
>   Collimator alignment
>   mR/mAs output
>   Half-Value layer
>   Focal spot resolution
>   kV accuracy
> *Other:*
>   Take x-ray of shields/aprons to detect leaks
>   Detailed re-take analysis
>   Fine-tune technique chart if necessary
>   Calibrate generator and control components

Table 3

Area of Examination	Film-Screen Speed Range
Extremities	100-200
Chest	200-400
Spine (sectional views)	400-800
Full spine (14 x 36)	600-1200

Table 4

Operating kVp	Minimum Total Filter (Inherent plus added)
Below 50 kVp	0.5 mm Aluminum
50-70 kVp	1.5 mm Aluminum
Above 70 kVp	2.5 mm Aluminum

Table 5 Technical Factors for the Production of Quality Radiographs

a) **Collimation.** Maximum collimation of the primary beam is used to expose only necessary areas and to exclude the eyes, breasts, and gonads whenever possible.

b) **Filtration.** Density equalizing filtration is used to minimize excess exposure to thinner body parts.

c) **Lead Shielding.** The breasts and gonads (male and female) are adequately protected with lead shields whenever possible.

d) **P-A Projection.** The posteroanterior projection is employed whenever possible to further reduce radiation exposure to the breast, eye, and thyroid.

e) **Rare-earth Screens.** Rare-earth screens with matching film of the same spectral sensitivity and in the 600-1200 speed category is used.

f) **Focal-Film Distance.** FFDs of greater than or equal to 72" are used.

g) **High kV.** Exposures frequently greater than 90kV are used to reduce radiation exposure.

h) **Adequate Grid.** Use of a 12:1 grid allows higher kV values to be employed and is optimal for scatter absorption in the 90-100 kV range. However, a 10:1 grid is acceptable.

i) **Technical Details**. Careful attention to radiographic and darkroom procedures is employed to minimize retake examinations.

3

Instrumentation

Chapter Outline

I. OVERVIEW

An instrument is a clinical tool that yields a measure. As such it may take on various forms. They all are intended to give one of three kinds of information about patient status or response to treatment. In general, they are: 1) perceptual measurements (e.g., reports of pain severity, satisfaction with life style); 2) functional measurements (e.g., range of motion, strength, activities-of-daily-living); and 3) physiological measurements (e.g., neurological assessment, serological changes).

The case history coupled with a discerning physical examination typically supplies most of the information necessary to make a diagnosis and determine a prognosis. Instrumentation serves to confirm a differential diagnosis, assess the severity of a condition or to monitor progress from a pre-established baseline. In order for the results from any instrument to be clinically useful, they must be appropriately applied and interpreted by the clinician, and the patient must be sincere and cooperative in performance.

Appropriate Use of Instruments

Instruments are all designed with various levels of sophistication and make use of underlying assumptions. Sapega[166] has observed that many clinical tools available today are capable of generating more measurements than can be meaningfully understood. The technological explosion in health care delivery has advanced far beyond valid clinical utility. Although the instruments themselves are not able to be validated, the application of the information they supply can be evaluated for their validity and usefulness.

The meaningful interpretation of changes in a subject's test results requires the reliability and validity of the procedures. The most effective means to ensure reliability is through test standardization and close attention to the correspondence of test conditions to those of the actual demands that the patient's lifestyle makes on his performance. The test clearly must be relevant to the individual's activities that have been impaired or to normative data, and should be able to discriminate healthy from unhealthy people.

Evaluating Instruments

Several qualities are found in common for instruments that ultimately prove to be clinically useful. Focusing on these qualities rather than on specific named instruments simplifies the task of evaluating instruments individually. They include the following:

1) Validity is the most clinically important quality. A test is valid when it accurately measures the desired function, and when that function is pertinent to the patient's condition.

2) Discriminability is determined by the ability to distinguish healthy from unhealthy individuals. In order to accomplish this, a normative data base consisting of studies of people from both groups is required. The relative frequency of false-positive (i.e., healthy persons who test positive) and false-negative tests (i.e., unhealthy persons who test negative) occurring for each group also helps to define a test's discriminability.

3) Accuracy of a measure is determined by comparison to a known value. Repeated use of some devices and the simple effects of passing time may cause loss of calibration which will alter accuracy.

4) Precision describes the variation of a measure across the range over which it is intended to be used. Both accuracy and precision can change over the possible ranges of test applications.

5) Reliability of a measure depends both on the accuracy of the instrument and the characteristics of the variable being measured.

For each category of instrument discussed below, knowledge of how each performs with respect to the above test qualities is presumed. Information of this kind is the minimum necessary, but may not be sufficient to achieve a rating above the classification of "Investigational."

Patient Motivation

Test results should be interpreted in conjunction with observations of the quality of patient performance and cooperation made while the test is being performed. As a result, only adequately trained personnel who can integrate clinically meaningful observations should perform most tests. Quality of patient performance, repeated measures testing [45, 82, 192] and correlation of findings with other clinical information [80] permit an accurate evaluation of patient motivation. Specific reasons for poor test performance include legitimate reduced capability, misunderstood instructions, apprehension of the test setting, fear of pain arising from the test, and questions of secondary gain.

II. DEFINITIONS

Accuracy: The property of a measurement which determines how closely the result will approximate the true value.

Anthropometry: The study of proportional relationships between the shape, weight and size of body segments.

Calibration: Periodic adjustment/maintenance of instrument components to yield minimum variation of measurements in contrast to a "Gold Standard" over a specified range of measurement.

Discriminability: The property of information derived from a test or a measurement that allows the practitioner to discern between groups of subjects: for example, healthy from unhealthy.

Gold Standard: A known value or attribute used to test veracity of instrumented measures to define the true state of the patient.

Instrument: A clinical tool that yields a measurement. For purposes of this section, standard diagnostic instruments used in the conduct of routine physical examination are omitted.

Motivation: Conscious or subliminal factors of attitude and belief which contribute to the rationale for a person to choose between self-reliance (coping), patient and claimant behaviors in contending with health related predicaments.

Physician Dependence: Patient behavior which transfers responsibility for health status to the care-giver.

Precision: The ability to obtain the same measurement of a function or structure repeatedly within a set margin of error across the possible range of test applications.

Reactivity: A test interaction effect causing an unintentional change in a patient's response when exposed to the repeated application of a test.

Reliability: The ability to obtain the same measurement of a stable function or structure upon repeated tests. Reliability depends both upon accuracy and precision which, for instruments, may be separately evaluated and adjusted for calibration.

Sensitivity: The ability to correctly identify positive test results among subjects who truly have a specific disorder. The likelihood of a positive test result in a person with a disorder (also true-positive rate, TPR).

Somatization: One of several contemporary terms (e.g., psychological overlay, supratentorial overlay, etc.) indicating that the patient's symptoms may be aggravated by or may arise from non-organic factors.

Specificity: The ability to correctly identify negative test results among subjects who truly do not have a specific disorder. The likelihood of a negative test in a patient without disorder (also true-negative rate, TNR).

Validity: The property of information derived from a test or a measurement that assures that it represents the function or structure that is intended.

III. LIST OF SUBTOPICS

Perceptual Measurements

A. Questionnaire Instruments
B. Screening Questionnaires
C. Pressure Algometry

Functional Measurements

A. Measures of Position/Clinical Anthropometry
1. Plumbline Analysis
2. Scoliometry
3. Photogrammetry
4. Moire Topography
5. Bilateral Weight Distribution
6. Automated Posture Measures

B. Measurement of Movement
1. Goniometers
2. Inclinometers
3. Optically Based Systems
4. Computer Assisted ROM Systems

C. Measurement of Strength
1. Manual Strength Testing
2. Isometric
3. Isokinetic
4. Isoinertial

Physiologic Measurements

A. Thermographic Recordings
1. Thermocouple Devices
2. Infrared Thermography

B. Galvanic Skin Response
1. Effectiveness
2. Acupuncture Point Finding

C. Electrophysiologic Recordings
1. Kinesiologic Surface EMG
2. Surface Electrodiagnostic Procedures
3. Needle Electrodiagnostic Procedures
4. Electrocardiography

D. Clinical Laboratory Procedures

E. Other Instrument Measures
1. Doppler Ultrasound
2. Plethysmography
3. Spirometry

IV. LITERATURE REVIEW

Perceptual Measurements

A. Questionnaires as Instruments:

Physical signs can be rather insensitive measures of a patient's disability.[162, 202] Standardized rating scales and questionnaires afford a simple means of appraising many aspects of patient life and health.[11] Instruments commonly used in the chiropractic community assess pain, activities-of-daily-living

(ADL), somatization, depression, and anxiety. Generally, questionnaires may be divided into two categories, self-reporting and practitioner-administered. Self-reporting questionnaires are often self-normalizing but suffer from reactivity which may result in an unintentional change in the patient's response when exposed to the same questions repeatedly.[11] Practitioner-administered questionnaires benefit from the involvement of a trained observer whose skill can help in interpreting the patient's response. In administering either format, several error sources should be considered including 1) patient motivation; 2) acquiescence to positively worded items; and 3) patient's seeking social approval.[189] Overall, functional questionnaires offer standardization of measurement, comprehensiveness, and generally good reproducibility and validity.[46]

There is no consensus on the use of a particular questionnaire for a specific clinical problem. For the measurement of the same clinical problem, different questionnaires may not yield interchangeable findings. Screening questionnaires may be used to obtain a broad patient overview in a comprehensive and timely manner.[221] With the recent intensive development in the outcome measurement field, future field standardization on use of questionnaires is to be expected.

Pressure Algometry

Pressure algometry is a comparatively new procedure which uses a pressure manometer to estimate pain threshold from applied pressures to the myofascial structures. Normative data[58, 59] shows that pressure pain thresholds are highly symmetrical and are generally lower in females than in males. Reeves et al.[220] have reported reliability coefficients ranging from 0.71 to 0.97. Pressure pain threshold levels are sensitive to a variety of treatment interventions.[203, 203b] Good inter-rater and test-retest reliability has been shown.

Functional Measurements

A. Measurement of Position/Clinical Anthropometry

1. Posture

Studies in ergonomics have shown that trunk, head and joint positions adopted during work can be used as an objective index for evaluating the intensity of physical work stress, mental concentration or manual dexterity.[6, 122] The choice of a particular position may be the most important factor contributing to whether an attempted physical activity is risky or safe. Individual instruments and automated measures are available to quantify posture or body segment position.

2. Plumbline analysis

The plumbline was one of the first tools to be used in chiropractic to analyze posture. The plumbline provides a visual frame of reference for the influence of the centers of gravity from each body segment, enabling the clinician to detect postural deviation, asymmetry, and suspect areas of postural stress. Patients are observed in the anterior, posterior, and lateral stances.[196] Effects of diurnal variations and differences in test methods on the interpretation of results have not been well studied.

3. Scoliometry

Various instruments are available to quantify the physical signs of scoliosis and may include a form of plumbline analysis. The most important measurement quantifies the deformity of the rib cage associated with axial rotation of the vertebrae. The prominence of the rib hump correlates with the severity of the curvature and may presage its progression.[160] The differences from side to side are measured in millimeters or in degrees of deformity. Pelvic and shoulder girdle unleveling may also be quantified with bubble level devices.

4. Photogrammetry

Photographic evidence is most often used to quantify postures selected by persons during specific tasks. Methods of measurement include static, video and opto-electronic systems. Three principal applications are made in clinical practice. They are: 1) recording of structural or topographical anomalies as a part of the baseline assessment data collected during the patient examination; 2) quantification of typical postures adopted by patients during functional performance tests for post-injury severity and return-to-work evaluations; and 3) work site ergonomic risk factor evaluations performed for industry.[30, 192] Quantitative knowledge of posture and velocities of motion are important to understand the physical stresses on musculoskeletal structures during work and recreational activities.

The main technical concerns that must be addressed in order to maintain confidence in the measures obtained from photogrammetry are similar to those considered in setting up radiographic equipment. They include calibrated alignment of the camera, image contrast, standardized postures for repeated measures and distortion effects. For static images, most may be resolved by standardizing camera distances, heights and lighting. For video and opto-electronic methods, more complex computerized methods are required to obtain reliable data. (See review on given distortion factors given in Chaffin and Andersson 1984.[30])

5. Moire topography

Moire topography is a static photographic technique modified to highlight body contours for the purpose of quantifying structural deformity, in the same manner as the methods of map making to denote elevation.[137, 213] Photographs are obtained of interference patterns cast onto the body surface by an angled light source passing through a grid. The relative number of resulting concentric contour lines on a Moire photograph are proportional to the elevation of a landmark with respect to a reference surface. Patient positioning is very important with this method of postural analysis, as the grid-to-patient distance relationship must be kept constant in order to achieve accurate follow-up evaluations. It is performed quickly and is reproducible, but the results are difficult to quantify and no good correlation to physical findings exists. Adequate interpretation is therefore lacking.

6. Bilateral weight distribution

Asymmetric posture and weight-bearing have been proposed as contributing factors in the development of degenerative joint disease, sacroiliac instability, chronic lumbar strain and other conditions.[36, 60, 87, 97, 136] Validity of these assumptions, including subtle postural asymmetries, remains to be demonstrated. The simplest means employed to determine if the loads transmitted throughout the skeleton are asymmetrical is through the use of bilateral weight scales or load cells positioned under each foot.[36, 91, 204] Recent biomechanical studies[85] suggest that postural balance may be useful in evaluating sacroiliac joint status and treatment. Inherent measurement variability and offset of postural sway necessitates careful attention to protocol.

7. Automated measurements of posture

Quantifying position in three dimensional space has been used as a research tool for several years. Several methods of spatial measurement are available including sonic, magnetic, photoelectric and electrogoniometric systems that locate the position of a point in space with respect to an arbitrary fixed reference point. Discussion of each is beyond the scope of this chapter primarily because they are not available for, nor useful in, general practice. Physical measurement systems that are available, for example three dimensional digitizers,[76] do not resolve fundamental problems of accuracy in landmark identification, characteristic of manual methods and can amplify them.[148]

B. Measurement of Movement

In the general course of patient care, range of motion is examined using goniometers, inclinometers and optical based systems. Most devices quantify the regional movement of a part and express it as an angular displacement about some center of rotation.

1. Goniometers

The degree of peripheral joint movement can be measured throughout active or passive ranges. Its usefulness is greatest in the extremities, particularly the small joints of the hands and feet. The reference point for measurement is the long axis of the part being measured and is determined by judgment. Accuracy is limited to a range of 10 to 15 degrees.[30] Usage for spinal measurements is no longer considered acceptable practice because of the advent of better methods.

2. Inclinometers

Inclinometers use the constant vertical direction of gravity as a reference and require only that a side rests against the body segment surface. Digital or analog and mechanical or electronic versions are available. Greater accuracy of measurement is available with ranges of 3 to 5 degrees being possible under typical clinical conditions.[127] Inclinometers are the more suitable instrument for assessing spinal function and are capable of separating components of motion, e.g., pelvic versus lumbar.

3. Optically based systems

Aside from research applications, the most prevalent clinical use of opto-electronic systems is in conjunction with the use of force plates for assessing gait abnormalities.[86, 154] Video-monitoring is often used in industrial practice to capture the salient features and at least semi-quantify motions and postures at the work station. Work related spine injuries, carpal tunnel syndrome and other cumulative trauma disorders are frequent areas of concern where these methods are used. The primary parameters of importance are joint angle, angular velocity and angular acceleration. Coupled with appropriate software and external load measurements, joint loads and patterns of behavior can provide information on relative risk of work related tasks.

C. Measurement of Strength

The term strength denotes the capacity for active development of muscle tension and through the resulting muscle force generates joint torque. Computerized muscle dynamometer systems quantify more variables than the average physician can properly interpret.[166] In the case of employment-related tests, the evaluation must closely simulate critical job tasks.[5]

The emphasis on computerized muscle-dynamometry systems (isometric, isokinetic, isotonic and isoinertial) has overshadowed earlier isometric and psychophysical testing methods. No single method of strength evaluation is decidedly superior or more valid for measuring muscular strength.[166] Each method also has a number of advantages and disadvantages. For valid interpretation of test results, the unique characteristics of each must be kept in mind. It has yet to be shown conclusively that testing can clearly predict that a patient can return to a certain activity level and will have less risk of reinjury under actual functional conditions. Only continued research and development of broader normative data bases than are now available will finally test the underlying assumptions currently used in these clinical applications.

1. Manual hand-held strength testing

Manual muscle strength testing provides only a rough approximation of capability[15, 64, 167, 207] and its use is limited. Accuracy in manual assessment requires differences in strength of 35% or more.[166] Hand-held dynamometers, while not eliminating all the problems of manual testing, provide greater degrees of accuracy and reliability.[19, 26, 177]

2. Instrumented strength measurement testing

Diagnostic assessment naturally falls into three categories: 1) preventative evaluation (as in employee job-matching); 2) post-injury evaluation; and 3) outcome monitoring following treatment.[5, 16, 81, 127, 149, 152, 166, 172, 195] Significant clinical information can be obtained toward these objectives, but careless interpretation of test data can result in inappropriate clinical decisions. Acute disorders are a contraindication to strength test protocols. The average discrepancy between symmetrical muscle groups for healthy populations has been reported as much as 12%.[71, 123, 135, 166, 217] When evaluating an individual's performance, differences of 20% or more may be needed to discriminate abnormalities.

a. Isometric testing

There are several technical concerns in the performance of isometric tests: 1) the inertial effects at the onset of the test; 2) patient fatigue; 3) patient posture; and 4) patient motivation. The objective of the test is to identify and record the maximum voluntary contraction force that can be sustained.[30] At this time, the tasks that can be adequately represented with isometric tests are sagittally symmetric. Up to 70% of work postures can be approximated symmetrically. Normative data for occupational classifications of lifting activities[29, 214] as well as for reciprocal trunk strength ratios[113, 131, 195] are available. Normative data is used to evaluate extremity strength for post-injury assessment or seasonal sports fitness.[166] Bilateral differences greater than 15-20% indicate abnormality.

The patient's motivation to supply a maximum effort can be assessed by repeated measurement and acceptable maximum effort protocols.[112, 141, 181] Quantitative knowledge of the patient's posture during the performance of the strength task is critical to any effort to relate the test result to joint loads or NIOSH standards.[5, 30, 166, 212]

b. Isokinetic testing

The primary measurement obtained is the torque generated which is only valid during the controlled part of the motion. The maximum voluntary effort will coincide with the greatest mechanical advantage of the joint for the motion that is being attempted.[10] There are two technical concerns with isokinetic measurements. They are: 1) gravitational effects; and 2) torque overshoot. Both may be corrected through computerized correction routines and damper settings. Standard isokinetic measurements are commonly taken at increments of 30 degrees per second using 2-6 repetitions with the maximum single torque value used as the measure of performance. As with isometric evaluation, the normal extensor/flexor trunk ratio falls when impairment is present.[16, 124, 128, 130, 188, 195] Kannus,[109] Nunn and Mayhew [144] feel the side-to-side comparison of extremity testing has some importance.

c. Isoinertial testing

While no testing method yet devised allows an assessment of free dynamic motion such as would occur at a work site or in sports, isoinertial equipment may come closer than others. Several authors have examined the ability to predict performance by controlling torque during movement.[99, 104, 105, 120, 121, 149, 185] Isoinertial systems can be made capable of monitoring position, velocity and torque simultaneously. Measures of regional coupled motions appear to hold promise in discriminating fatigue effects from healthy movement.[149] Likewise, velocity measurements appear to be sensitive to lumbar spine disorders. Normative data is available for a number of occupational subgroups including sedentary workers.[74]

Physiologic Measurements

A. Thermographic Recordings

Body heat loss to the environment takes place passively by convection, conduction and radiation. Regional body temperature is governed by the interaction of central autonomic control mechanisms[165] and multisegmental spinal vasomotor reflexes.[67] Regional variations of sympathetic thermoregulation produce a complex pattern of temperature distribution including cephalocaudal, diurnal and circadian patterns.[78] Accurate measure requires accommodation of the skin to room temperature, which should be kept at between 33.5 to 34 C.[93] For reproducible measures, the patient needs to establish constant patterns of work and rest and follow-up testing should be performed at the same time of day.[159] Measurements of skin temperature and the amount of heat radiated from anatomically symmetrical regions yields useful information about the relative circulatory volume to each part. Areas of increased cutaneous temperature have been ascribed to vasodilation occurring during a migraine headache,[205] inflammation[1, 52, 95, 114, 115, 116, 146] or muscle spasm.[40, 51, 110] Decreased cutaneous temperature may reflect vasoconstriction, vascular obstruction, or fibrous and fatty replacement.[106] An abundance of literature is available documenting employment of thermography as a screening tool; e.g., detection of deep vein thrombosis, identification of allergic reactions,[9] qualification of vascular phenomena, and the identification of pain.[151, 175] The clinical value of the data, however, remains uncertain.

1. Thermocouple devices

Several thermocouple devices have been marketed to be used for the manual determination of local paraspinal temperature variations.[43, 155, 197] While sometimes still used, these types of paraspinal measures have not been shown to have good discriminability, and both their validity and reliability of measurement is highly doubtful.[31, 197]

2. Telethermography

Measurement of skin temperature differences across the torso, head and extremities is a highly controversial procedure that has been proposed as a means of evaluating functional changes from somatic lesions. Various forms of "gold standard" comparison have been used including surgical confirmation of disc herniation and percentage agreement or statistical correlation with other more widely accepted diagnostic procedures. Normative data are available; for example, see Chang et al., 1985,[31] Feldman and Nickolff [55] 1984, Goodman et al., 1986,[75] and Uematsu et al., 1988.[198] A number of efforts to evaluate diagnostic truth from telethermographic measures have been made.[77, 94, 198, 199] Unfortunately, a high proportion of the writings on the topic reflect opinion or fail to account for sample population factors such as prevalence, bias or experimental blinding procedures.

The results of comparative studies of thermography and other diagnostic procedures for nerve root entrapments are quite varied.[52, 68, 158] Where some studies claim that thermography has little diagnostic and uncertain prognostic value in the evaluation of low back pain and radiculopathy,[134, 183] others praise its sensitivity and positive predictive value.[28, 198] Thermographic images have been used in the diagnosis of myofascial pain syndromes and their respective pain referral zones. Perhaps the strongest evidence for use of telethermography is for cases of suspected neurodystrophy.[150,20] There has been a high correlation between the thermographically defined referral zones and those as described in the literature. Additional zones, not previously identified, have also been recognized.[47] Meta-analysis attempting to resolve the question of clinical utility for thermography has concluded that the procedure cannot be recommended as routine since its role remains unclear.[88]

Hubbard[94b] has written an interesting commentary on various criticisms of the thermography literature for lumbar radiculopathy concluding with the need for more studies published in the "mainstream" literature with attention to the political climate and valid criticism.

B. Galvanic Skin Response (GSR)

Devices to detect differences in paraspinal regional electrical skin resistance have been employed by the chiropractic profession for many decades. Loci of lowered skin resistance were thought to be related to areas of cutaneous hyper or hyposympathetic activity which, themselves, would be due to a putative vertebral subluxation. Other devices have been employed to detect punctate areas to lowered skin resistance putatively corresponding to acupuncture points (i.e., "point finders"). A final category consists of an apparatus designed to measure digital (hand) GSR, thought to reflect global levels of sympathetic nervous system activity, and, by influence, general levels of arousal.

These devices are subject to a high degree of intra- and inter-subject variability calling into question their reliability. Older class II studies are seriously in need of update and replication with modern instrumentation and more rigorous research methodology. Recent Class II studies have cast serious doubt on the reliability and validity of GSR in assessment of spinal dysfunction.[70,140]

C. Electrophysiologic Recordings

Several variables affect all electrophysiologic recordings: 1) the size and location of the recording electrode; 2) the configuration of the electrode position relative to the structure being recorded; 3) characteristic resistance of the tissues; 4) the pathophysiology of the patient's problem and 5) artifacts.

1. Electrodiagnosis

Several specialized procedures are available to evaluate select neuromuscular functions. These include measures of myoelectric activity during muscular loading, fatigue studies, conduction velocity tests, H-wave and F-wave responses, and evoked potentials. Generally these studies can be simply grouped as either 1) stimulation studies; or 2) electromyography (EMG).[37] The clinical procedures are sometimes divided according to whether needle or surface electrodes are used.

Surface electrode studies may be used in many cases, but are traditionally applied to the examination of nerve conduction velocities, reflex studies and kinesiological evaluations.[23,126] In kinesiologic applications, up to 16% of the surface recordings from the upper leg muscles, for example, is from co-contraction activity.[49] Surface electrodes may be used with repetitive stimulation to examine suspected myoneural junction disorders. Somatosensory evoked potentials (EP) are performed with surface electrodes. EP serve to discern between peripheral and cord (dorsal column) lesion sites.[79] Needle electrode studies are classically termed electromyography. This technique may be used in all varieties of electrodiagnostic studies, but it is required to detect denervation, myoneural junction disorders, cerebellar and brainstem tremors, anterior cord disease and motor unit potentials. To obtain accurate information about single motor units, needle electrodes are necessary.

a. Nerve stimulation studies

Nerve stimulation studies can be performed using either surface or needle electrodes. Basic information may be gained about the neuromuscular peripheral sensory and motor components using conduction velocity and reflex responses of the nerve (i.e., H-reflex and F-waves). Practically, this information may be used to evaluate the nerve trunk integrity as well as significant compression, or temporal dispersion from entrapment or metabolic neuropathy. Both sensory and motor studies permit analysis of wave form, amplitude and duration of the impulse.[98] Nerve compression from lumbar root lesions can be quantified.[44,53,79,211] While nerve conduction velocity is a poor index for radicular syndromes, F-waves and H-reflexes are more useful. Similar use can be made for study of complaints from the upper extremity.[79,193] Sensitivity and specificity for each of the following electrodiagnostic procedures are well studied. Sequencing of tests often increases the diagnostic yield. Timing of tests performed with respect to the onset of symptoms is important since their appearance and disappearance can be temporally dependent.[79]

Evoked, transforaminal responses (surface or needle): Peripheral motor nerve fibers of major nerve trunks from the extremities may be evaluated by use of the F-wave of Maglodery. Adequate assessment requires a sequence of supramaximal stimuli with measure of several response latencies. These signals may be absent in diseases of compression affecting the anterior horn or peripheral nerve.

For lesions involving the peripheral motor or sensory fibers from L5/S1 or S1/S2, the Hoffman reflex may be used. A series of progressively increasing subthreshold to suprathreshold stimuli are used to evaluate sensory and motor fiber responses.

Nerve conduction studies (surface or needle NCV): Motor nerves can be evaluated for site and severity of lesions from mechanical or pathological causes. Stimulation of major nerve trunks at a series of sites along their path can locate the region affected. Characteristic wave form and relative conduction velocity changes may also be important to differentiate between causes of nerve damage. Sensory nerve conduction is studied in a similar fashion.

Somatosensory evoked potentials (Surface or Needle SSEP): Similar to conduction velocities, these procedures stimulate the peripheral nerve either at accessible nerve trunks or by dermatomal sensory nerve endings. Responses may be monitored along the nerve pathway traversing the IVF, cord, brainstem and cortex.

b. **Electromyography**

Kinesiologic studies: A surface measurement that monitors myoelectric volitional responses can be used to examine superficial layer muscle recruitment and fatigue. When calibrated against known exertional efforts, biomechanical estimates of muscle tensions for simple isometric tasks can be made.[219] Clinical applications to the evaluation of spine related disorders has been proposed under the heading of surface paraspinal scanning EMG[69] using either post-style or adhesive tape-on electrodes. With the exception of flexion-relaxation[2, 176, 195] and spectral density parameters like mean/median frequency shifts[20, 54, 164] during isometric contraction using tape-on electrodes, clinical usefulness is limited because the discriminability of these procedures has not been fully evaluated. Myoelectric monitoring during simple postural tasks shows common patterns of behavior but these are easily influenced by subtle changes in posture and other sources of error.[96] Triano and Luttges[194] found that an ensemble of flexion and postural tasks might discriminate healthy subjects from unhealthy patients, whereas single postures

alone were insufficient. Lumbar disc and nonspecific backache tend to have overall higher electrical activity but are confounded by a high sensitivity to positional variation.[4]

Comparison of right/left myoelectric amplitudes during static postures remain to be validated as being discriminable. Acute spinal symptoms may be associated with alterations in muscular tone (e.g., hypotonus, hypertonus, spasm). However, the meaning of measurements associated with them is uncertain and does not significantly contribute to therapeutic decision making.[46] In chronic back pain, matters are even worse with conflicting evidence as to whether changes in paraspinal muscle tone can be found.[2, 38, 39, 41, 133, 143, 174] Six other groups have found differences based only on more complex spine loading tasks and multiple testing procedures.[32, 118, 142, 184, 194, 195]

Motor unit potentials: Needle electrode EMG is used to measure single motor unit potentials. The characteristics of the duration, amplitude and phases of the action potential are examined for abnormalities suggesting disease including: synchronization; fibrillation potentials; positive sharp waves; fasciculation; and long duration, large amplitude polyphasic potentials. Appropriate interpretation can be conclusive for myopathies; radiculopathy; metabolic; myoneural junction; and central nervous system diseases.[14, 126, 178, 182, 187]

2. Electrocardiography

Electrocardiography (ECG) is very useful in the diagnosis of various heart diseases and the differentiation of noncardiac disorders such as thyroid, renal, pulmonary and electrolyte disorders. They also serve to differentiate spondylogenic symptoms that emulate heart disease, such as found in cervical angina.[210] Anecdotal and uncontrolled reports have been provided by many researchers and clinicians about improvement within patients having both ischemic and arrhythmic disorders of the heart following correction of spinal lesions.

D. Clinical Laboratory Procedures

For the present purposes, laboratory procedures will be arbitrarily sectioned into three hierarchical concerns: 1) the differential diagnosis of symptoms produced by somatic lesions from referred symptoms; 2) testing for contraindications to manipulative therapy in conjunction with evidence from other physical and examination findings; and 3) nutritional evaluation and monitoring.

1. Differential diagnosis of somatic and referred symptoms

Disorders with somatic reference of pain in the spinal region include peptic ulcer, aneurysm, pylorospasm, colitis, diverticulitis, abdominal carcinomas, prostatic carcinoma and obstructive uropathy, among others.[22] Appropriate laboratory procedures encompass the full set of services including hematology, serology, and urinalysis.[111, 209]

2. Contraindications to manipulative treatment

Under certain pathologic circumstances undue manipulative force may result in increased joint irritation, nerve compression, vertebral collapse, or hemorrhage. It is doubtful that absolute contraindications to manipulation of pathologic tissues/structures would be disagreed upon by many. They include vertebral malignancy, tuberculosis, osteomyelitis, infectious arthritis, acute vertebral fracture, extreme osteoporosis, metabolic bone disease, and extensive disc prolapse with evidence of severe nerve damage.[102, 132, 186] Common laboratory tests used for some of these conditions have been reported[60, 169] and are detailed in the chapter on clinical laboratory.

3. Nutritional evaluation and monitoring

The clinical usefulness of nutrition and the rational approach of nutritional counselling as therapy for malnutrition, chronic undernutrition,[25] overnutrition,[170] functional disease and some organic disorders has historically been of interest to chiropractors. Variance of individual nutritional needs are hotly contested issues.[3, 25, 27 33, 62, 83, 117, 139, 168, 179, 218] Periodic laboratory testing becomes valuable as a means of monitoring patient response and affirming diagnosis. The outcome of nutritional and pharmaceutical therapies prescribed for certain conditions is monitored by laboratory analysis. These include infection, cardiovascular disease, arteriosclerosis, anemia, osteoporosis, renal disease, and diabetes.[21, 48, 50, 1, 72, 90, 100, 101, 107, 119, 147, 153, 161, 170, 171, 215]

Functional disorders are often misunderstood and misdiagnosed entities. A few of these have been found to have measurable biochemical alterations that allow easier diagnosis and monitoring but remain poorly described. Examples of the types of functional disorders for which laboratory evaluation is found to be useful include hypoglycemia, carbohydrate malabsorption, hypothyroid, and functional hypoadrenia.[24, 90, 103, 180, 206] Further validation studies and statistical analyses are needed.

E. Other Instrument Measures

Several other types of examining instruments are in use within the chiropractic profession. As none of these are widespread, only the fundamentals of their use will be described.

1. Non-invasive vascular measures

Both plethysmography and doppler ultrasonic measures allow objective evaluation of vascular disorders by quantifying segmental limb blood pressures, velocities or pulse wave forms.

Doppler ultrasound:

Doppler ultrasound is the most simple and versatile method available for screening examinations of suspected vascular disease.[13, 125] Frequency shifts of ultrasound reflected from moving blood cells are detected. Simple hand held devices are adequate to screen peripheral vessels; however, doppler spectral analysis (Duplex scanning) is more accurate for cerebrovascular and visceral arterial disease.

For lower extremity claudication, doppler will identify significant occlusive arterial disease with a high degree of reproducibility.[216] Special procedures of value include the ankle/arm index[157] and lower extremity, multi-segmental pressure analysis. The latter examines for a pressure gradient greater than 30 mm Hg across appropriate intervals.[66] Hemodynamic deficit may be further evaluated using hyperemia procedures.

Plethysmography:

The plethysmograph quantifies the relative tissue volume of the distal extremities. This method has been used by Figar and Krausova[56, 57] to portray improvement in manipulative treatment of radicular syndromes involving the sixth to eighth cervical segments.

2. Spirometry

Estimation of vital capacity, total lung capacity, expiratory flow rate, maximum voluntary ventilation and forced expiratory volume are important in the evaluation and clinical follow-up of lung disorders.[63] It also serves to assess the severity of pulmonary involvement in patients with severe scoliosis. Monitoring of pulmonary function in patients with asthma, upper respiratory infection and chronic pulmonary disease[7, 17, 18, 22, 42, 73, 145, 156, 208] has periodically been reported as being responsive to change from treatment of the related spinal lesions. Good controlled studies are needed to evaluate the nature of manipulative therapy for these conditions.

V. ASSESSMENT CRITERIA

Procedure Ratings (System I)

Established: Accepted as appropriate by the practicing chiropractic community for the given indication in the specified patient population.

Promising: Given current knowledge, this technology appears to be appropriate for the given indication in the specified patient population. As more evidence and experience accumulates, this interim rating will change. This connotes provisional acceptance but permits a greater role for the level of current clinical use.

Equivocal: Current knowledge exists to support a given indication in the specified patient population, though value can neither be confirmed or denied. As more evidence and experience accumulates, this interim rating will change. Expert opinion recognizes a need for caution in general application.

Investigational: Evidence is insufficient to determine appropriateness. Further study is warranted. Use for a given indication in the specified patient population should be confined largely to research protocols. As more evidence and experience accumulates this interim rating will change.

Doubtful: Given current knowledge, this appears to be inappropriate for the given indication in the specified patient population. As more evidence and experience accumulates this interim rating will change.

Inappropriate: Regarded by the practicing chiropractic community as unacceptable for the given indication in the specified patient population.

Quality of Evidence

The following categories of evidence are used to support the ratings.

Class I:
Evidence provided by one or more well-designed controlled clinical trials; or well-designed experimental studies that address reliability, validity, positive predictive value, discriminability, sensitivity, and specificity.

Class II:
Evidence provided by one or more well-designed uncontrolled, observational clinical studies such as case control, cohort studies, etc.; or clinically relevant basic science studies that address reliability, validity, positive predictive value, discriminability, sensitivity and specificity; and published in refereed journals.

Class III:
Evidence provided by expert opinion, descriptive studies or case reports.

Suggested Strength of Recommendations Ratings

Type A. Strong positive recommendation. Based on Class I evidence or overwhelming Class II evidence when circumstances preclude randomized clinical trials.

Type B. Positive recommendation based on Class II evidence.

Type C. Positive recommendation based on strong consensus of Class III evidence.

Type D. Negative recommendation based on inconclusive or conflicting Class II evidence.

Type E. Negative recommendation based on evidence of ineffectiveness or lack of efficacy based on Class I or Class II evidence.

Safety and effectiveness

Safety: a judgment of the acceptability of risk in a specified situation, e.g., for a given health problem, by a provider with specified training (at a specific stage of the disorder, etc.).

Effectiveness: producing a desired effect under conditions of actual use.

VI. RECOMMENDATIONS

All recommendations are made based upon the assumptions that the operator/examiner is appropriately trained, versed in the technical issues affecting the qualities of safety, validity, discriminability, accuracy, precision and reliability of the measures. Standardized test protocols and periodic instrument calibration is important to ensure clinical utility of the information. Interpretation should be made by the attending clinician in all cases.

Perceptual Measurements

A. Questionnaires as Instruments

Questionnaire instruments are safe and effective. Several instruments have been fully validated, are widely used and well established. Their use is supported by both Class I (modified to the discipline of measurement) and Class II evidence.

> 3.1.1 Strength of recommendation: Type A.
> **Consensus Level: 1**

B. Screening Questionnaire

Their use is safe and effective, supported by Class II and III evidence.

> 3.1.2 Strength of recommendation: Type C.
> **Consensus Level: 1**

C. Pressure Algometry

Pressure algometry is safe and effective when contrasted with normative values for region and gender. It is a new procedure that is not yet in wide use but is promising. Its use is supported by Class II and Class III evidence.

> 3.1.3 Strength of recommendation: Type B.
> **Consensus Level: 1**

Functional Measurements

A. Measurement of Position/Clinical Anthropometry (Posture)

1. Plumbline Analysis
Plumbline analysis is safe and effective when used to assess upright posture. It can be administered by persons with mini-

mal training but should be interpreted by a professional health care provider. The procedure is widely used, established and supported by both Class II and Class III evidence.

3.2.1 Strength of recommendation: Type B.
Consensus Level: 1

2. Scoliometry

Scoliometry is safe and effective and can be administered by persons with minimal training but should be interpreted by a professional health care provider. The procedure is well established and supported by both Class I and Class II evidence.

3.2.2 Strength of recommendation: Type A.
Consensus Level: 1

3. Photogrammetry Methods

Photogrammetry methods are safe and effective means to quantify topographical or structural anomaly and work postures. Training is necessary to avoid error sources and assure reliability of measures. The procedures are well established and supported by evidence in Classes I, II and III.

3.2.3 Strength of recommendation: Type A.
Consensus Level: 1

4. Moire Topography

Moire topography is safe and can be administered by persons with minimal training but requires oversight on technical procedures. It is of limited effectiveness. The procedure is promising only as a qualitative screening method supported by Class II and Class III evidence.

3.2.4 Strength of recommendation: Type B.
Consensus Level: 1

5. Bilateral Weight Distribution

Bilateral weight scales are safe but their effectiveness is unknown and are rated as equivocal. Class II & III evidence is available.

3.2.5 Strength of recommendation: Type C.
Consensus Level: 1

6. Automated Measurements of Posture

Automated methods have received limited acceptance and are rated as promising. They are safe to administer but their effectiveness is limited by the training and practice of the operator. Fundamental difficulty in landmark identification and limited information on reliability restricts the use to screening purposes. Their use is supported by Class II and Class III evidence.

3.2.6 Strength of recommendation: Type B.
Consensus Level: 1

B. Measurement of Movement

1. Goniometers

Goniometers are widely used, safe and effective. They are established to measure peripheral joint motion although the margin of error remains high. Class I and Class II evidence supports their use.

3.3.1 Strength of recommendation: Type A.
Consensus Level: 1

2. Inclinometers

Inclinometers are established for measurements of spinal motion. Their common use is supported by Class I and Class II evidence and is safe and effective.

3.3.2 Strength of recommendation: Type A.
Consensus Level: 1

3. Optically Based Systems

Optically based systems are established for evaluating specific gait abnormalities or risky positions related to work tasks. They are safe and effective when evaluated by specially trained personnel and are supported by Class II evidence.

3.3.3 Strength of recommendation: Type B.
Consensus Level: 1

4. Computer Assisted Range of Motion Systems

Computer assisted range of motion systems provide improved levels of precision and reproducibility. They are safe, effective and non-invasive. They require specialized training and should be interpreted by a qualified health care provider. Clinical applications are promising. Class II & III evidence is available.

3.3.4 Strength of recommendation: Type B.
Consensus Level: 1

C. Measurement of Strength

1. Manual Strength Testing

Manual strength testing is widely used, safe and largely ineffective for strength differences less than 35%. Hand held load cells may assist in finding smaller differences in extremity muscle strengths. It is established as a screening procedure and is supported by Class I and Class II data.

3.4.1 Strength of recommendation: Type A.
Consensus Level: 1

2. Isometric Strength Testing

Isometric strength testing is an established procedure that is effective for limited applications involving employment evaluation and post-injury assessment where relevant standards can be determined. The methods are safe when performed by trained personnel who can make appropriate clinical judgments with respect to patient limitations during the procedure and when contraindications are observed. Class I and Class II data are available.

3.4.2 Strength of recommendation: Type A.
Consensus Level: 1

3. Isokinetic Strength Testing

Isokinetic strength testing is widely used, safe for non-acute disorders and effective for making bilateral comparisons or contrasting performance to normative data. The procedures are well established in sports applications and promising for post-injury use after the acute phase of treatment has passed. Class II and Class III evidence supports its use.

3.4.3 Strength of recommendation: Type B.
Consensus Level: 1

4. Isoinertial Strength Testing

Isoinertial strength testing is a promising procedure for employment selection and post-injury applications. It is safe for non-acute disorders when carried out by trained personnel. Class II and Class III evidence has been reported.

3.4.4 Strength of recommendation: Type C.
Consensus Level: 1

Physiologic Measurements

A. Thermographic Recordings

1. Thermocouple Devices

Thermocouple devices are still in use. While they are safe, there is no evidence to support a claim of effectiveness. Their use is rated doubtful and is supported by Class II and Class III evidence.

3.5.1 Strength of recommendation: Type D.
Consensus Level: 3
(See Section IX [3.10.1] for minority opinion)

2. Infrared Thermography

Infrared thermography is a safe procedure of intense controversial effectiveness. Its use requires specially trained personnel and specially adapted surroundings. Its rating as equivocal/promising is supported by continuing controversy from Class II and Class III evidence.

3.5.2 Strength of recommendation: Type C because of the controversy.
Consensus Level: 3
(See Section IX [3.10.2] for minority opinion)

B. Galvanic Skin Response

These types of measurement are safe, but generally ineffective as a result of questions remaining on reliability and validity from Class II and Class III types of evidence. For general arousal studies they are considered investigational.

3.6.1 Strength of recommendation: Type D.
Consensus Level: 1

For acupuncture point finding and for assessing spine related disorders, they are considered as doubtful.

3.6.2 Strength of recommendation: Type E.
Consensus Level: 1

C. Electrophysiologic Recordings

All of the electrodiagnostic methods are safe when carried out by specially trained personnel. Interpretation should be carried out only by physicians with extensive training in the technical and clinical considerations that can readily confound the findings.

1. Kinesiologic Surface (Scanning) EMG

Kinesiologic surface (scanning) EMG is a rapidly proliferating, safe procedure that has not been shown effective with the exception of limited use for flexion/relaxation and mean/median frequency shifting measures. Generally, its use remains investigational. Specific procedures of flexion/relaxation and mean/median frequency shift evaluation are considered promising based on Class II and Class III evidence.

3.7.1 Strength of recommendation - scanning surface EMG: Type C.
Consensus Level: 2

3.7.2 Strength of recommendation - flexion/relaxation and mean/median frequency shift measures: Type B.
Consensus Level: 1

2. Surface Electrodiagnostic Procedures (NCV, F-Wave, H-Reflex, SSEP)

Surface electrodiagnostic procedures (NCV, F-wave, H-reflex, SSEP) are established procedures effective for examination of peripheral nerve disorders and are supported by Class I and Class II evidence. Somatosensory evoked potentials are established for limited applications to peripheral nerve disorders and lesions affecting the long sensory tracks of the spinal cord.

3.7.3 Strength of recommendation: Type A.
Consensus Level: 1

3. Needle Electrodiagnostic Procedures (EMG, NCV, F-wave, H-reflex, SSEP)

Needle electrodiagnostic procedures (EMG, NCV, F-wave, H-reflex, SSEP) are widely used, established procedures that are affective in assessing functional effects of pathology affecting the central and peripheral nervous system and muscle. Class I and Class II evidence is available.

3.7.4 Strength of recommendation: Type A.
Consensus Level: 1

4. Electrocardiography

ECG is a widely used, safe, effective and established procedure for aiding in the differential diagnosis of complaints that may be cardiopulmonary in origin. Interpretation requires specialized training. Class I and Class II evidence is available.

3.7.5 Strength of recommendation: Type A.
Consensus Level: 1

D. Clinical Laboratory Procedures

Clinical laboratory testing is an established approach that is widely used, safe and effective when used in differential diagnosis. Test procedures require appropriate technical instrumentation operated by specially trained and certified staff as determined by law. Equipment must be kept calibrated and standardized. Quality assurance procedures must be followed to ensure accuracy and reliability. Class I, II and III evidence is available.

3.81   Strength of recommendation: Type A.
Consensus Level: 1

E. Other Instrument Measures

1. Doppler Ultrasound

Doppler measures are well established, safe and effective as means to quantify the presence of vascular disease. Special training is necessary and results should be interpreted by a trained health care provider. Both Class II and Class III data are available.

3.9.1   Strength of recommendation: Type B.
Consensus Level: 1

2. Plethysmography

Plethysmography is used on occasion. It is safe and effective when tissue volume changes and a symptom or peripheral vascular differential diagnosis is needed. Use for these purposes is well established. Special training is necessary and results should be interpreted by a trained health care provider. Its effectiveness as a monitor of treatment of spine disorders is not determined and use for this purpose should be considered investigational. Class II and Class III data are available.

3.9.2   Strength of recommendation - differential diagnosis: Type B.
Consensus Level: 1

3.9.3   Strength of recommendation - monitor spine disorders: Type D.
Consensus Level: 1

3. Spirometry

Pulmonary function testing is established as a method to assess effect of severe scoliosis and the differential diagnosis of lung disease. These uses are backed by Class I and Class II evidence. The procedures are safe and effective when performed by appropriately trained personnel.

3.9.4   Strength of recommendation: Type A.
Consensus Level: 1

VII. COMMENTS, SUMMARY OR CONCLUSION

Measurement instruments used in chiropractic practice are important not only in the initial assessment of the patient but also in the ongoing evaluation of their response to a particular intervention. The instrument used, therefore, must be applicable, appropriate, reliable, and valid. This necessitates that the clinician utilizing a particular instrument clearly understand the intended use and the limitation of the selected instrument.

This paper attempts to outline the instruments available to the practitioner and rates them according to the results of studies and reports in the scientific and clinical literature. It is expected that many of the aforementioned recommendations may in fact change as a result of ongoing investigations.

In order for the interpretation of changes in a subject's test results to be meaningful, the reliability and validity of the procedures used must be high. The test clearly must be relevant to the individual's activities that have been impaired, to normative data, or both, and should be able to discriminate healthy from unhealthy people. Careful attention to standardized test protocols is essential if replication of meaningful results is to occur.

VIII. REFERENCES

1. Agarwal A, Lloyd KN, Dovey P: Thermography of the spine and sacroiliac joints in spondylitis. *Rheum Phys Med* 1970, 10:349.

2. Ahern DK, Follick MJ, Council JR, Laser-Wolston N, Litchman H: Comparison of lumbar paravertebral EMG patterns in chronic low-back pain patients and non-patient controls. *Pain* 1988, 34:153.

3. Albanese AA: Calcium nutrition in the elderly: maintaining bone health to minimize fracture risk. *Postgrad Med* 1978, 63:167.

4. Arena J, Sherman R, Buno G, Young T: Electromyographic recordings of 5 types of low-back pain subjects and non-pain controls in different positions. *Pain* 1989, 37: 57-65.

5. Ayoub MA: Design of a pre-employment screening program. In: Kvalseth TO (ed). *Ergonomics of workstation design.* London, Butterworths, 1983, 152-8.

6. Ayoub MA: Ergonomic deficiencies: I. Pain at work. *J Occup Med* 1990, 32:52.

7. Ayres SM: Pulmonary function studies. In: Holman CW, Muschenheim C (eds): *Bronchopulmonary diseases and related disorders.* Hagerstown, Harper & Row, 1972.

8. Bailey HW, Beckwith DO: Short leg and spinal anomalies. *J Am Osteopath Assoc* 1937, 13:4.

9. Baillie AJ, Biagioni PA, Forsyth A, Garioch JJ: Thermographic assessment of patch-test responses. *Br J Dermatol* 1990, 122:351.

10. Baltzopoulos V, Brodie DA: Isokinetic dynamometry applications and limitations. *Sports Med* 1989, 8:101.

11. Barlow DH, Hayes S, Nelson R: *The scientist practitioner: research and accountability in clinical and educational settings.* New York, Pergamon Press, 1984, 112-124.

12. Barnes WS: The relationship of motor unit activation to isokinetic muscular contraction at different contractile velocities. *Phys Ther* 1980, 60:1152.

13. Barnes R: Noninvasive diagnostic assessment of peripheral vascular disease. Circulation 83 [Suppl I], 1991, 20-27.

14. Basmajian JV, DeLuca CJ: *Muscles alive: their function revealed by electromyography.* 5th ed. Baltimore, Williams & Wilkins, 1985.

15. Beasley WC: Influence of method on estimates of normal knee extensor force among normal and postpolio children. *Phys Ther Rev* 1956, 36:21.

16. Beimborn DS, Morrissey MC: A review of the literature related to trunk muscle performance. *Spine* 1988, 13:655.

17. Bergofsky EH, Turnio GM, Fishman AP: Cardiorespiratory failure in kyphoscoliosis. *Medicine* 1959, 38:263.

18. Bjure J, Grimby G, Kasalicky J, Lindh M, Nachemson A: Respiratory impairment and airway closure in patients with untreated idiopathic scoliosis. *Thorax* 1970, 25:451.

19. Bohannan RW: Hand-held dynamometry: stability of muscle strength over multiple measurements. *Clinical Biomech* 1986, 2:74.

20. Bolecek C, Steiner C, Guzelsu N: Evaluation of conservative treatment of low-back pain via electromyography and pain quantification. In: *Electromyographic Kinesiology Excerpta Medica*, New York, 1990, 191-194.

21. Born BA: Nutritional aspects in the prevention and treatment of arteriosclerosis. *ACA J Chiropr* 1972, 9:S53.

22. Braunwald E, Isselbacher KJ, Petersdorf RG, Wilson JD, Martin JB, Fauci AS (eds): *Harrison's principles of internal medicine*. New York, McGraw-Hill, 1987.

23. Brown WF: *The physiological and technical basis of electromyography*. Boston, Butterworths, 1984.

24. Buehler MT: The hypoglycemic state. *ACA J Chiropr* 1971, 8:S33.

25. Busse EW: How mind, body, and environment influence nutrition in the elderly. *Postgrad Med* 1978, 63:118.

26. Byl NN, Richards S, Asturias J: Intrarater and interrater reliability of strength measurements of the biceps and deltoid using a hand held dynamometer. *J Orthop Sports Phys Ther* 1988, 9:399.

27. Caliendo MA, Sanjur D, Wright J, Cummings G: Nutritional status of preschool children. *J Am Diet Assoc* 1977, 71:20.

28. Chafetz N, Wexler CE, Kaiser JA: Neuromuscular thermography of the lumbar spine with CT correlation. *Spine* 1988, 13:922.

29. Chaffin D: Ergonomics guide for the assessment of human static strength. *Am Ind Hyg Assoc J* July 1975, 505-511.

30. Chaffin DB, Andersson GBJ: *Occupational Biomechanics*, Wiley Interscience Publishers, New York, 1988, 117-122.

31. Chang L, Abernathy M, O'Rourke D, Dittberner M, Robinson C: The evaluation of posterior thoracic temperatures by telethermography, thermocouple, thermistor and liquid crystal thermography. *THERM* 1985, 1: 95-101.

32. Chapman AE, Troup JDG: The effect of increased maximal strength on the integrated electrical activity of lumbar erectores spine. *Electromyography* 1969, 9:263.

33. Cichoke AJ: Protein malnutrition and introduction of low-cost protein-rich supplements. *ACA J Chiropr* 1972, 9:S11.

34. Clarke GR: Unequal leg length - an accurate method of detection and some clinical results. *Rheum Phys Med* 1972, 11:385.

35. Cleveland RH, Kushner DC, Ogden MC, Herman TE, Kermond W, Correia JA. Determination of leg length discrepancy. A comparison of weight-bearing and supine imaging. *Invest Radiol* 1988, 23:301.

36. Coggins WN: *Basic techniques and systems of body mechanics*. Florrissant, Elco, 1975.

37. Cohen HL, Brumlik JD: *Manual of electroneuromyography*. 2nd ed, Hagerstown, Harper & Row, 1976.

38. Cohen MJ, Swanson GA, Naliboff BD, Schandler SL, McArthur DL: Comparison of electromyographic response patterns during posture and stress tasks in chronic low-back pain patterns and control. *J Psychosom Res* 1986, 30:135.

39. Collins GA, Cohen MJ, Naliboff BD, Schandler SL: Comparative analysis of paraspinal and frontalis EMG, heart rate and skin conductance in chronic low-back pain patients and normals to various postures and stress. *Scand J Rehab Med* 1982, 14:39.

40. Cooper P, Randall WC, Hartzman AB: Vascular convection of heat from active muscle to overlying skin. *J Appl Physiol* 1959, 14:207.

41. Corlett E, Manecica I, Guillau P: The relationship between EMG activity of the sacrospinalis and reported back discomfort. *Euro J Applied Physiol.* 1983, 50:213.

42. Davis D: Respiratory manifestations of dorsal spine radiculitis simulating cardiac asthma. *Ann Intern Med* 1950, 32:954.

43. DeBois EF: *The mechanism of heat loss and temperature regulation*. Stanford, Stanford University Press, 1937.

44. Deschuytere J, Rosselle N: Diagnostic use of monosynaptic reflexes in L5 and S1 root compression. In: Desmedt JE (ed): *New developments in electromyography and clinical neurophysiology*. 1973, Vol. 3, Basel, S. Karger.

45. Deutsch S: *B-200 back evaluation system*. Hillsborough, Isotechnologies, 1989-90.

46. Deyo R: Measuring the functional status of patients with low-back pain. *Chiropractic Technique* 1990, 2(3): 127-136.

47. Diakow PR: Thermographic imaging of myofascial trigger points. *J Manip Physiol Ther* 1988, 11:114.

48. Dold WR: Anemia investigation and classification. *ACA J Chiropr* 1976, 13:S35.

49. Dowling JJ, Kennedy SR: The quantitative assessment of EMG crosstalk in human soleus and gastrocnemius muscles. Thirteenth annual meeting of the American Society of Biomechanics. Vermont, August, 1989.

50. Dudley WN: Triglycerides and sucrose. *ACA J Chiropr* 1972, 9:S79.

51. Dudley WN: Preliminary findings in thermography of the back. *ACA J Chiropr* 1978, 15:S83.

52. Duensing F, Becker P, Rittmeyer K: Thermographic findings in lumbar disc protrusions. *Arch Psychiatr Nervenkr* 1973, 217:53.

53. Eisen A, Schomer D, Melmed C: An electrophysiological method for examining lumbosacral root compression. *Can J Neurol Sci* 1977, 4:117.

54. Emley M, Klein A, Mackler L, Roy S, De Luca C: Comparison of spinal mobility and strength to EMG spectral parameters in identifying low-back pain. In: *Electromyographical Kinesiology Excerpta Medica,* New York, 1990, 171-174.

55. Feldman F, Nickoloff: Normal thermographic standards for the cervical spine and upper extremities. *Skeletal Radiol* 1984, 12:235-249.

56. Figar S, Krausova L: A plethysmographic study of the effects of chiropractic treatment in vertebrogenic syndromes. *ACTA Univ Carol Med (Suppl)* 1965, 21:84.

57. Figar S, Krausova L, Levit K: Plethysmographic examination following treatment of vertebrogenic disorders by manipulation. *ACTA Neuroveg* 1967, 29:618.

58. Fisher AA: Pressure threshold meter: Its use for quantification of tenderspots. *Arch Phys Med Rehab 1986,* 67 (11): 836-838.

59. Fisher AA: Pressure algometry over normal muscles: Standard values, validity and reproducibility of pressure threshold. *Pain* 1989, 1: 115-126.

60. Fisk JW: *A practical guide to management of the painful neck and back - diagnosis, manipulation, exercises, prevention*. Springfield, Charles C. Thomas, 1977, 10.

61. Forshee GK: Arterio and atherosclerosis with relation to vitamin D. *ACA J Chiropr* 1971, 8:S81.

62. Frank GC, Voors AW, Schilling PE, Berenson GS: Dietary studies of rural school children in a cardiovascular survey. *J Am Diet Assoc* 1977, 71:31.

63. Freedman S: Design of respiratory circuits and spirometry. In: Laszlo G, Sudlow MF (eds): *Measurement in clinical respiratory physiology*. London, Academic Press, 1983.

64. Frese E, Brown M, Norton B: Clinical reliability of manual muscle testing. Middle trapezius and gluteus medius muscles. *Phys Ther* 1987, 67(7): 1072-1076.

65. Friberg O, Nurminen M, Korhonen K, Soininen E, Manttari T: Accuracy and precision of clinical estimation of leg length inequality and lumbar scoliosis: comparison of clinical and radiological measurements. *Internat Disabil Studies* 1988, 10:49.

66. Fronk A, Coel M, Bernstein E: The importance of combined multisegmental pressure and doppler flow velocity studies in the diagnosis of peripheral arterial occlusive disease. *J Surg* 1978, 84: 840-847.

67. Fuhrer MJ: Effects of stimulus site on the pattern of skin conductance responses evoked from spinal man. *J Neurol Neurosurg Psychiatr* 1975, 38:749.

68. Gerow G, Callton M, Meyer JJ, Demchak JJ, Christiansen J: Thermographic evaluation of rats with complete sciatic nerve transection. *J Manip Physiol Ther* 1990, 13:257.

69. Gientempo P, Kent C: Establishing medical necessity for paraspinal EMG scanning. *Texas J Chiropractic*, January 1990.

70. Giesen JM, Center DB, Leach RA: An evaluation of chiropractic manipulation as a treatment of hyperactivity in children. *J Manip Physiol Ther* 1989, 12(5):353-363.

71. Gleim GW, Nicholas JA, Webb JN: Isokinetic evaluation following leg injuries. *Phys Sportsmed* 1978, 68:74.

72. Goldman SR: Pathogenesis of the diabetic syndrome. *ACA J Chiropr* 1967, 4:S22.

73. Goldman SR: A structural approach to bronchial asthma. *Bull EuroChiropr Union* 1972, 21:66.

74. Gomez T, Beach G, Cooke C, Hrudey W, Goyert P: Normative database for trunk range of motion, strength, velocity, and endurance with the isostation B-200 lumbar dynamometer. *Spine* 1991, 16:15.

75. Goodman PH, Murphy MG, Siltanen GL, Kelley MP, Rucker L: Normal temperature asymmetry of the back and extremities by computer-assisted infrared imaging. *THERM* 1986, 1:195-202.

76. Gosselin G: Diagnostic tools for the sports chiropractor. *SOMA* 1987, October, 23.

77. Green J, Coyle M, Becker C, Reilly A: Abnormal thermographic findings in asymptomatic volunteers. *THERM* 1986, 2: 13-15.

78. Halberg F: Chronobiology. *Annu Rev Physiol* 1969, 31:675.

79. Haldeman S: The electrodiagnostic evaluation of nerve root function. *Spine* 1984, 9(1): 42-48.

80. Hazard RG, Bendix A, Fenwick JW: Disability exaggeration as a predictor of functional restoration outcomes for patients with chronic low-back pain. *Spine* 1991, 16(9), 1062-1067.

81. Hazard RG, Fenwick JW, Kalisch SM, Redmond J, Reeves V, Reid S, Frymoyer JW: Functional restoration with behavioral support - A one-year prospective study of patients with chronic low-back pain. *Spine* 1989, 14:157.

82. Hazard RG, Reid S, Fenwick J, Reeves V: Isokinetic trunk and lifting strength measurements: Variability as an indicator of effort. *Spine* 1988, 13:54.

83. Head MK, Weeks RJ, Gibbs E: Major nutrients in the type A lunch. *J Am Diet Assoc* 1973, 63:620.

84. Hellsing AL: Leg length inequality. A prospective study of young men during their military service. *Upsala J Med Sci* 1988, 93:245.

85. Herzog W, Nigg B, Read L: Quantifying the effects of spinal manipulation on gait using patients with low-back pain. *J Manip Pysiol Ther* 1988, 11(3): 151-157.

86. Herzog W, Nigg B, Read L, Olsson E: Asymmetries in ground reaction force patterns in normal human gait. *Med Sci Sports Exerc* 1989, 21(1): 110-114.

87. Hildebrandt RW: *Chiropractic spinography - a manual of technology and interpretation.* Des Plains, Hilmark Publication, 1977.

88. Hoffman R, Kent D, Deyo R: Diagnostic accuracy and clinical utility of thermography for lumbar radiculopathy: a Meta-analysis. *Spine* 1991, 16, 623-638.

89. Hoikka V, Ylikoski M, Tallroth K: Leg-length inequality has poor correlation with lumbar scoliosis. A radiological study of 100 patients with chronic low-back pain. *Arch Orthop Trauma Surg* 1989, 108:173.

90. Hollen WV: Clinical carbohydrate evaluation. *ACA J Chiropr* 1969, 6:S73.

91. *Hoppenfeld S: Scoliosis: a manual of concept and treatment.* Philadelphia, Lippincott, 1967.

92. Horsfield D, Jones SN: Assessment of inequality in length of the lower limb. *Radiography* 1986, 52:223.

93. Houdas Y, Guieu JD: Environmental factors affecting skin temperatures. *Bibl Radiol* 1974, 6:157.

94. Hubbard JE, Hoyt C: Pain evaluation by electronic infrared thermography: correlations with symptoms, EMG, myelogram and CT scan. *THERM* 1985, 1: 26-35.

94b. Hubbard JE: Thermal imaging of radiculopathy: a review. Clinical Proceedings. Academy Neuromuscular Thermography, Orlando, FL. September 1986.

95. Huskisson EC, Berry H, Browett J, Wykeham Balme H: Measurement of inflammation. *Ann Rheum Dis* 1973, 32:99.

96. Iacono C: EMG scanning norms: Caveat emptor. *Biofeedback and Self-Regulation* 1991, 16(3): 227-241.

97. Illi FW: The phylogenesis and clinical import of the sacroiliac mechanism. *J Can Chiropr Assoc* 1965, 9:9.

98. Jabre JF, Hackett ER: *EMG manual.* Springfield, Thomas, 1983.

99. Jacobs I, Bell DG, Pope J: Comparison of isokinetic and isoinertial lifting tests as predictors of maximal lifting capacity. *Europ J Appl Physiol Occup Physiol* 1988, 57:146.

100. Jamison JR: Dietary control of mild essential hypertension. *J Manip Physiol Ther* 1987, 10:101.

101. Jamison JR: Dietary intervention in the clinical prevention of ischemic heart disease. *J Manip Physiol Ther* 1990, 13:247.

102. Jaquet P: *An introduction to clinical chiropractic.* Geneva, Jaquet and Grinard, 1976.

103. Jessen AR: Diagnosis of thyroid dysfunction. *ACA J Chiropr* 1967, 4:S49.

104. Jiang BC, Smith JL, Ayoub MM: Psychophysical modelling of manual materials-handling capacities using isoinertial strength variables. *Hum Factors* 1986, 28:691.

105. Jiang BC, Smith JL, Ayoub MM: Psychophysical modelling for combined manual materials-handling activities. *Ergonomics* 1986, 29:1173.

106. Jones CH: Physical aspects of thermography in relation to clinical techniques. *Bibl Radiol* 1974, 6:1.

107. Jowsey J: Osteoporosis. *Postgrad Med* 1976, 60:75.

108. Judovich B, Bates W: *Pain syndromes - diagnosis and treatment.* 4th ed. Philadelphia, F.A. Davis, 1954.

109. Kannus P: Ratio of hamstring to quadriceps femoris muscles' strength in the anterior cruciate ligament insufficient knee. Relationship to long-term recovery. *Phys Ther* 1988, 68:961.

110. Karpman HL, Knebel A, Semel CJ, Cooper J: Clinical studies in thermography: II. application of thermography in evaluating musculoligamentous injuries of the spine - a preliminary report. *Arch Environ Health* 1970, 20:412.

111. Kieffer JD: Laboratory procedures in the low-back syndrome. *ACA J Chiropr* 1965, 2:17.

112. Khalil TM, Goldberg ML, Asfour SS, Moty EA, Rosomoff RS, Rosomoff HL: Acceptable maximum effort (AME) a psychophysical measure of strength in back pain patients. *Spine* 1987, 12:372.

113. Kibler WB, Chandler TJ, Uhl T, Maddux RE: A musculoskeletal approach to the preparticipation physical examination. Preventing injury and improving performance. *Am J Sports Med* 1989, 17:525.

114. Kimmel E: Electro-analytical instrumentation. *ACA J Chiropr*, April, 1966, 3:9.

115. Kimmel E: Electro-analytical instrumentation. *ACA J Chiropr*, May, 1966, 3:9.

116. Kimmel E: Electro-analytical instrumentation. *ACA J Chiropr*, June, 1966, 3:11.

117. Kohrs MB, O'Neil R, Preston A, Eklund D, Abrahams O: Nutritional status of elderly residents in Missouri. *Am J Clin Nutri* 1978, 31:2186.

118. Kravitz E, Moore ME, Glaros A. Paralumbar muscle activity in chronic low-back pain. *Arch Phys Med Rehabil* 1981, 62:172.

119. Kritchevsky D: How aging affects cholesterol metabolism. *Postgrad Med* 1978, 63:133.

120. Kroemer KHE: An isoinertial technique to assess individual capacity. *Hum Factors* 1983, 25:493.

121. Kroemer K: Testing individual capability to lift materials. Repeatability of a dynamic test compared with static testing. *J Safety Res* 1985, 16:1.

122. Kvalseth TO (ed.): *Ergonomics of workstation design* London, Butterworths, 1983.

123. Lakomy HKA, Williams C: Measurement of isokinetic concentric and eccentric muscle imbalance. *Int J Sports Med* (Suppl) 1984, 5:40.

124. Langrana NA, Lee CK, Alexander H, Mayott CW: Quantitative assessment of back strength using isokinetic testing. *Spine* 1984, 9:287.

125. Lawrence D (Ed): *Fundamentals of Chiropractic Diagnosis and Management.* Baltimore, Williams and Wilkins, 1991, 256-264.

126. Ludin HP: *Electromyography in practice.* Stuttgart, Georg Thieme Verlag, 1980.

127. Mayer TG, Gatchel RJ: *Functional restoration for spinal disorders: the sports medicine approach.* Philadelphia, Lea & Febiger 1988, p 208.

128. Mayer TG, Gatchel RJ, Kishino N, Keeley J, Mayer H, Capra P, Mooney V: A prospective short-term study of chronic low-back pain patients utilizing novel objective functional measurement. *Pain* 1986, 25:53.

129. Mayer TG, Gatchel RJ, Maher H, Kishino ND, Keeley J, Mooney V: A prospective two year study of functional restoration in industrial low-back pain injury. An objective assessment procedure. *JAMA* 1987, 258:1763.

130. Mayer TG, Smit SS, Keeley J, Mooney V: Quantification of lumbar function. Part 2: Sagittal plane trunk strength in chronic low-back pain patients. *Spine* 1985, 10:765.

131. McNeill T, Warwick D, Andersson G, Schultz A: Trunk strengths in attempted flexion, extension, and lateral bending in healthy subjects and patients with low-back disorders. *Spine* 1980, 5:529.

132. Mennell J McM: *Back pain - diagnosis and treatment using manipulative techniques.* Boston, Little Brown, 1960.

133. Miller DJ: Comparison of electromyographic activity in the lumbar paraspinal muscles of subjects with and without chronic low-back pain. *Phys Ther* 1985, 65:1347.

134. Mills GH, Davies GK, Getty CJ, Conway J: The evaluation of liquid crystal thermography in the investigation of nerve root compression due to lumbosacral lateral spinal stenosis. *Spine* 1986, 11:427.

135. Mira AJ, Markley K, Greer RB III: A critical analysis of quadriceps function after femoral shaft fracture in adults. *J Bone Joint Surg* 1980, 62A:61.

136. Mitchell FL, Pruzzo NL: Investigation of voluntary and primary respiratory mechanisms. *J Am Osteopath Assoc* 1971, 70:1109.

137. Moreland MS, Pope MH, Armstrong GWD eds.: *Moire fringe topography and spinal deformity.* New York, Pergamon Press, 1981.

138. Moseley CF: A straight line graph for leg length discrepancies. *Clin Orthop* 1978, 136:33.

139. Munroe HN, Young VR: Protein metabolism in the elderly: observations relating to dietary needs. *Postgrad Med* 1978, 63:143.

140. Nansel DD, Jansen RD: Concordance between Galvanic Skin Response and spinal palpation findings in pain-free males. *J Manip Physiol Ther* 1988, 11(4):267-272.

141. Niebuhr BR, Marion R: Detecting sincerity of effort when measuring grip strength. *Am J Phys Med* 1987, 66:16.

142. Nouwen A: EMG biofeedback used to reduce standing levels of paraspinal muscle tension in chronic low-back pain. *Pain* 1983, 17:353.

143. Nouwen A, Bush C: The relationship between paraspinal EMG and chronic low-back pain. *Pain* 1984, 20:109.

144. Nunn KD, Mayhew JL: Comparison of three methods of assessing strength imbalances at the knee. *J Orthop Sports Phys Ther* 1988, 10:134.

145. O'Donovan D: The possible significance of scoliosis of the spine in the causation of asthma and allied allergic conditions. *Ann Allergy* 1951, 9:184.

146. Owen E, Holt GA: Thermographic patterns in sacroiliitis and ankylosing spondylitis. American Thermographic Society, New York, 1973.

147. Palmateer DC, Hollen WV: Urinary tract calculi diagnosis and treatment. *ACA J Chiropr* 1971, 8:S25.

148. Panjabi MM, Goel VK, Walter SD: Errors in kinematic parameters of a planar joint: guidelines for optimal experimental design. *J Biomechanics* 1982, 15:537.

149. Parnianpour M, Li F, Nordin M, Kahanovitz N: A database of isoinertial strength tests against three resistance levels in sagittal, frontal, and transverse planes in normal male subjects. *Spine* 1989, 14:409.

150. Perelman RB, Adler D, Humphreys M: Reflex sympathetic dystrophy: A thermographic evaluation. *Acad. Neuromuscular Therm Clin Proceedings.* Orlando, Florida, Sept 1986.

151. Pochaczevsky R: Thermography in posttraumatic pain. *Am J Sports Med* 1987, 15:243.

152. Pollock ML, Leggett SH, Graves JE, Jones A, Fulton M, Cirulli J: Effect of resistance training on lumbar extension strength. *Am J Sports Med* 1989, 17:624.

153. Pressman R: Calcium and neglected minerals. *ACA J Chiropr* 1971, 8:S45.

154. Prodromas C, Andriacchi T, Galante J: A relationship between gait and clinical changes following high tibial osteotomy. *JBJS* 1985, 67(8): 1188-1196.

155. Pullella SF, Andre J, Bell L, Blackmon C, Jenness ME, Martin PA, Nordstrom D, Riekeman C, Shaw A, VanSkyhock G: Correlative study of various instruments and procedures in chiropractic. *ACA J Chiropr* 1974, 11:S197.

156. Purse FM: Manipulative therapy of upper respiratory infections in children. *J Am Osteopath Assoc* 1966, 65:964.

157. Quigley F, Paris I, Duncan H: A comparison of doppler ankle pressures and skin perfusion pressure in subjects with and without diabetes. *Clin Physiology* 1991, 11:21-25.

158. Raskin M: *Thermography in low-back diseases. Medical thermography: theory and clinical applications.* Los Angeles, Brentwood, 1976.

159. Reinberg : Circadian changes in the temperature of human beings. *Bibl Radiol* 1975, 6:128.

160. Roaf R: *Scoliosis.* Baltimore, Williams & Wilkins, 1966.

161. Robinson R: Calcium and vitamins C and D in nutrition of bone, muscle, and nerve. *ACA J Chiropr* 1965, 2:14.

162. Roland M, Morris R: A study of the natural history of back pain, Part I: development of a reliable and sensitive measure of diasability in low-back pain. *Spine* 1983, 8:141.

163. Roland M, Morris R: A study of the natural history of low-back pain, Part II: development of guidelines for trials of treatment in primary care. *Spine* 1983, 8:145.

164. Roy SH, DeLuca CJ, Casavant DA: Lumbar muscle fatigue and chronic lower back pain. *Spine* 1988, 14:992-1001.

165. Ruch TC, Patton HD, Woodbury JW, Towe AL: *Neurophysiology.* Philadelphia, Saunders, 1965.

166. Sapega AA: Muscle performance evaluation in orthopaedic practice. *J Bone Joint Surg* 1990, 72A:1562.

167. Saraniti AJ, Gleim GW, Melvin M, Nicholas JA: The relationship between subjective and objective measurements of strength. *J Orthop Sports Phys Ther* 1980, 2:15.

168. Sawyer CE: Nutritional disorders. In: Lawrence D (ed): *Fundamentals of chiropractic diagnosis and management.* Baltimore, Williams & Wilkins, 1991.

169. Schafer RE (ed): *Basic chiropractic procedural manual.* DesMoines, American Chiropractic Association, 1977.

170. Schneider HA, Anderson CE, Coursin DB: *Nutritional support of medical practice.* Hagerstown, Harper & Row, 1977.

171. Schroeder RM: Diseases related to the pathologic biochemistry of calcium, phosphorus, and alkaline phosphatase metabolism. *ACA J Chiropr* 1975, 12:S13.

172. Seeds RH, Levene JA, Goldberg HM: Abnormal patient data for the isostation B100. *J Orthop Sports Phys Ther* 1988, 10:121.

173. Seeman DC: *C1 subluxations: short leg and pelvic distortions. The upper cervical monograph* 1978, 2:5, p 1.

174. Sherman RA: Relationships between strength of low-back muscle contraction and reported intensity of chronic low-back pain. *Am J Phys Med* 1985, 64:190.

175. Sherman RA, Barja RH, Bruno GM: Thermographic correlates of chronic pain: analysis of 125 patients incorporating evaluations by a blind panel. *Arch Phys Med Rehabil* 1987, 68:273.

176. Sihoven T, Partanen J, Hanninen O, Soimakallio S: Electric behavior of low-back muscles during lumbar pelvic rhythm in low-back pain patients and healthy controls. *Arch Phys Med Rehabil* 72: Dec. 1991.

177. Silverman JL, Rodriquez AA, Agre JC: Reliability of a hand-held dynamometer in neck strength testing. *Arch Phys Med Rehabil* (Suppl) 1989, 70:94.

178. Simpson JA; Neuromuscular diseases. In: Remond A (ed) *Handbook of electroencephalography and clinical neurophysiology.* Amsterdam, Elsevier, 1973.

179. Sims LS, Morris PM: Nutritional status of preschoolers. *J Am Diet Assoc 1974,* 64:492.

180. Sisson JA: *Handbook of clinical pathology.* Philadelphia, JB Lippincott, 1976.

181. Smith GA, Nelson RC, Sadoff SJ, Dadoff AM: Assessing sincerity of effort in maximal grip strength tests. *Am J Phys Med Rehabil* 1989, 68:73.

182. Smorto MP, Basmajian JV: *Electrodiagnosis: a handbook for neurologists.* New York, Harper & Row, 1977.

183. So YT, Aminoff MJ, Olney RK: The role of thermography in the evaluation of lumbosacral radiculopathy. *Neurology* 1989, 39:1154.

184. Soderberg GL, Barr JO: Muscular function in chronic low-back dysfunction. *Spine* 1983, 8:79.

185. Stevenson JM, Andrew GM, Bryant JT, Greenhorn DR, Thomson JM: Isoinertial tests to predict lifting performance. *Ergonomics* 1989, 32:157.

186. Stoddard A: *Manual of osteopathic practice.* New York, Harper & Row, 1969.

187. Taylor A: The significance of grouping motor unit activity. *J Physiol* (London) 1962, 162:259.

188. Thorstensson A, Arvidson A: Trunk muscle strength and low-back pain. *Scand J Rehabil Med* 1982, 14:69.

189. Topf M: Response sets in questionnaire research. *Nursing Res* 1986, 35:119.

190. Triano J: The Chiropractic Rehabilitation Practice. In: *Spine Rehabilitation.* Guyer, R (ED) (In Press).

191. Triano J: Objective electromyographic evidence for the use and effects of lift therapy. *J Manip Physiol Ther* 1983, 6:13.

192. Triano J, Baker J, McGregor M, Torres B: Optimizing measures on maximum voluntary contraction. *Spine Rehab* (Submitted 1991).

193. Triano JJ, Humphreys CR: Patient monitoring in the conservative management of cervical radiculopathy. *J Manip Physiol Ther* 1987, 10:94.

194. Triano JJ, Luttges M: Myoelectric paraspinal response to spinal loads: Potential for monitoring low-back pain. *J Manip Physiol Ther* 1985, 8:137.

195. Triano JJ, Schultz AB: Correlation of objective measure of trunk motion and muscle function with low-back disability ratings. *Spine* 1987, 12:561.

196. Triano J, Skogsbergh D, Kowalski M: The use of instrumentation by chiropractors. In: Haldeman S (ed): *Modern Developments in the Principles and Practice of Chiropractic.* Appleton-Lange, 1992 (in press).

197. Trott PH, Maitand GD, Gerrard B: The neurocalometer: a survey to assess its value as a diagnostic instrument. *Med J Aus* 1972, 1:464.

198. Uematsu S: Quantification of thermal asymmetry. Part 1; Normal values and reproducibility. *J Neurosurg* 1988, 69: 552-555.

199. Uematsu S, Hendler U, Hungerford, et al.: Thermography and electromyography in the differential diagnosis of chronic pain syndromes and reflex sympathetic dystrophy. *Electro Clin Neurophysiol* 1981, 21: 165-182.

200. Uematsu S, Jankel WR, Edwin DH, Kim W, Kozikowski J, Rosenbaum A, Long DM: Quantification of thermal asymmetry. Part 2. Application in low-back pain and sciatica. *J Neurosurg* 1988, 69:556.

201. Uricchio JV: Reflex sympathetic dystrophy and causalgia. *Acad. Neuromuscular Therm Clin Proceedings.* Orlando, Florida, Sept 1986.

202. Vallfors B: Acute, subacute and chronic low-back pain. Clinical symptoms, absenteeism and working environment. *Scand J Rehabil Med* (Suppl) 1985, 185:1.

203. Vernon H: Applying research-based assessments of pain and loss of function to the issue of developing standards of care in chiropractic. *Chiropractic Technique* 1990, 2(3):121-126.

203b. Vernon H, Aker P, Burns S, Viljakanen S, Short L: Pressure pain threshold evaluation of the effect of a spinal manipulation in the treatment of chronic neck pain. *J Manip Physiol Ther* 1990, 13(1): 13.

204. Vernon H, Grice A: The four quadrant weight scale: a technical and procedural review. *J Manip Physiol Ther* 1984, 3:165.

205. Walshe FMR: *Diseases of the nervous system described for practitioners and students.* 10th ed, Baltimore, Williams and Wilkins, 1963.

206. Walther DS: *Applied kinesiology - the advanced approach in chiropractic.* Pueblo Systems, D.D., 1976.

207. Watkins MP, Harris BA, Kozlowski BA: Isokinetic testing in patients with hemiparesis. A pilot study. *Phys Ther* 1984, 64:184.

208. Weber B, Smith JP, Briscoe WA, Friedman SA, King TK: Pulmonary function in asymptomatic adolescents with idiopathic scoliosis. *Am Rev Respir Dis* 1975, 111:389.

209. Wickes D: Laboratory evaluation. In: Cox JM: *Low-back pain -mechanism, diagnosis and treatment.* 5th ed. Baltimore, Williams & Wilkins, 1990.

210. Wickes DJ: Cardiovascular disorder in ambulatory patients. In: Lawrence D (ed): *Fundamentals of chiropractic diagnosis and management.* Baltimore, Williams & Wilkins, 1991.

211. Wilbourn A, Aminoff M: AAEE minimomograph #32: The electrophysiologic examination in patients with radiculopathies. *Muscle Nerve* 1988, 11(11): 1099-1114.

212. Williams M, Stutzman L: Strength variation through the range of joint motion. *Phys Ther Rev* 1959, 39:145.

213. Willner S: Moire topography for the diagnosis and documentation of scoliosis. *Acta Orthop Scand* 50(3): 295-302, 1979.

214. Work Practices Guide for Manual Lifting. NIOSH technical report; *USDHHS* 1981, #81-122.

215. Wozny PJ: Iron and Anemias. *ACA J Chiropr* 1975, 12:S135.

216. Wright J, Cruickshank J, Kontis S, et al.: Aortic compliance measured by non-invasive doppler ultrasound: description of a method and its reproducibility. *Clin Sci* 1990, 78: 463-468.

217. Wyatt MP, Edwards AM: Comparison of quadriceps and hamstring torque values during isokinetic exercise. *J Orthop Sports Phys Ther* 3:48.

218. Ziegler EE, O'Donnel AM, Stearns G, Nelson SE, Burmeister LF, Fomon SJ: Nitrogen balance studies with normal children. *Am J Clin Nutr* 1977, 30:939.

219. Bean JC, Chaffin DB: Biomechanical model calculation of muscle contraction forces: A double linear programming method. *J Biomechanics* 1988, 21(1) :59-66.

220. Reeves JL, Jaeger B, Graff-Radford SB: Reliability of the pressure algometer as a measure of myofascial trigger point sensitivity. *Pain* 1986, 24:313-321.

221. Ebrall, PS: A chiropractic screening health questionnaire: A pilot study concerned with quality standard of practice. *J. Aust. Chiropractor's Assoc.* 1990; 20; 122-8.

IX. MINORITY OPINIONS

Physiologic Measurements

Thermographic Recordings

Thermocouple Devices

Thermocouple devices are commonly used in chiropractic practice. They are safe in a clinical setting. Their use is rated as equivocal and this rating is supported by Class II evidence.

3.10.1 **Strength of recommendation:** Type C.
(For majority recommendation, see 3.5.1.)

Physiologic Measurements

Thermographic Recordings

Infrared Thermography

Infrared thermography is a safe and effective procedure. Its use requires specially trained personnel, specially adapted surroundings and explicit protocols. Its use is considered to be promising as supported by Class II and Class III evidence.

3.10.2 **Strength of recommendation:** Type B.
(For majority recommendation, see 3.5.2.)

4

Clinical Laboratory

Chapter Outline

I. OVERVIEW

A chiropractic practitioner who accepts a patient for any professional reason has a duty and responsibility to perform an appropriate clinical evaluation on that patient for the purpose of assessing the patient's current health status and identifying if the patient is a proper subject for chiropractic care. Such a clinical evaluation necessarily involves diagnostic procedures which aid in arriving at a clinical impression.

The purpose of this chapter is to identify and provide guidelines for the appropriate use of clinical laboratory procedures in chiropractic practice. The role of the clinical laboratory in diagnosis, screening, and patient management is discussed as well as the principles of appropriate test selection and use. Guidelines for clinical laboratory test interpretation are presented and recommendations for appropriate use of commonly requested clinical laboratory tests are described.

Definitions useful to the practitioner as applied to laboratory testing are provided in Section II. Section III lists all topics covered in the Recommendations section. Section IV reviews literature relevant to clinical application of laboratory procedures for the doctor of chiropractic.

Additionally, investigational procedures are briefly discussed.

Literature for well-established standard procedures are listed in the references, but detailed test descriptions are not possible in the space available. The bulk of this information appears in the Section VI recommendations. It has been divided for the purposes of clinical relevance into four sections:

A. General recommendations regarding use of laboratory procedures in chiropractic practice.
B. Detailed guidelines for ordering commonly used tests.
C. Investigational laboratory procedures.
D. Inappropriate laboratory procedures.

The Reference Section (Section VIII) is organized by topic to allow the reader to access relevant material upon which this chapter is based.

Lastly, this chapter contains an appendix that characterizes useful examples of clinical laboratory guidelines for the investigation of spinal disorders, common visceral pain disorders, as well as examples of focused organ/health problem profiles.

II. DEFINITIONS

Screening: The application of a test to detect a potential illness or condition in a person who has no known signs or symptoms of that illness or condition. Screening is performed on "at risk" populations in order to determine appropriate intervention(s).

Case Finding: Laboratory testing of health care seeking patients for disorders that may be unrelated to their chief complaint.

Accuracy: The property of a measurement which determines how closely the result will approximate the true value.

Precision: A measurement of the agreement between repeated measurements; an indication of the random error. The term may be interchanged with the term "reliability."

Prevalence: The total number of cases of a disorder in existence at a certain time in a designated area.

False-Negative Rate (FNR): The likelihood of a negative test in a patient with a disorder.

False-negative rate =

$$\frac{\text{number of patients with a disorder with negative test}}{\text{number of patients with a disorder}}$$

False-Negative Result: A negative result in a patient with a disorder.

False-Positive Rate (FPR): The likelihood of a positive test in a patient without a disorder.

False-positive rate =

$$\frac{\text{number of patients without a disorder with positive test}}{\text{number of patients without disorder}}$$

False-Positive Result: A positive result in a person who does not have the disorder.

"Gold Standard" Test: An accepted reference test or procedure that is used to define the true state of the patient's health.

Likelihood Ratio: A measure of discrimination by a test result. A test result with a likelihood ratio of greater than 1.0 raises the probability of a disorder and is often referred to as a "positive" test result. A test result with a likelihood ratio of less than 1.0 lowers the probability of a disorder and is often called a "negative" test result.

Likelihood ratio =

$$\frac{\text{probability of result in person with disorder}}{\text{probability of result in person without disorder}}$$

LIKELIHOOD RATIO FOR A POSITIVE TEST RESULT:

$$\text{Likelihood ratio (+)} = \frac{\text{sensitivity}}{1 - \text{specificity}}$$

LIKELIHOOD RATIO FOR A NEGATIVE TEST RESULT:

$$\text{Likelihood ratio (−)} = \frac{1 - \text{sensitivity}}{\text{specificity}}$$

Negative Test Result: A test result that occurs more frequently in patients who do not have a disorder than in patients who do have the disorder.

Odds: The odds of an event is another way to express its probability.

$$\text{Odds} = \frac{\text{probability of event}}{1 - \text{probability of event}}$$

Positive Test Result: A test result that occurs more frequently in patients with a disorder than in patients without the disorder.

Post-Test Probability: The probability of disorder after the results of a test have been learned (also posterior probability or post-test risk).

Predictive Value Negative: Probability of a disorder being absent if a test is negative.

Predictive Value Positive: Probability of a disorder being present if a test is positive.

Pretest Probability: The probability of disorder before a test is done (also prior probability or pretest risk).

Probability: An expression of opinion, on a scale of 0 to 1.0, about the likelihood that an event will occur.

Sensitivity: The likelihood of a positive test result in a person with a disorder (also true-positive rate, TPR).

$$\text{Sensitivity} = \frac{\text{number of patients with disorder with positive test}}{\text{number of patients with disorder}}$$

Specificity: The ability to correctly identify negative test results among subjects who truly do not have a specific disorder. The likelihood of a negative test in a patient without the disorder (also true-negative rate, TNR).

$$\text{Specificity} = \frac{\text{number of patients without disorder with negative test}}{\text{number of patients without disorder}}$$

True-Negative Result: A negative test result in a patient who does not have a disease.

True-Negative Rate: See specificity.

True-Positive Rate: See sensitivity.

III. LIST OF SUBTOPICS

A. General Recommendations

1. The Role of Clinical Laboratory Procedures in Chiropractic Practice
2. Laboratory Selection
3. Office Laboratories
4. Proper Patient Preparation
5. Specimen Collection and Preservation
6. The Need for Laboratory Testing
7. Laboratory Test Selection in Diagnosis
8. Laboratory Test Selection in Screening
9. Laboratory Test Selection in Patient Management
10. Interpretation of Laboratory Reference Values
11. Integration of Clinical Laboratory Data with Other Examination Findings
12. Communication of Laboratory Procedures to the Patient
13. Recording Laboratory Procedures
14. Consultation on Laboratory Procedures
15. Use of Focused Organ/Health Problem-Oriented Test Profiles
16. Use of Investigational Laboratory Tests
17. Novel Application of Established Laboratory Procedures in Chiropractic Practice

B. Guidelines for Ordering Commonly Utilized Laboratory Tests

1. Routine Urinalysis
2. Complete Blood Count
3. Erythrocyte Sedimentation Rate
4. Biochemical Profiles
5. Plasma Glucose
6. Serum Urea Nitrogen and Creatinine
7. Serum Calcium
8. Serum Inorganic Phosphorus
9. Serum Total Protein and Albumin
10. Serum Cholesterol
11. Serum Alkaline Phosphatase
12. Serum Prostatic Acid Phosphatase
13. Serum Prostate-Specific Antigen
14. Serum Aspartate Aminotransferase
15. Serum Creatine Kinase
16. Thyroid Function Tests
17. Serum Uric Acid
18. Rheumatoid Factor
19. Anti-Nuclear Antibody Test
20. HLA-B27 Test
21. C-Reactive Protein Test
22. Serum Potassium Test
23. Serum Sodium Test
24. Serum Iron and Total Iron-Binding Capacity Test
25. Fecal Occult Blood Test
26. Serum Ferritin Test

C. Investigational Clinical Laboratory Procedures

1. Analysis of Trace Minerals in Hair
2. Live Cell Analysis
3. Biochemical Biopsy
4. Determination of "Optimal" Reference Values

D. Inappropriate Clinical Laboratory Procedures

1. Cytotoxic Testing for Food Allergies
2. Reams Testing and Interpretation of Urine

E. Appendix

IV. LITERATURE REVIEW

The literature search for this topic utilized the MEDLINE database on CD-ROM from 1980 to the present for articles using the medical subject heading terms relevant to guidelines for the selection and interpretation of laboratory tests. In addition, the CHIROLARS database was searched for articles related to the use of laboratory diagnosis in chiropractic practice. A manual search of the *Chiropractic Research Archives Collection* was also accomplished. From these sources bibliographies were compiled which contained both journal articles and textbooks.

Materials were selected for inclusion if they contained information on the usefulness of clinical laboratory tests in patient care. Included was information on the principles of test selection and interpretation of procedures commonly used in chiropractic practice. Priority was given to well-designed studies published in peer-reviewed journals. Second priority was given to review articles and textbooks.

Role of Laboratory Diagnosis

The role of clinical laboratory diagnosis in chiropractic has evolved since the inception of the profession to where currently, laboratory diagnosis courses are taught at all accredited chiropractic colleges. In addition, the majority of jurisdictions in North America allow some form of access to laboratory tests (Lamm 1989).

The chiropractic practitioner, as a portal of entry health care provider, has the responsibility to perform an appropriate clinical examination for the purpose of assessing a patient's current health status and identifying if the patient is a proper subject for chiropractic care. The clinical laboratory can, at times, provide useful information when the findings from the clinical examination are insufficient to answer the questions at hand. The decision to order a test is made on the assumption that the results will appreciably reduce the uncertainty surrounding a given clinical question and significantly change the pre-test probability that a disorder is present.

Use of Laboratory Tests

Laboratory procedures can be used as screening devices to identify "at risk" patients who may be prone to illness that can be prevented or diminished by early detection and care. For example, routine measurement of cholesterol can be useful in determining which patients should start on preventive management for atherosclerotic cardiovascular disease. The prob-

lem with screening, though, is the number of false-positive results it produces. As the prevalence of a disorder in a population falls, the percentage of false-positive results rises dramatically, so there are five to ten false-positive results for every true-positive one. In order to deal with this situation, many attempts have been made to develop guidelines for selection of appropriate patients and tests for early detection (Eddy, 1991).

A second reason for using clinical laboratory tests is to provide assistance in establishing diagnostic hypotheses. The laboratory may be particularly helpful in sorting out whether a patient's clinical complaints are due to a functional or organic disorder.

To rule out a disorder, very sensitive tests are most effective in reducing the probability of that disorder. Very specific tests are most effective in raising the probability of the presence of a disorder and thus are useful for ruling in diagnoses. Such tests when abnormal can confirm the presence of a disorder.

The intelligent selection of an appropriate laboratory test depends on choosing the proper test for the purpose intended. The purpose of the test is affected by the practitioner's estimate of the pretest likelihood that a disorder is present based on an assessment of the available clinical information. The use of a test to exclude or confirm a diagnosis should indicate that the practitioner's best estimate after a careful evaluation of the patient's problem is that the diagnosis in question is either relatively unlikely or probable, respectively. When these principles are followed, the conclusions reached from laboratory test results are likely to be correct and lead to appropriate action (Panzer 1991).

Laboratory tests are used for patient management which includes monitoring patient's response to care, the need for care, and determination of prognosis. Compared with tests for screening and diagnosis, tests used for monitoring are more likely to have abnormal results, show a change from previous test values, cause a change in patient care, and be followed up with repeat testing. Determining the optimal frequency for monitoring patients with repeat tests or procedures cannot be based solely on the presence of the disorder but requires the application of principles of normal physiology, knowledge of the tests or procedures used to monitor the disorder, and awareness of factors other than the disorder that may influence the test result.

Laboratory Test Characteristics

Each laboratory test or procedure possesses a set of characteristics that reflects the information expected in patients with and without the disorder in question. These test characteristics provide clinicians with answers to two fundamental questions: 1) If the disorder is present, what is the likelihood that the test result will be abnormal (positive)? And, 2) if the disorder is not present, what is the likelihood that the result will be normal (negative)? The answer to the first question defines the sensitivity of the test and the answer to the latter defines its specificity.

An ideal test is one for which there is no overlap in the range of results among patients with and without the disorder in question. Few tests are ideal. Usually there is an overlap of results among patients with or without a specific disorder. Each point along the distribution of results that overlap defines a set of operating characteristics for the test. As the point used to define an abnormal result (cutoff point) is moved in the direction of patients with the disorder, the sensitivity decreases. As it is moved in the direction of patients without the disorder, the reverse is true. Some tests may be used both to exclude or to confirm a disorder by altering the criteria for a positive test according to the purpose of the test.

Knowledge of test characteristics is important in deciding which test to select for a given purpose. The process of confirming a disorder requires a test whose specificity is high. When two or more tests are available for this purpose, the one with the highest specificity is ordinarily preferred. When a test is used either for the purpose of screening or to exclude a diagnostic possibility, it must be sensitive. When two or more such tests are available, that with the highest sensitivity is ordinarily preferred. Multiple tests are most helpful when: 1) all are normal, thus tending to exclude the disorder, and 2) when all are abnormal thus tending to confirm the presence of the disorder. Multiple tests are least helpful when one is positive and the others are normal. If two or more tests are highly sensitive and the primary purpose of the test is to exclude a disorder the gain in sensitivity obtained by ordering more than one test may be offset by the increase in false-positive results.

Reference Ranges for Tests

The limits of normal for most analytical tests are determined by measurements done on a large number of subjects and defined as the range encompassed by two standard deviations from the mean value. There are several limitations inherent in this conventional definition. First, the definition excludes approximately 2.5 percent of the subjects whose values lie at the extremes of the distribution curve, rendering them abnormal but presumably not ill. Second, for most measurable biological substances, the distribution curve of test results is skewed rather than symmetric and the method used to express the reference range does not precisely define the central 95 percent of subjects. Third, the reference population used to calculate the limits is not necessarily free of illness. It is assumed that with a large enough sample, the impact of subjects with disease will be diluted. This assumption has been shown to be invalid for many chemistry determinations. The result is often the reporting of reference limits that are too broad. Fourth, few laboratories adjust the reference range for the many factors that may influence the test results other than disease; these include age, sex, weight, diet, time of day, activity, and position of the subject when the specimen is drawn. Last, and most important, the uniform method used to define the reference range does not recognize the many purposes that the test may serve. This range will differ according to whether the clinician is concerned with confirming a condition or excluding one. Although this traditional approach suffers from the above limitations, alternative approaches which create narrower reference ranges should follow acceptable methods in determining those ranges.

Laboratory Test Interpretation

To ensure proper interpretation of the results of laboratory tests, it is important to consider a prior estimate of the likelihood of the presence of a disorder suspected to be present from the history and clinical examination. This is referred to as a pretest probability or prevalence. When the pretest probability is high, a positive result tends to confirm the presence of a disorder, but an unexpected negative result is not particularly helpful in ruling the condition out. When the pre-test probability is low, a normal result tends to exclude the condition, but an unexpectedly positive result is not particularly helpful in confirming the disorder.

If the sensitivity, specificity, and prevalence of the condition are known, then one may easily calculate the effect of the test result on the probability of a correct diagnosis. This is referred to as predictive value or post-test probability (Gottfried, 1982).

Commonly Utilized Laboratory Procedures

This chapter contains information on commonly utilized laboratory tests. These tests were selected based upon an informal survey of test utilization by a representative sample of doctors of chiropractic. Each test is described as it relates to its usefulness in screening, diagnosis and patient management. A critical review of the literature on the utility of each test was performed to provide a basis for guideline recommendations.

V. ASSESSMENT CRITERIA

Procedure Ratings (System I)

Established: Accepted as appropriate by the practicing chiropractic community for the given indication in the specified patient population.

Promising: Given current knowledge, this appears to be appropriate for the given indication in the specified patient population. As more evidence and experience accumulates, this interim rating will change. This connotes provisional acceptance but permits a greater role for the current level of clinical use.

Equivocal: Current knowledge exists to support a given indication in a specified patient population, though value can neither be confirmed or denied. As more evidence and experience accumulates this interim rating will change. Expert opinion recognizes a need for caution in general application.

Investigational: Evidence is insufficient to determine appropriateness. Further study is warranted. Use for a given indication in a specified patient population should be confined to research protocols. As more evidence and experience accumulates this interim rating will change.

Doubtful: Given current knowledge, this appears to be inappropriate for the given indication in the specified patient population. As more evidence and experience accumulates, this interim rating will change.

Inappropriate: Regarded by the practicing chiropractic community as unacceptable for the given indication in the specified patient population.

Quality of Evidence:

The following categories of evidence are used to support the ratings.

Class I:

Evidence provided by one or more well-designed, controlled clinical trials; or well-designed experimental studies that address reliability, validity, positive predictive value, discriminability, sensitivity, and specificity.

Class II:

Evidence provided by one or more well-designed uncontrolled, observational clinical studies such as case-control, cohort studies, etc.; or clinically relevant basic science studies that address reliability, validity, positive predictive value, discriminability, sensitivity, and specificity; and are published in refereed journals.

Class III:

Evidence provided by expert opinion, descriptive studies or case reports.

Suggested Strength of Recommendation Ratings:

Type A. Strong positive recommendation. Based on Class I evidence or overwhelming Class II evidence when circumstances preclude randomized clinical trials.

Type B. Positive recommendation based on Class II evidence.

Type C. Positive recommendation based on strong consensus of Class III evidence.

Type D. Negative recommendation based on inconclusive or conflicting Class II evidence.

Type E. Negative recommendation based on evidence of ineffectiveness or lack of efficacy based on Class I or Class II evidence.

VI. RECOMMENDATIONS

A. General

1. The Role of Laboratory Procedures in Chiropractic Practice

The appropriate use of clinical laboratory procedures in chiropractic practice is for diagnosis, screening, and patient management.

Comment: Clinical laboratory tests are used by the practitioner to (1) aid in the diagnostic process; (2) screen for early recognition of preventable health problems ; and (3) monitor patient progress and outcomes. It is inappropriate to utilize clinical laboratory procedures for other purposes (e.g., for defensive testing or economic gain).

4.1.1 **Rating:** Established
Evidence: Class III
Consensus Level: 1

2. Laboratory Selection

It is recommended that the practitioner who uses the services of a clinical laboratory should be aware of the laboratory's scope of services, recognition (licensure and accreditation), and reputation.

4.1.2 **Rating:** Established
Evidence: Class III
Consensus Level: 1

3. Office Laboratories

The practitioner who performs office laboratory procedures should carry out testing in a manner which meets state and/or federal regulations, and is consistent with quality laboratory practice.

Comment: State and federal regulations define the scope of testing, qualification of laboratory personnel, and the need and extent of quality assurance and proficiency testing.

4.1.3 **Rating**: Established
Evidence: Class III
Consensus Level: 1

4. Proper Patient Preparation

The practitioner should make sure the patient is adequately prepared for laboratory testing, verifying that the patient understands any special instructions to assure adequate specimens necessary to generate valid laboratory results.

4.1.4 **Rating:** Established
Evidence: Class III
Consensus Level: 1

5. Specimen Collection and Preservation

The practitioner should assure that in-office laboratory specimens are appropriately collected and preserved.

4.1.5 **Rating:** Established
Evidence: Class III
Consensus Level: 1

6. The Need for Laboratory Testing

Laboratory procedures may be appropriate when the information available from the history, clinical examination, and previous evaluation is considered insufficient to address the clinical questions at hand.

Comment: The decision to order and/or perform a given test or procedure is made on the assumption that the results will appreciably reduce the uncertainty surrounding a given clinical question and significantly change the pre-test probability that the disorder is present.

4.1.6 **Rating:** Established
Evidence: Class I, II, III
Consensus Level: 1

7. Laboratory Test Selection in Diagnosis

The practitioner should select a laboratory test(s) appropriate for the purpose of ruling out a specific condition(s) or confirming a strong clinical suspicion by considering the sensitivity and specificity of the test(s) and estimating the likelihood of the condition(s) (pretest probability) based on his or her assessment of the available clinical information.

4.1.7 **Rating:** Promising
Evidence: Class I, II, III
Consensus Level: 1

8. Laboratory Test Selection in Screening

The use of laboratory tests for screening purposes should include selection of a highly sensitive laboratory test(s) and the appropriate application of the test(s) to health problem(s) which are common, have significant morbidity/mortality and are preventable and/or amenable to effective care.

4.1.8 **Rating:** Established
Evidence: Class I, II, III
Consensus Level: 1

9. Laboratory Test Selection in Patient Management (Monitoring)

The reproducibility (precision) of the test is the most important characteristic when selecting laboratory tests for monitoring.

Comment: The optimal frequency for monitoring patients cannot be predicted solely on the basis of knowledge of the disorder or the effectiveness of chiropractic care. It requires the application of normal physiology, knowledge of the natural history of the underlying disorder, tests or procedures used to monitor the disorder and awareness of factors other than the disorder that may influence the test results.

4.1.9 **Rating:** Established
Evidence: Class II, III
Consensus Level: 1

10. Interpretation of Laboratory Reference Values

The practitioner should have an understanding of "normality" as it applies to conventional laboratory reference values in order to appropriately interpret laboratory results.

4.1.10 **Rating:** Established
Evidence: Class I, II, III
Consensus Level: 1

11. Integration of Clinical Laboratory Data with Other Examination Findings

Clinical laboratory data should be integrated with results from other examinations as part of the clinical decision-making process when monitoring the patient's clinical status.

4.1.11 **Rating:** Established
Evidence: Class I, II, III
Consensus Level: 1

12. Communication of Laboratory Procedures and Results to the Patient

The practitioner should effectively discuss with the patient the purposes, possible complications, and clinical significance of the results of laboratory studies conducted or ordered.

4.1.12 **Rating:** Established
Evidence: Class III
Consensus Level: 1

13. Recording Laboratory Results:

Clinical laboratory results should be recorded in the patient case record.

4.1.13 **Rating:** Established
Evidence: Class III
Consensus Level: 1

14. Consultation on Laboratory Procedures

The practitioner should seek assistance when uncertain about appropriate test selection, patient preparation, and/or interpretation of laboratory results.

4.1.14 **Rating:** Established
Evidence: Class III
Consensus Level: 1

15. Use of Focused Organ/Health Problem-Oriented Test Profiles

The use of profiles which focus on an organ system and/or health problem in a symptomatic patient can be considered a cost-effective and efficient procedure for generating appropriate laboratory data to help confirm or rule out a diagnosis or clinical impression.

4.1.15 **Rating:** Established
Evidence: Class I, II, III
Consensus Level: 1

16. Use of Investigational Laboratory Tests

Laboratory tests which are considered to be investigational should be used in clinical settings only when part of an acceptable research protocol which is supervised by the staff of a recognized research institution.

Comments: Research protocols for the evaluation of investigational clinical laboratory tests should take into consideration the actual need for the tests, the inherent properties of the tests, the population characteristics to which the tests are applied, the existence of gold standard tests, the required study population size, and the tests' discrimination abilities relative to sensitivity, specificity, and predictive value (Adams, 1990). Research protocols should be approved by an institutional review board.

4.1.16 **Rating:** Established
Evidence: Class I, II, III
Consensus Level: 1

17. The Novel Application of Established Laboratory Procedures in Chiropractic Practice

Novel application of established laboratory procedures should not be used in chiropractic practice as a substitute for conventional application of laboratory procedures in the clinical decision-making process.

Comment: Novel applications of established tests should be evaluated by appropriate research methods. If used in a patient care setting, informed consent is necessary.

4.1.17 **Rating:** Established
Evidence: Class I, II, III
Consensus Level: 1

B. Guidelines for Ordering Commonly Utilized Laboratory Procedures

1. Guidelines for Ordering a Urinalysis
a. **Outpatient Screening/Case-Finding**
   i. A urinalysis is not indicated in asymptomatic individuals whose history and physical examination findings are within the normal ranges for age and sex.
   ii. In specific subsets of the population with higher prevalence of renal disease, urinary tract infections, liver disease, and diabetes mellitus, the urinalysis may be useful to identify those who are significantly at risk, including but not limited to the following:
      • Pregnancy
      • Elderly (> 60 years) men and women
      • Obese individuals with a positive family history of diabetes mellitus
      • Individuals taking hepato- or nephrotoxic drugs
      • Individuals routinely exposed to toxic chemicals in the work or home environment
b. **Diagnosis**
   i. The urinalysis is indicated in patients where there are clinical findings suggestive of urinary tract infections, renal disease, diabetes mellitus, and liver disease. The urinalysis should include physical, chemical, and microscopic evaluation.
   ii. The urinalysis may be useful in patients with previous positive findings for proteinuria, microhematuria, bacteriuria, pyuria, or diabetes mellitus.

c. **Monitoring**
   i. Repeat urinalysis is not indicated in patients in whom no abnormality is suspected.
   ii. Repeat urinalysis may be useful in the following:
      • Documenting evidence of response to treatment for urinary tract infections, renal disease, and diabetes mellitus
      • Patients in whom there is concern that treatment has not been effective
      • Patients taking medications which are hepato- or nephrotoxic
      • Individuals routinely exposed to toxic chemicals
      • Pregnancy

4.2.1 **Rating:** Established
Evidence: Class I, II, III
Consensus Level: 1

2. Guidelines for Ordering a Complete Blood Count (CBC)
a. **Outpatient Screening/Case-Finding**
   i. CBCs are not indicated in asymptomatic individuals whose history and physical examination findings are within reference for age and sex.
      • Routine use of CBCs in populations of low disease prevalence have a low diagnostic yield
   ii. In specific subsets of the population with higher prevalence of anemia, the CBC may be useful to identify those who are significantly anemic because of poor nutrition or undiagnosed chronic illness, including but not limited to the following:
      • Pregnant women in whom there is a suspicion that iron supplementation or nutrition has not been adequate
      • The elderly (> 75 years old)
      • Recent immigrants from Third World countries, especially persons at increased risk of malnourishment
      • Individuals on diets which are nutritionally unbalanced
b. **Diagnosis of Suspected Abnormality**
   i. The CBC is useful in the diagnosis of infection or primary hematological disorders.
      • The CBC is indicated in patients in whom there are clinical findings suggestive of anemia, including fatigue, mucous-membrane pallor, sore tongue, peripheral neuropathy, abnormal bleeding, or findings suggestive of polycythemia
   ii. The CBC may be useful in conditions that may be associated with anemia and/or abnormal leukocyte counts, such as rheumatoid arthritis, ma-

lignancy (e.g., lymphoma)and renal insufficiency.

iii. The CBC may be useful when fever is present or when infection is suspected, especially when other confirmatory findings are absent.

c. **Monitoring**

i. Repeat CBCs are not indicated in patients in whom no abnormality is suspected.

ii. Repeat CBCs may be useful in the following:
- Patients in whom there is concern that treatment has not been effective
- Documenting evidence of response to treatment for anemia
- Patients with infection not improving clinically under collaborative care
- Patients with leukopenia (leukocyte count is less than 4,500/µl)
- Patients taking cytotoxic medications

4.2.2 **Rating:** Established
Evidence: Class I, II, III
Consensus Level: 1

3. Guidelines for Ordering the Erythrocyte Sedimentation Rate (ESR) Test

a. **Outpatient Screening/Case-Finding**

i. The ESR is not indicated in asymptomatic persons.

ii. An ESR should be ordered/performed selectively and interpreted with caution in patients whose symptoms are not adequately explained by a careful history and physical examination.
- Significant infections or inflammatory or neoplastic disease are unlikely in such patients, and the ESR must be markedly elevated to be diagnostically useful.
- Extreme elevation of the ESR seldom occurs in patients with no evidence of serious disease.

b. **Diagnosis**

i. The ESR is useful for the diagnosis of temporal arteritis (giant cell arteritis) and polymyalgia rheumatica.
- A normal ESR virtually excludes the diagnosis of temporal arteritis in most patients who are suspected of having the disease.
- When there is strong clinical evidence for temporal arteritis and the ESR is normal, further efforts to diagnose temporal arteritis are required.

ii. A careful history and physical examination are the most reliable means of making a diagnosis of rheumatoid arthritis. In patients with an equivocal examination, an ESR may be indicated and an abnormal result is a clue to the presence of this disease.

iii. The ESR may be indicated in the differential diagnosis of solitary bone lesions.

iv. The ESR may be indicated in the diagnosis of metastatic breast cancer.

v. The ESR may be indicated as a means of excluding suspected vertebral osteomyelitis.

vi. The ESR may assist in the differential diagnosis of certain infectious, inflammatory, and malignant disorders.

vii. The ESR may provide assistance in distinguishing spinal pain of organic origin from mechanical origin.

c. **Monitoring**

i. The ESR is useful for monitoring temporal arteritis and polymyalgia rheumatica.

ii. The judicious use of the ESR combined with other clinical and laboratory observations may be of value in patients with rheumatoid arthritis and systemic lupus erythematosis.

iii. The ESR may be indicated for monitoring patients with Hodgkin's disease.

iv. The ESR may be indicated for monitoring patients with acute rheumatic fever.

4.2.3 **Rating:** Established
Evidence: Class I, II, III
Consensus Level: 1

4. Guidelines for Ordering Biochemical Profiles

a. **Outpatient Screening/Case-Finding**

i. Biochemical profiles are not routinely indicated for screening asymptomatic patients.

ii. Selected components of biochemical profiles may be indicated for screening and/or case-finding in adults: serum glucose, cholesterol and creatinine.

iii. Specific components of biochemical profiles that are not indicated for screening include the following: serum calcium, alkaline phosphatase, uric acid, sodium, potassium, chloride, AST, lactic dehydrogenase (LDH), total protein, albumin, and total bilirubin.

iv. In cases where current technology and/or cost prohibit selective test ordering, biochemical profiles should be used with caution because of a greater likelihood of false-positive findings in low disease-prevalent populations.

4.2.4 **Rating:** Established
Evidence: Class I, II, III
Consensus Level: 1

5. Guidelines for Ordering a Serum or Plasma Glucose Test.

a. **Outpatient Screening/Case-Finding**

i. A serum or plasma glucose test is not routinely indicated to screen for diabetes mellitus in asymptomatic, nonpregnant adults.

ii. A serum or plasma glucose test may be indicated in individuals who are at increased risk for diabetes mellitus.

- Risk factors for diabetes mellitus include age (> 50 years), family history in a first degree relative, personal history of gestational diabetes, body weight that exceeds generally accepted standards by at least 25 percent, or membership in an ethnic group that has a high prevalence of diabetes.

iii. A serum or plasma glucose test is recommended for all pregnant women to screen for gestational diabetes.

- A serum or plasma glucose test obtained after a 50-gram glucose load is the preferred screening procedure.

b. **Diagnosis**

i. A fasting or random plasma glucose measurement is useful for the diagnosis of diabetes mellitus in persons who present with symptoms of hyperglycemia (rapid weight loss, polyuria, polydipsia) and/or diabetes (for example, peripheral neuropathy or peripheral vascular disease).

- An oral glucose tolerance test may be indicated to confirm equivocal tests.

ii. In patients with clinical findings of hypoglycemia, a serum or plasma glucose should be ordered.

- The true hypoglycemia syndrome refers to the presence of adrenergic (sweating, tremor, tachycardia, anxiety, and hunger) or neuroglycopenic (dizziness, headache, clouded vision, blunted mental acuity, confusion, abnormal behavior, coma) signs and symptoms in the presence of a low serum or plasma glucose concentration.

c. **Monitoring**

i. A plasma or serum glucose test is not optimal as the primary modality for monitoring glycemia in insulin-dependent (Type I) diabetic patients with diabetes.

- Daily self-monitored blood glucose measurement, along with periodic (3-4 times per year) measurement of glycated hemoglobin (glycosylated hemoglobin) are appropriate monitoring evaluations

ii. In non-insulin dependent (Type II) diabetes, laboratory performed plasma or serum glucose testing may be indicated every three months.

- Self-monitored blood glucose measurement may be indicated one or two times per day to assess glycemia
- Glycated hemoglobin measurements are indicated at least two times per year to provide an index of mean glucose levels as a measure of overall chronic glucose control

iii. Laboratory performed fasting and postprandial plasma glucose measurements are indicated in diet-treated gestational diabetes every one to two weeks from time of diagnosis until 30 weeks' gestation, and once or twice weekly thereafter.

4.2.5 **Rating:** Established
Evidence: Class I, II, III
Consensus Level: 1

6. Guidelines for Ordering Serum Urea Nitrogen and Creatinine Test

a. **Outpatient Screening/Case-Finding**

i. Serum urea nitrogen and creatinine tests are not indicated in asymptomatic individuals whose history and physical examination findings are within reference ranges.

ii. Individuals who have a higher likelihood of developing renal dysfunction may benefit from measuring serum urea nitrogen and creatinine concentrations

- Patients with hypertension, diabetes mellitus, congestive heart failure, cirrhosis, prostatic hypertrophy, exposure to nephrotoxic agents, taking diuretics, eating a high-protein diet, and over 75 years of age, are candidates for these tests.

b. **Diagnosis**

i. Serum urea nitrogen and creatinine tests are useful in the diagnosis of renal disorders.

- These tests are indicated in patients with clinical findings suggestive of renal dysfunction, such as pallor, anemia, anorexia, unexplained weight loss, polyuria, urinary hesitancy, nocturia, renal colic, dehydration, retinopathy, hypertension, skin lesions of vasculitis, and/or an abnormal urinalysis (high specific gravity, proteinuria, hematuria, pyuria, presence of crystals and/or casts).

ii. Measuring serum urea nitrogen and creatinine concentration, or creatinine alone, may be useful in hypertension or diabetes patients.

iii. Conditions in which both the serum urea nitrogen and creatinine concentration may be indicated include but are not limited to the following:

- Gastrointestinal bleeding, complicated by some degree of renal insufficiency
- A suspected diagnosis of water intoxication
- Syndrome of inappropriate antidiuretic hormone secretion

c. **Monitoring**

i. Measuring serum urea nitrogen and serum creatinine concentration, or creatinine alone, may be useful for the following conditions and at the following frequencies:

- Uncomplicated hypertensive patients, every one to two years
- Chronic renal disease, every four to six months
- Patients in acute renal failure, every one to two days

4.2.6 **Rating:** Established
Evidence: Class I, II, III
Consensus Level: 1

7. Guidelines for Ordering a Serum Calcium Test

a. Outpatient Screening/Case-Finding

i. The serum calcium test is not indicated in asymptomatic individuals whose history and physical examination findings are within reference limits for age and sex.

ii. The use of serum calcium as a screening test for occult metabolic bone disease or malignancy will result in a low diagnostic yield.

- For most of these conditions, the post-test probability of disease after abnormal calcium results is not sufficiently high to warrant the inclusion of calcium determinations in a screening profile.

b. Diagnosis

i. The serum calcium test is useful in the evaluation of patients who present with clinical evidence of hypercalcemia (anorexia, nausea, constipation, polyuria, polydipsia, bone pain, and mental or neurologic aberrations) or hypocalcemia (paresthesis, muscle cramps, tetany, weakness, convulsions).

ii. The serum calcium test may be useful in the evaluation of patients with hypertension, renal calculi, peptic ulcer disease, metabolic bone disease, malignant disorders, history of previous neck surgery, alcoholism, and acid-base imbalance.

c. Monitoring

i. Repeat serum calcium measurement is not indicated in patients in whom no abnormality is suspected.

ii. Serum calcium may be used to follow the course of hypercalcemia and hypocalcemic disorders and their response to care.

- A serum calcium level should be interpreted with knowledge of the serum albumin level

4.2.7 **Rating:** Established
Evidence: Class II, III
Consensus Level: 1

8. Guidelines for Ordering a Serum Inorganic Phosphorus Test

a. Outpatient Screening/Case-Finding

i. The serum inorganic phosphorus test is not indicated in asymptomatic individuals whose history and physical examination findings are within reference limits for age and sex.

ii. The use of serum inorganic phosphorus as a screening test for various malignant, inflammatory, bony, renal and metabolic disorders will result in a low diagnostic yield.

- For most of these conditions, the post-test probability of disease after abnormal inorganic phosphorus results is not sufficiently high to warrant the inclusion of inorganic phosphorus determinations in a screening profile.

b. Diagnosis

i. The serum inorganic phosphorus test is useful in the evaluation of patients suspected of having metabolic bone disease, renal disorders, endocrine disorders, and acid-base imbalance.

c. Monitoring

i. Repeat serum inorganic phosphorus measurement is not indicated in patients in whom no abnormality is suspected.

ii. Serum inorganic phosphorus may be used to follow the course of hyperphosphatemic and hypophosphatemic disorders and their response to care.

- A serum inorganic phosphorus level should be interpreted with knowledge of the serum urea nitrogen level.

4.2.8 **Rating:** Established
Evidence: Class II, III
Consensus Level: 1

9. Guidelines for Ordering Serum Total Protein and Albumin Test

a. Outpatient Screening/Case-Finding

i. The serum total protein and albumin tests are not indicated in asymptomatic individuals whose history and physical examination findings are within reference limits for age and sex.

ii. The use of serum total protein and albumin as screening tests for malnutrition, protein loss or breakdown, and impaired protein synthesis will result in a low diagnostic yield.

b. Diagnosis

i. The serum total protein and albumin tests may be useful in the evaluation of patients with suspected malnutrition, liver disorders, renal disease, malabsorption, recurrent infections, blood dyscrasias, and malignancies such as multiple myeloma.

- Results which fall outside the reference range for these tests may require a protein electrophoresis determination and/or immunoelectrophoresis.

c. **Monitoring**

i. Repeat serum total protein and albumin measurements are not indicated in patients in whom no abnormality is suspected.

ii. Serum total protein and albumin determinations have limited value in monitoring disorders associated with changes in serum protein levels.

4.2.9 **Rating:** Established
Evidence: Class II, III
Consensus Level: 1

10. Guidelines for Ordering a Serum Cholesterol Test

a. **Outpatient Screening/Case-Finding**

i. A total serum cholesterol measurement is recommended at least once in early adulthood and at intervals of five or more years up to age 70.

• The LDL and HDL cholesterol and serum triglyceride levels should be measured in persons with an elevated total serum cholesterol.

ii. In patients who demonstrate risk factors for coronary artery disease, a serum total cholesterol is indicated to assess cardiac risk.

• Risk factors for coronary artery disease include: being male or postmenopausal female, positive family history, smoker, hypertension, history of hyper-cholesterolemia, low HDL-cholesterol levels, diabetes mellitus, previous stroke, peripheral vascular disease, or severe obesity.

b. **Diagnosis**

i. The total serum cholesterol is useful in the diagnosis of patients with coronary artery disease and peripheral vascular disease.

ii. The total serum cholesterol may be useful in the diagnosis of nephrotic syndrome, pancreatitis, and liver disease.

c. **Monitoring**

i. Total serum cholesterol may be used to follow up hypercholesterolemic related disorders and their response to care.

4.2.10 **Rating:** Established
Evidence: Class I, II, III
Consensus Level: 1

11. Guidelines for Ordering a Serum Alkaline Phosphatase Test

a. **Outpatient Screening/Case-Finding**

i. The serum alkaline phosphatase test is not indicated in asymptomatic individuals whose history and physical examination findings are within reference limits for age and sex.

ii. The use of serum alkaline phosphatase as a screening test for unsuspected skeletal and hepatobiliary diseases provides a low diagnostic yield.

• The pretest probability is low in the general population for those disorders most strongly associated with an elevated alkaline phosphatase.

• The serum alkaline phosphatase test is not specific for any particular disorder or sensitive enough to identify most patients with any single disease.

b. **Diagnosis**

i. The serum alkaline phosphatase may be useful in the evaluation of patients who present with clinical evidence of a skeletal disorder with increased osteoblastic activity, and are suspected of having either Paget's disease of bone (osteitis deformans), osteomalacia, primary bone tumors, metastatic bone tumors or primary hyperparathyroidism.

• Clinical evidence may include backache, bone pain, bone swelling, abnormal plain film bone radiographs, and bone scans.

ii. The serum alkaline phosphatase test may be useful in the evaluation of patients who present with clinical evidence of a hepatobiliary disorder such as cholelithiasis with obstruction, drug-induced cholestasis, metastatic tumor or space-occupying lesion in the liver, cirrhosis, hepatitis, and alcoholism.

• Clinical evidence may include fever, nausea, vomiting, abdominal pain, jaundice, certain medication use, and abnormal liver function tests.

iii. The serum alkaline phosphatase test may exhibit abnormal results in a number of other disorders.

• These conditions include intestinal disorders, malignancy, malnutrition, congestive heart failure, renal disorders, thyroid dysfunction, diabetes mellitus, and physiological influences (age, pregnancy, non-fasting patient).

c. **Monitoring**

i. Repeat serum alkaline phosphatase measurement is not indicated in patients in whom no abnormality is suspected.

ii. Periodic determinations of serum alkaline phosphatase may be used to follow the course of a disorder and its response to care.

4.2.11 **Rating:** Established
Evidence: Class I, II, III
Consensus Level: 1

12. Guidelines for Ordering Serum Prostatic Acid Phosphatase

a. **Outpatient Screening/Case-Finding**

i. The serum prostatic acid phosphatase test is not indicated in asymptomatic individuals whose history and physical examination findings are within reference limits for age and sex.

ii. The use of serum prostatic acid phosphatase as a screening test for unsuspected cancer of the prostate provides a low diagnostic yield.

- Assays for serum prostatic acid phosphatase are not sufficiently sensitive to detect prostatic carcinoma in 70 to 80 percent of patients with localized disease (Stage A or B) or 5 to 15 percent of patients with metastatic prostatic disease.
- Specificity is low because nearly every method devised for detecting prostatic acid phosphatase exhibits cross-reactivity with other acid phosphatase isoenzymes found widely in human tissues.

b. **Diagnosis**

i. The serum prostatic acid phosphatase test may be useful in the evaluation of patients with clinical evidence of prostatic carcinoma.

- Patients may present with obstructive symptoms (hesitancy, diminished urine stream, dribbling, intermittency), lumbar and/or sacral pain, and have induration or nodular irregularities of the prostate discovered by digital rectal examination.

c. **Monitoring**

i. Repeat serum prostatic acid phosphatase measurement is not indicated in patients in whom no abnormality is suspected.

ii. Serum prostatic acid phosphatase measurement may be used to monitor cancer patients for recurrence after prostatectomy or other ablative care.

4.2.12 **Rating:** Established
Evidence: Class I, II, III
Consensus Level: 1

13. Guidelines for Ordering Serum Prostate-Specific Antigen (PSA)

a. **Outpatient Screening/Case-Finding**

i. The serum prostate-specific antigen (PSA) test is not indicated in asymptomatic individuals whose history and physical examination findings are within reference limits for age and sex.

ii. The use of serum PSA as a screening test for unsuspected cancer of the prostate provides a low diagnostic yield.

- Serum PSA measurements are not sufficiently sensitive to be used alone as a screening test.
- The specificity of PSA is limited, due to elevations of the antigen occurring in men with benign prostatic hyperplasia or prostatitis.

b. **Diagnosis**

i. The serum prostate-specific antigen is a useful test in the evaluation of patients with clinical evidence of prostatic carcinoma.

- Serum PSA measurement is a useful addition to rectal examination and ultrasonography in the detection of prostate cancer.
- PSA is more sensitive but less specific than prostatic acid phosphatase for prostatic cancer.

c. **Monitoring**

i. Repeat serum prostate-specific antigen measurement is not indicated in patients in whom no abnormality is suspected.

ii. Serum PSA measurements may be useful to detect recurrences of prostate cancer.

iii. Serum PSA measurements may be useful in monitoring the response to care for prostate cancer.

4.2.13 **Rating:** Established
Evidence: Class I, II, III
Consensus Level: 1

14. Guidelines for Ordering a Serum Aspartate Aminotransferase (AST) Test

NOTE: This test was formerly known as glutamic-oxaloacetic transaminase (SGOT).

a. **Outpatient Screening/Case-Finding**

i. The serum AST is not indicated in asymptomatic individuals whose history and physical examination findings are within reference limits for age and sex.

ii. The use of serum AST as a screening test for liver disorders, cardiac disease, and skeletal muscle disorders will result in a low diagnostic yield.

b. **Diagnosis**

i. The serum AST test may be useful in the evaluation of patients with suspected liver disorders.

c. **Monitoring**

i. Repeat serum AST measurement is not indicated in patients in whom no abnormality is suspected.

ii. Serum AST may be used to follow the course of various liver disorders and their response to care.

4.2.14 **Rating:** Established
Evidence: Class I, II, III
Consensus Level: 1

15. Guidelines for Ordering Serum Creatine Kinase (CK)

NOTE: This test was formerly known as Creatine Phosphokinase (CPK).

a. **Outpatient Screening/Case-Finding**

i. The serum creatine kinase (CK) test is not indicated in asymptomatic individuals whose history and physical examination findings are within reference limits for age and sex.

ii. The use of the serum creatine kinase (CK) as a screening test for cardiac, skeletal muscle, and central nervous system disorders will result in a low diagnostic yield.

b. **Diagnosis**

i. The serum creatine kinase (CK) test is useful in the evaluation of patients who present with clinical evidence of acute myocardial infarction.
- Fractionation and measurement of CK isoenzymes (CK-MB primarily) augments total CK results.

ii. The serum creatine kinase (CK) test may be useful in the differential diagnosis of chest pain, hypothyroidism and in the detection of skeletal muscle disorders that are not of neurogenic origin, such as Duchenne Muscular Dystrophy.

c. **Monitoring**

i. Measurement of serial levels of serum CK and CK-MB isoenzymes are used to monitor care in acute myocardial infarction.

ii. Total serum CK may be used to follow patients with certain primary myopathies.

4.2.15 **Rating:** Established
Evidence: Class I, II, III
Consensus Level: 1

16. Guidelines for Ordering Thyroid Function Tests
a. **Outpatient Screening/Case-Finding**

i. Routine testing for thyroid disorders is not indicated in asymptomatic individuals.

ii. Case-finding is indicated in women over 50 years of age who have general symptoms that could be associated with thyroid dysfunction.

b. **Diagnosis**

i. The sensitive thyrotropin assay (sTSH) is useful in the evaluation of patients of either sex who present with clinical evidence of thyroid dysfunction.
- If sTSH is not available, the Free T3, Free T4, or Free T4 Index can be used in the evaluation of suspected hyperthyroidism.
- For the diagnosis of hypothyroidism, the Free T4 or Free T4 Index, followed by a serum thyrotropin (TSH) test, is acceptable. For patients suspected of having thyroiditis, antithyroid antibody studies may be useful.

c. **Monitoring**

i. The sTSH test is indicated for monitoring patient response to care.

4.2.16 **Rating:** Established
Evidence: Class I, II, III
Consensus Level: 1

17. Guidelines for Ordering a Serum Uric Acid Test
a. **Outpatient Screening/Case-Finding**

i. The serum uric acid test is not indicated in asymptomatic individuals whose history and physical examination findings are within reference limits for age and sex.

ii. The use of serum uric acid as a screening test for gout will provide a low diagnostic yield.
- On the basis of established prevalences, if asymptomatic individuals were screened, those with an elevated uric acid have only a 5 percent chance of having gout

iii. For case finding, with a pretest probability of 10 percent (prevalence of gout in the U.S. is estimated at 0.3%), the probability that a correct diagnosis will be derived from a positive test is less than 50%.

b. **Diagnosis**

i. The serum uric acid test is useful in the evaluation of patients who present with clinical evidence of monoarticular arthritis and are suspected of having gout.
- Gout is a disorder of purine metabolism where the presence of an elevated serum uric acid level is but one of several criteria necessary for diagnosis.

ii. The serum uric acid test may be elevated in a number of disorders other than gout which affect urate production or excretion, or both.
- These conditions include: (1) increased nucleic acid turnover related to hematological disorders, malignancy and psoriasis; (2) reduced excretion due to renal dysfunction, certain drugs, and organic acidosis, and (3) miscellaneous causes such as arteriosclerosis and hypertension.

iii. Serum uric acid measurement is not useful as a test for renal function because the reference range is wide and the rise in uric acid in renal dysfunction is not constant.

c. **Monitoring**

i. Repeat serum uric acid measurement is not indicated in patients in whom no abnormality is suspected.

ii. Periodic determinations of serum uric acid may be useful in monitoring patients under care for gout.

iii. Serial serum uric acid analyses are sometimes of value in estimating prognosis in toxemia of pregnancy.

4.2.17 **Rating:** Established
Evidence: Class I, II, III
Consensus Level: 1

18. Guidelines for Ordering a Rheumatoid Factor Test
a. **Outpatient Screening/Case-Finding**

i. The rheumatoid factor test is not indicated in asymptomatic individuals whose history and physical examination findings are within reference ranges for age and sex.

ii. The use of rheumatoid factor as a screening test for rheumatoid arthritis will result in a low diagnostic yield.

- If the rheumatoid factor test is ordered when there is little likelihood of rheumatoid arthritis (e.g., low-back pain) and where the pretest probability is low (1 percent), the predictive value will be very low.

iii. For case finding, with a pretest probability of 10 percent (prevalence of rheumatoid arthritis in the U.S. is estimated at 0.5% to 3%), the probability that a correct diagnosis will be derived from a positive test is less than 50%.

iv. Many more false-positive results as compared to true-positive results will occur from screening.

- There is less than a one in five chance in a screening program that an individual with a positive rheumatoid factor test will have rheumatoid arthritis.

b. **Diagnosis of Rheumatoid Arthritis and Related Disorders**

i. The rheumatoid factor test is useful in the evaluation of patients who present with clinical evidence of symmetric polyarthritis and are suspected of having rheumatoid arthritis.

- Seronegative patients suspected of having rheumatoid arthritis should be retested in six months.

ii. The usefulness of the rheumatoid factor test among patients already known to have rheumatoid arthritis is primarily prognostic. Patients with high titers of rheumatoid factor tend to have more severe disease, subcutaneous nodules, vasculitis, and poorer long-term prognosis. However, individual patients will vary with these manifestations.

iii. Rheumatoid factor is positive in a significant subset of patients with other rheumatic and nonrheumatic diseases, but its presence or absence weighs little in the diagnosis of the majority of such diseases.

- The disappearance of the rheumatoid factor in a patient with Sjogren's syndrome may herald the onset of lymphoma.
- The rheumatoid factor is frequently positive in cryoglobulinemia.

c. **Monitoring**

i. Repeat rheumatoid factor tests are not indicated in patients in whom rheumatoid arthritis is not suspected.

ii. The use of the rheumatoid factor test to guide treatment in patients with rheumatoid arthritis is not recommended. There is little evidence to

suggest that an individual rheumatoid arthritis patient with a highly positive rheumatoid factor test will fare better if treated earlier or more aggressively.

iii. The rheumatoid factor test is not a generally accepted measure of improvement in rheumatoid arthritis.

4.2.18 **Rating:** Established
Evidence: Class I, II, III
Consensus Level: 1

19. Guidelines for Ordering the Anti-Nuclear Antibody Test (ANA)

a. **Outpatient Screening/Case-Finding**

i. The ANA test is not indicated in asymptomatic individuals whose history and physical examination findings are within reference ranges for age and sex.

ii. The use of the ANA as a screening test for systemic lupus erythematosus, drug-induced lupus, or mixed connective tissue disease where a moderate pretest probability is low will result in a low diagnostic yield.

b. **Diagnosis**

i. The ANA test is useful in the evaluation of patients suspected of having systemic lupus erythematosus, drug-induced lupus, or mixed connective tissue disease where a moderate pretest probability is estimated based on the clinical criteria present.

ii. A positive test, while nonspecific, increases the post-test probability of disease.

- A positive ANA test (titer > 1:40) should be followed up with more specific tests such as anti-nDNA and precipitating antibodies (against RNP, Sm, Ro/SS-A).
- However, in a patient over 70 years of age, a titer of 1:40 may be insignificant, and repeat measurement should be obtained to see if the titer increases or is stable.

iii. A negative ANA test result is extremely powerful in reducing the probability of these diseases.

- In patients who have high probability of systemic lupus erythematosus based on clinical criteria but who have a negative antinuclear antibody assay, a determination for anti-Ro or antiphospholipid antibodies may be helpful.

c. **Monitoring**

i. Repeat measurements of antinuclear antibodies were not indicated in patients in whom connective tissue disease is not suspected.

ii. The ANA test can be used as an aid in the assessment of systemic lupus erythematosus disease activity and as a guide for treatment.

4.2.19 **Rating:** Established
Evidence: Class I, II, III
Consensus Level: 1

20. Guidelines for Ordering the HLA-B27 Test
a. **Outpatient Screening/Case-Finding**
  i. The HLA-B27 test is not indicated in asymptomatic individuals whose history and physical examination findings are within reference ranges for age and sex.
  ii. The use of the HLA-B27 as a screening test for ankylosing spondylitis in patients presenting with low-back pain will result in a low diagnostic yield.
b. **Diagnosis**
  i. The HLA-B27 test is not useful for confirmation of the diagnosis of spondyloarthropathies (e.g., ankylosing spondylitis and Reiter's syndrome) when adequate clinical and radiologic criteria are present.
  ii. However, the HLA-B27 test may be useful in patients with low-back pain of insidious onset, minimal tenderness over the sacroiliac joints, normal spinal movement and chest expansion and equivocal radiographic findings where the pretest probability is close to 50 percent for ankylosing spondylitis.
    • A positive HLA-B27 test increases the likelihood of ankylosing spondylitis significantly and a negative result lowers the likelihood.
  iii. The HLA-B27 test may be useful in children with spondyloarthropathy, especially those with a history of juvenile chronic polyarthritis, to help establish the diagnosis of ankylosing spondylitis.
  iv. The HLA-B27 test may be useful in helping to differentiate incomplete Reiter's syndrome from seronegative rheumatoid arthritis and gonococcal arthropathy.
c. **Monitoring**
  i. The HLA-B27 test is not useful for monitoring spondyloarthropathies including the establishment of prognosis, genetic counseling, and patient management.

4.2.20 **Rating:** Established
Evidence: Class I, II, III
Consensus Level: 1

21. Guidelines for Ordering the C-Reactive Protein (CRP) Test
a. **Outpatient Screening/Case Finding**
  i. The CRP is not indicated in asymptomatic persons.
  ii. The CRP test should be used selectively and interpreted with caution in patients with symptoms that are not explained by a careful history and physical examination.
    • Significant infections or inflammatory or neoplastic disease is unlikely in such patients, and the CRP must be markedly elevated or positive to be diagnostically useful.
b. **Diagnosis**
  i. Measurement of CRP by quantitative methods provides the most clinically useful information.
  ii. The CRP is useful for the diagnosis of temporal arteritis (giant cell arteritis) and polymyalgia rheumatica.
  iii. A CRP test may be indicated in patients suspected of rheumatoid arteritis where clinical examination findings are equivocal.
  iv. Measurement of CRP may be useful in the differential diagnosis of peripheral joint pain.
  v. The CRP may be indicated in the differential diagnosis of solitary bone lesions.
  vi. The CRP may be indicated in the diagnosis of metastatic breast cancer.
  vii. The CRP may be indicated as a means of excluding suspected vertebral osteomyelitis.
  viii. The CRP may assist in the differential diagnosis of certain infectious, inflammatory, and malignant disorders.
  ix. The CRP may provide assistance in distinguishing spinal pain of organic from mechanical origin.
c. **Monitoring**
  i. Measurement of CRP by quantitative methods provides the most clinically useful information.
  ii. The CRP is indicated for monitoring temporal arteritis and polymyalgia rheumatica.
  iii. The judicious use of the CRP test combined with other clinical and laboratory observations may be of value in patients with rheumatoid arthritis and systemic lupus erythematosis.
  iv. The CRP may be indicated for monitoring patients with Hodgkin's disease.
  v. The CRP may be indicated for monitoring patients with acute rheumatic fever.

4.2.21 **Rating:** Established
Evidence: Class I, II, III
Consensus Level: 1

22. Guidelines for Ordering a Serum Potassium Test
a. **Outpatient Screening/Case-Finding**
  i. A serum potassium test is not indicated in asymptomatic individuals whose history and physical examination are within reference limits for age and sex.
  ii. Measurement of serum potassium levels is not useful in general screening of ambulatory care patient populations.

b. **Diagnosis**
   i. Serum potassium measurement is useful in patients with chronic renal disease, including diabetic renal insufficiency.
   ii. Serum potassium measurement is useful in patients with hypertension to detect primary hyper-aldosteronism.
      • Measurements should be made at time of diagnosis and before initiation of care.
   iii. Serum potassium measurement is useful in patients with symptoms or signs suggestive of renal tubular acidosis.
   iv. Serum potassium measurement is useful in patients with signs and symptoms suggestive of altered serum potassium concentration, including generalized or proximal weakness, new atrial tachyarrhythmias, nocturia, polyuria, or ileus.

c. **Monitoring**
   i. Serum potassium measurement is indicated one to two times a year in patients with diabetic renal disease.
   ii. Serum potassium measurement is indicated in hypertensive patients receiving diuretic therapy.
   iii. Serum potassium measurement may be useful every six months in diuretic-treated patients concurrently receiving digitalis.
   iv. Serum potassium measurements may be useful in patients with renal dysfunction, cardiac arrhythmias, diarrhea, dehydration, and metabolic acidosis in whom there is a change in clinical status.

4.2.22 **Rating:** Established
   Evidence: Class I, II, III
   Consensus Level: 1

23. Guidelines for Ordering a Serum Sodium Test

a. **Outpatient Screening**
   i. A serum sodium test is not indicated in asymptomatic individuals whose history and physical examination are within reference limits for age and sex.
   ii. Measurement of serum sodium levels is not useful in general screening of ambulatory care patient populations.

b. **Diagnosis**
   i. Serum sodium measurement may be indicated in patients with the following signs or symptoms:
      • Rapid change in weight
      • Rapid change in fluid balance (severe vomiting, diarrhea, polyuria)
      • Rapid change in mental status
      • Clinical evidence of dehydration or volume depletion

   ii. Serum sodium concentration is not indicated in hypertensive patients to identify primary aldosteronism.

c. **Monitoring**
   i. Serum sodium measurement may be useful as an index of hydration, especially in elderly persons or others who may fail to ingest adequate quantities of water to maintain water balance.
   ii. Serum sodium measurement may be useful in patients with chronic renal insufficiency at the following frequencies:
      • At the time of change in clinical status
      • When serum creatinine reaches 7 to 8 mg/dL; thereafter, every two to three months
   iii. Serum sodium measurement may be indicated in most patients at the time of change in clinical status, especially change in mental or neurologic status, fluid balance, weight, or dehydration or volume depletion.

4.2.23 **Rating:** Established
   Evidence: Class I, II, III
   Consensus Level: 1

24. Guidelines for Ordering Serum Iron and Total Iron Binding Capacity (TIBC) Tests

a. **Outpatient Screening/Case-Finding**
   i. The serum iron and total iron binding capacity (TIBC) tests are not indicated in asymptomatic individuals whose history and physical examination findings are within reference limits for age and sex.
   ii. In individuals with a moderate to high pretest probability of iron deficiency (e.g., pregnant women, premenopausal female with hemorrhagia, premature infants, and the malnourished) a serum iron and TIBC may be useful.
   iii. Measurement of serum iron and TIBC may be useful in screening for iron overload.

b. **Diagnosis**
   i. Measurement of serum iron and TIBC are useful in patients whose complete blood count results are consistent with a microcytic hypochromic anemia.
      • Calculation of transferrin saturation from the serum iron and TIBC may provide additional diagnostic information.
   ii. Patients who present with clinical features of iron deficiency may benefit from measurement of serum iron and TIBC tests.
   iii. Serum iron and TIBC measurements may be useful in the differential diagnosis of microcytic hypochromic anemias.
   iv. Measurement of serum iron and TIBC may be useful in the confirmation of iron overload.

c. **Monitoring**

   i. Measurement of serum iron and TIBC have limited value in monitoring the management of patients with iron deficiency anemia.

     • A complete blood count (CBC) and an absolute reticulocyte count are useful tests to monitor the management of iron-deficiency anemia.

4.2.24 **Rating:** Established
Evidence: Class I, II, III
Consensus Level: 1

25. Guidelines for Ordering a Fecal Occult Blood Test

a. **Outpatient Screening/Case-Finding**

   i. Screening with fecal occult blood tests is not indicated for asymptomatic patients under 40 years of age.

   ii. For persons 40 years and older who have familial polyposis coli, inflammatory bowel disease, or a history of colon cancer in a first-degree relative, screening with fecal occult blood tests is recommended annually.

     • Due to the nature of gastrointestinal bleeding, it is recommended that three consecutive samples be obtained.

     • Screening for colorectal cancer with air-contrast barium enema or colonoscopy in addition to annual fecal occult blood tests is recommended every 3 to 5 years.

   iii. Screening with fecal occult blood tests is recommended annually for persons 50 years of age and older.

     • Every 3 to 5 years, in addition to the annual fecal occult blood test, a sigmoidoscopic examination should be performed.

b. **Diagnosis**

   i. Patients with significant colorectal symptoms (abdominal pain, localized tenderness, diarrhea or constipation, gastrointestinal bleeding) should have a fecal occult blood test performed as part of a colorectal examination.

   ii. A fecal occult blood test result should be interpreted with caution.

     • The influence of diet and nutritional supplements (Vitamin C and iron) should be considered as possible causes of false-positive and false-negative results.

     • Further evaluation of patients with a positive occult blood test may include an air contrast barium enema plus colonoscopy.

4.2.25 **Rating:** Established
Evidence: Class II, III
Consensus Level: 1

26. Guidelines for Ordering a Serum Ferritin Test

a. **Outpatient Screening/Case-Finding**

   i. The serum ferritin test is not indicated in asymptomatic individuals whose history and physical examination findings are within reference limits for age and sex.

   ii. In individuals with a moderate to high pretest probability of iron deficiency and with CBC and serum iron/TIBC levels within reference ranges, the serum ferritin test may be useful in detecting the early stages of iron depletion.

b. **Diagnosis**

   i. Measurement of serum ferritin is useful in anemic patients who are suspected of having iron depletion but have equivocal serum iron and TIBC test results.

   ii. Serum ferritin measurements may be useful in the differentiation of anemia of chronic disease from iron deficiency anemia.

     • A CRP determination should be performed along with serum ferritin to identify possible effects of chronic disease state on ferritin results.

   iii. Measurement of serum ferritin may be useful in the detection of iron overload.

c. **Monitoring**

   i. Serum ferritin measurement may be useful in the determination of the end-point to oral iron therapy.

   ii. Measurement of serum ferritin may be useful in monitoring iron status of patients with chronic renal disease.

   iii. Serum ferritin measurement may be useful in monitoring the rate of iron accumulation in iron overload.

4.2.26 **Rating:** Established
Evidence: Class I, II, III
Consensus Level: 1

C. Investigational Clinical Laboratory Procedures

1. Analysis of Trace Minerals in Hair

a. **Outpatient Screening/Case Finding**

   i. Hair analysis is not indicated for screening of nutritional status in asymptomatic individuals.

   ii. In specific subsets of the population who are at risk for nutritional imbalances, the use of hair analysis has not been found to be superior to traditional methods of assessing nutritional status.

b. **Diagnosis**

   i. Hair analysis for trace minerals is not indicated in the determination of nutritional imbalances.

     • Measurement of some elements (e.g., iron) have not been found to be superior to traditional methods of assessment.

ii. Hair analysis suffers from many problems with interpretation of results
- Hair mineral content can be affected by shampoo, bleaches, hair dyes and other environmental factors.
- The level of certain minerals can be affected by color, diameter, rate of growth of an individual's hair and the season of the year.
- Most commercial hair analysis laboratories have not validated their analytical techniques.
- Reference ranges for hair minerals have not been adequately established.
- For most elements no correlation has been established between hair levels and other known indicators of nutritional status.

iii. Hair analysis may be useful in experimental studies of nutritional status.
- More human and animal studies are needed to validate this technique.

c. **Monitoring**
i. Repeat hair analysis for trace minerals is not indicated.
ii. The beneficial effects of nutritional therapy based on hair analysis have not been adequately documented.

4.3.1 **Rating:** Investigational
Evidence: Class I, II, III
Consensus Level: 1

2. Live Cell Analysis
a. **Outpatient Screening/Case Finding**
i. Live cell analysis is not indicated for screening health problems including nutritional imbalances in asymptomatic patients.
ii. In specific subsets of the population who are "at risk" for various health problems, the use of live cell analysis has not been found to be superior to traditional laboratory procedures utilized in case finding.

b. **Diagnosis**
i. Live cell analysis is not indicated in the determination of organ pathologies, infections, immune status or nutritional status.
- Blood indicators which live cell analysis claims are useful in diagnosing health problems have not been validated by adequate scientific studies
ii. Additional studies on the use of dark field microscopy for various diagnoses are needed.

c. **Monitoring**
i. Repeat live cell analysis for various health conditions is not indicated.
ii. The beneficial effects of patient care based on live cell analysis results have not been adequately documented.

4.3.2 **Rating:** Investigational
Evidence: Class III
Consensus Level: 1

3. Biochemical Biopsy: (Multiple Test Analysis Including Protein Electrophoresis and Isoenzyme Fractionation with Predictive Interpretation of Results)
Biochemical biopsy utilizes a comprehensive approach to laboratory testing where a multitest biochemical test profile is ordered along with isoenzyme fractionation of common enzymes and a serum protein electrophoresis. It may also include other serum protein analyses and complete blood count. The rationale behind the use of this approach is detection of early pathologies in the subclinical phase.

a. **Outpatient Screening/Case Finding**
i. Biochemical biopsy is not indicated for screening of health problems in asymptomatic patients.
ii. This approach has not met the criteria as an effective screening procedure. The biochemical biopsy may not be sensitive enough to detect early pathology and is indiscriminate as is currently applied to patients with health problems that don't fit the criteria for screening.
- This approach increases the probability of test results being outside the reference range and generates a significant number of false-positive results which leads the clinician to follow up on these laboratory abnormalities.
iii. Additional research is needed to determine the validity of this approach.

b. **Diagnosis**
i. The biochemical biopsy approach to testing is not useful for diagnosis of specific health problems and/or vague multisystem patient complaints.
ii. The role of the biochemical biopsy as an aid to diagnosis requires further scientific investigation.

c. **Monitoring**
i. Repeat determinations of the laboratory tests in the biochemical biopsy is not indicated.
ii. The beneficial effects of the biochemical biopsy approach to testing on patient management and health outcomes has not been documented.

4.3.3 **Rating:** Investigational
Evidence: Class I, II, III
Consensus Level: 1

4. Determination of "Optimal" Reference Values for Laboratory Tests without Following Acceptable Procedures for the Establishment of Reference Ranges.
a. **Outpatient Screening/Case Finding**
i. This approach to interpretation of lab reference values results is not recommended for screening and/or case findings in asymptomatic patients.

b. **Diagnosis**

i. The optimal reference value approach to the interpretation of lab values is not useful in the diagnosis of specific health problems and nutritional imbalances because of its unusual way of determining reference ranges and because this approach does not take into consideration biological, analytical and statistical variations.

- The reference ranges are determined by measurements performed on a large number of subjects and arbitrarily defined as the range encompassed by two standard deviations.
- The distribution curve of test results is skewed rather than symmetric.
- The population used to calculate reference ranges is not necessarily healthy.

ii. Further research is necessary to determine the validity of this approach to the establishment of laboratory reference ranges.

c. **Monitoring**

i. Utilizing the optimal value approach to laboratory interpretation is not useful in monitoring changes in patients' health status.

4.3.4 **Rating:** Investigational
Evidence: Class I, II, III
Consensus Level: 1

D. Inappropriate Clinical Laboratory Procedures

1. Cytotoxic Testing for Food Allergies

a. Based on the data derived from controlled investigations, there is poor test reliability.

b. This test has not been shown to produce results that can be consistently correlated with other examination findings.

c. This test lacks an acceptable scientific rationale, lacks sensitivity and specificity and lacks evidence of clinical effectiveness.

4.4.1 **Rating:** Inappropriate
Evidence: Class I, II, III
Consensus Level: 1

2. Reams Testing and Interpretation of Urine

a. There is no clinical or scientific evidence for the use of this procedure in chiropractic or other related health science literature.

b. This test has not been shown to produce results that can be consistently correlated with examination findings.

c. This test lacks an acceptable scientific rationale, lacks sensitivity and specificity and lacks evidence of clinical effectiveness.

4.4.2 **Rating:** Inappropriate
Evidence: Class III
Consensus Level: 1

VII. COMMENTS, SUMMARY OR CONCLUSION

This chapter attempts to provide a conceptual model for the appropriate use of clinical laboratory test in chiropractic practice. The application of this model takes place with the development of clinical practice guidelines which are explicit yet clinically adaptable.

The true test of the effectiveness of these guidelines will come with their ability to be implemented and cause a positive effect to occur on health practices and patient outcomes.

Finally, the recommendations suggested here must be subject to periodic review and revision.

VIII. REFERENCES

The Role of Clinical Laboratory Tests in Chiropractic Practice

Adams AH: Determining the usefulness of diagnostic procedures and tests. *Chiropractic Technique* 1990; 2(3): 90-93.

Gottfried EL, Gerard SK: Selection and interpretation of laboratory tests and diagnostic procedures. In: AH Samily, RG Douglas, Jr., JA Barondess, (eds.): *Textbook of Diagnostic Medicine.* Philadelphia: Lea & Febiger, 1987: 19-38.

Jaquet P: The importance of laboratory methods in chiropractic diagnosis. *Annals of the Swiss Chiropractors Association.* Vol. V, 1971.

Lamm L: Chiropractic scope of practice. *Am J Chiro Med* 1989; 2(4): 155-159.

Vear HJ: Scope of chiropractic practice. In: HJ Vear, (ed.): *Chiropractic Standards of Practice and Quality of Care.* Gaithersburg, Maryland: Aspen Pub., 1992: 49-67.

Wertman BG, et al.: Why do physicians order laboratory tests? A study of laboratory test request and use patterns. *J Am Med Assoc* 1980; 243: 2080-2.

Principles of Appropriate Laboratory Test Selection and Use

Baer D, et al.: Regulation of physician's office laboratories. *Medical Laboratory Observer* 1988; September: 26-32.

Black ER, et al.: Characteristics of diagnostic tests and principles for their use in quantitative decision making. In: RJ Panzer, ER Black, and PF Griner, eds. *Diagnostic Strategies for Common Medical Problems.* Philadelphia: American College of Physicians, 1991: 1-16.

Eddy DM: How to think about screening. In: DM Eddy, (ed.): *Common Screening Tests.* Philadelphia: American College of Physicians, 1991: 1-21.

Griner PF, et al.: Selection and interpretation of diagnostic tests and procedures. Principles And Applications. *Ann Intern Med* 1981; 94: 553-600.

Kassirer JP: Our stubborn quest for diagnostic certainty. A cause of excessive testing. *N Engl J Med* 1989; 320(22): 1489-1491.

Sox HC, Jr: Probability theory in the use of diagnostic tests. In: HC Sox Jr., (ed.): *Common Diagnostic Tests, Use and Interpretation.* Philadelphia: American College of Physicians, 1987: 1-17.

Woolf SH, Kamerow DB: Testing for uncommon conditions. The heroic search for positive test results. *Arch Intern Med* 1990; 150: 2451-2458.

Principles of Laboratory Test Interpretation

Gottfried EL, Wagar, EA: Laboratory Testing: A Practical Guide. *Disease-A-Month* 1983; 29(11):1.

Panzer RI, et al.: Interpretation of Diagnostic Tests and Strategies for Their Use in Quantative Decision Making. In: RJ Panzer, ER Black, and PF Griner, (eds.): *Diagnostic Strategies for Common Medical Problems.* Philadelphia: American College of Physicians, 1991: 17-28.

Skenzel LP: How physicians use laboratory tests. *JAMA* 1978; 239: 1077-1080.

Speicher CE, Smith JW: Interpretation of strategies. In: CE Speicher and JW Smith, *Choosing Effective Laboratory Tests.* Philadelphia: WB Saunders Co., 1983: 37-46.

Statland BE, Winkel P: Selected pre-analytical sources of variation. In: Z Grasbeck and T Alstrom, (eds.): *Reference Values in Laboratory Medicine. The Current State of the Art.* New York: John Wiley and Sons, 1981: 127-141.

Guidelines for Ordering Commonly Utilized Laboratory Tests

Routine Urinalysis

Free AH, Free HM: Urinalysis: Its proper role in the physician's office. *Clinics in Laboratory Medicine* 1986; 6(2): 253-266.

Keil DP, Moskowitz MA: The Urinalysis: A Critical Appraisal. *Medical Clinics of North America* 1987; 71(4): 607-624.

Pels RJ, et al.: Dipstick urinalysis screening of asymptomatic adults for urinary tract disorders, II. bacteriuria. *JAMA* 1989; 262(9): 1221-1224.

Sheets D, Lyman JL: Urinalysis. *Emergency Medicine Clinics of North America* 1986; 4(2): 263-280.

Woolhander S, et al.: Dipstick urinalysis screening of asymptomatic adults for urinary tract disorders I. hematuria and proteinuria. *JAMA* 1989; 262 (9): 1215-1219.

Complete Blood Count (CBC)

Frye EB, Hubbell FA, Akin BV, Rucker L: Usefulness of routine admission complete blood counts on a general medical service. *J Gen Intern Med* 1987; 2:373-6.

Rich EC, Crowson TW, Connelly DP: Effectiveness of differential leukocyte count in case finding in the ambulatory care setting. *JAMA* 1983; 249:633-6.

Ruttiman S, Clemencon D., DuBach U: Usefulness of complete blood counts as a case-finding tool in medical outpatients. *Ann Intern Med* 1992; 116: 44-50.

Shapiro MF, Greenfield S: The complete blood count and leukocyte differential count. an approach to their rational application. *Ann Intern Med* 1987; 106: 65-74.

Erythrocyte Sedimentation Rate (ESR)

Bedell SE, Bush BT: Erythrocyte sedimentation rate from folklore to facts. *Amer J Med* 1985; 78: 1001-1009.

Cunha BA: Interpreting the ESR: An advanced course. *Diagnosis* 1983; Feb. 62-69.

Lewis SM: *Erythrocyte sedimentation rate and plasma viscosity.* Broadsheet 94: June 1980. Association of Clinical Pathologists, London.

Sox HC: The erythrocyte sedimentation rate. Guidelines for rational use. *Ann Intern Med* 1986; 103: 515-523.

Biochemical Profiles

Cebul RD, Beck JR: Biochemical profiles: application in ambulatory screening and preadmission testing of adults. *Ann Intern Med* 1987; 106: 403-13.

Hubbell FA, Frye EB, Akin BV, Rucker L: Routine admission laboratory testing for general medical patients. *Med Care* 1988; 26: 619-30.

Sackett DL: The usefulness of laboratory tests in health screening programs. *Clin Chem* 1973; 19: 366-72.

Witte DL, Angstadt DS, Schweitzer JK: Chemistry profiles in wellness programs: test selection and participant outcomes. *Clin Chem* 1988; 34: 1447-50.

Plasma Glucose

National Diabetes Data Group. Classification and diagnosis of diabetes mellitus and other categories of glucose intolerance. *Diabetes* 1979; 28: 1039-57.

Service FI, O'Brien PC, Rizza RA: Measurements of glucose control. *Diabetes care* 1987; 10: 225-37.

Singer DE, et al.: Screening for diabetes mellitus. *Ann Intern Med.* 1988; 109: 639-49.

Singer DE, et al.: Tests of glycemia in diabetes mellitus. *Ann Intern Med* 1989; 110: 125-87.

Serum Urea Nitrogen and Creatinine

Baum N, Dichoso CC, Carlton CE, Jr: Blood urea nitrogen and serum creatinine: Physiology and interpretations. *Urology,* 1975; 5:583.

Beck LH, Kassirer JP: Serum electrolytes, serum osmolality, blood urea nitrogen. In: HC Sox, Jr., (ed.): *Common Diagnostic Tests: Use and Interpretation.* 2nd ed. Philadelphia: American College of Physicians, 1990: 367-389.

Checchio MD, Como AJ: Electrolytes, BUN creatinine: Who's at risk? *Ann Rev Med* 1988; 39:465-90.

Serum Calcium

Juan D: Hypocalcemia: Differential diagnosis and mechanisms. *Arch Inter Med* 1979; 139: 1167-71.

Lafferty FW: Primary hyperparathyroidism: Changing clinical spectrum, prevalence of hypertension, and discriminant analysis of laboratory tests. *Arch Intern Med* 1981; 141: 1761-1766.

Mundy G: Calcium homeostasis: *Hypercalcemia and Hypocalcemia,* 2nd ed. London: Martin Dunitz Ltd., 1990.

Wong ET, Freier EF: The differential diagnosis of hypercalcemia: An algorithm for more effective use of laboratory tests. *JAMA* 1982; 247: 75-80.

Serum Inorganic Phosphorus

Knochel JP: The clinical status of hypophosphatemia: An update. *N Engl J Med* 1985; 313:447.

Yu GC, Lee DB: Clinical disorders of phosphorus metabolism. *West J Med* 1987; 147: 569-576.

Serum Total Protein and Albumin

Whicher JT and Spencer C: When is serum albumin worth measuring? *Ann Clin Biochem* 1987; 24: 572-580.

Whicher JT et al.: The laboratory investigation of paraproteinanemia *Ann Clin Biochem* 1987; 24: 119-132.

Serum Cholesterol

Garber AM, Sox HC, Littenberg B: Screening asymptomatic adults for cardiac risk factors: the serum cholesterol level. *Ann Intern Med* 1989; 110: 622-39.

Krahn M, Naylor CD, Basinski AS, Detsky AS: Comparison of an aggressive (U.S.) and a less aggressive (Canadian) policy for cholesterol screening and treatment. *Ann Intern Med*; 115: 248-55.

Report of the national cholesterol education program expert panel on the detection, evaluation, and treatment of high blood cholesterol in adults. *Arch Intern Med* 1988; 148: 36-39.

Schucker B, Bradford RH: Screening for High Blood Cholesterol. *Clinics in Laboratory Medicine* 1989; 9(1): 29-36.

Serum Prostatic Acid Phosphatase

Carson JL et al.: Diagnostic accuracy of four assays of prostatic acid phosphatase. *JAMA* 1985; 253: 665-9.

Heller JE: Prostatic acid phosphatase: Its current clinical status. *J Urol* 1987; 137: 1091-1093.

U.S. preventative services task force. Screening for prostate cancer. In: *Guide to Clinical Preventative Services.* Baltimore, Maryland: Williams & Wilkins; 1989: 63.

Watson RA, Tang DB: The predictive value of prostatic acid phosphatase as a screening test for prostatic cancer. *N Engl J Med* 1980; 303-487.

Serum Prostate-Specific Antigen (PSA)

Brawer MK: Laboratory studies for the detection of carcinoma of the prostate. *Urologic Clinics of North America* 1990; 17(4): 759-768.

Catalona WJ, Smith DS, Ratliff TL, et al.: Measurement of prostate specific antigen in serum as a screening test for prostate cancer. *N Engl J Med* 1991; 324: 1156-61.

Chadwick DJ et al.: Pilot study of screening for prostate cancer in general practice. *Lancet* 1991; 338: 613-616.

Fiorelli RL et al.: Early detection of Stage A prostate carcinoma: combined use of prostate-specific antigen and transrectal ultra-sonography. *JAOA* 1991; 91(9): 863-870.

Serum Asparatate AminoTransferase (AST)

Chopra G, Griffin PH: Laboratory tests and diagnostic procedures in evaluation of liver disease. *Am J Med* 1985; 79(8): 221-30.

Clermont RJ and Chalmers TC: The transaminase tests in liver disease. *Medicine* 1967; 46: 199-207.

Kools AM, Bloomer JR: Abnormal liver function tests. how to assess their importance in asymptomatic patients. *Postgraduate Medicine* 1987; 81(6): 45-51.

Serum Creatinine Kinase (CK)

Lee TH, Goldman L: Serum enzyme assays in the diagnosis of acute myocardial infarction. In HC Sox, (ed.): *Common Diagnostic Tests, Use and Interpretation,* 2nd ed. Philadelphia: American College of Physicians, 1990: 35-66.

Klatt EC, Wasef ES, Wong ET: Creatinine kinase in a biochemical test panel. The high cost of a seemingly inexpensive test. *American Journal of Clinical Pathology,* 1982; 77(3): 280-284.

Lott JA, Wolf PL: *Clinical Enzymology, A Case-Oriented Approach.* New York: Field, Rich and Associates, Inc. 1986.

Thyroid Function Tests

DeLos Santos ET, Mazzaferri EL: Thyroid Function Tests. Guidelines for Interpretation in Common Clinical Disorders. *Postgraduate Medicine* 1989; 85(5): 333-352.

Feldkamp CS, McKenna MI: Contemporary approach to thyroid disease -emphasizing use of high-sensitivity thyrotropin assays. *Henry Ford Hosp Med J* 1991; 39(1): 25-29.

Helfand M, Crapo LM: Screening for thyroid disease. *Ann Intern Med* 1990; 112(11): 840-849.

Surks MI et al.: American thyroid association guidelines for use of laboratory tests in thyroid disorders. *JAMA* 1990; 263(11): 1529-1532.

Serum Uric Acid

Wallace SL et al.: Preliminary criteria for the classification of the acute arthritis of primary gout. *Arthritis Rheum* 1977; 20: 895-900.

Rheumatoid Factor

Lichtenstein MJ, Pincus T: How useful are combinations of blood tests in "rheumatic panels" in diagnosis of rheumatic diseases? *J Gen Intern Med* 1988; 3: 435-42.

Shmerling RH, Delbanco TL: The rheumatoid factor: An analysis of clinical utility. *Amer J Med* 1991; 91: 528-534.

Wolfe F, Cathey MA, Roberts FK: The latex test revisited. Rheumatoid factor testing in 8,287 rheumatic disease patients. *Arthritis Rheum* 1991; 34: 951-60.

Anti-Nuclear Antibody (ANA) Test

Fritzler MJ: Antinuclear antibodies in the investigation of rheumatic diseases. *Bull Dis* 1985; 35: 1-10.

Richardson B, Epstein SV: Utility of the fluorescent antinuclear antibody test in a single patient. *Ann Intern Med* 1981; 95: 333-8.

White RH, Robbins DL: Clinical significance and interpretation of antinuclear antibodies. *West J Med* 1987; 147: 210-213.

HLA-B27

Baron M, Zendel I: HLA-B27 testing in ankylosing spondylitis: An analysis of the pretesting assumptions. *J Rheumatol* 1989; 16: 631-6.

Hawkins BR et al.: Use of the B27 test in the diagnosis of ankylosing spondylitis: A statistical evaluation. *Arthritis and Rheumatism* 1981; 24(5): 743-746.

Khan MA, Khan MK: Diagnostic value of HLA-B27 testing in ankylosing spondylitis and Reiter's syndrome. *Ann Intern Med;* 96: 70-6.

C-Reactive Protein

Kushner I, Volanakis JE, Gewurz H: C-reactive protein and the plasma response to tissue injury. *Annals of the New York Academy of Sciences,* 1982; 389.

Marchand A, Van Lente F: How the laboratory can monitor acute inflammation. *Diagnostic Medicine,* 1984; Nov/Dec., 57-66.

Okamura J. et al.: Potential clinical applications of C-reactive protein. *Journal of Clinical Laboratory Analysis* 1990; 4:231-235.

Pepys MB: C-reactive protein fifty years on. *Lancet,* 1981; March 21: 653-657.

Powell LJ. C-reactive protein: A review. *Am J Med Tech* 1979; 45(2):138-142.

Serum Potassium

Beck LH, Kassirer J: Serum electrolytes, serum osmolality, blood urea nitrogen, and serum creatinine. In HC Sox, Jr., (ed.): *Common Diagnostic Tests, Use and Interpretation,* 2nd ed., Philadelphia: American College of Physicians, 1990: 367-389.

Martin M, Hamilton R, West MF: Potassium *Emergency Medicine Clinics of North America* 1986; 4(1):131-144.

Narina RG, et al.: Diagnostic strategies in disorders of fluid, electrolyte and acid-base homeostasis. *Am J Med,* 1982; 72:496-520.

Serum Sodium

Beck LH, Kassirer J: Serum electrolytes, serum osmolality, blood urea nitrogen, and serum creatinine. In HC Sox, Jr., ed. *Common Diagnostic Tests, Use and Interpretation,* 2nd ed., Philadelphia: American College of Physicians, 1990: 367-389.

Janz T: Sodium *Emergency Medicine Clinics of North America,* 1986; 4(1): 115-130.

Narina RG, et al.: Diagnostic strategies in disorders of fluid, electrolyte and acid-base homeostasis. *Am J Med,* 1982; 72:496-520.

Serum Iron and Total Iron Binding Capacity

Cavill J, Jacobs A and Worwood M: Diagnostic methods for iron status. *Ann Clin Biochem* 1986; 23:168-171.

Fairbanks VF: Laboratory testing for iron status. *Hospital Practice, Supplement 3* 1991; 26:168-171.

Psaty BM, et al.: The value of serum iron studies as a test for iron-deficiency anemia in a country hospital. *J Gen Intern Med,* 1987; 2:160-167.

Fecal Occult Blood Test

Brandeau ML, Eddy D: The workup of the asymptomatic patient with a positive fecal occult blood test. *Medical Decision Making* 1987; 7(1):32-46.

Eddy D: Screening for colorectal cancer. *Ann Intern Med* 1990; 113: 373-84.

Knight K, Fielding J, Battista R: Occult blood testing for colorectal cancer. *JAMA* 1989; 261(4):586-93.

Serum Ferritin

Fairbanks VF: Laboratory testing for iron status. *Hospital Practice Supplement 3* 1991; 26:17-24.

Patterson C, et al.: Iron deficiency anemia in the elderly: The diagnostic process. *Can Med Assoc J* 1991; 144(4):435-440.

Hair Analysis

Taylor A: Usefulness of measurement of trace elements in hair. *Ann. Clin. Biochem.* 1986; 23: 364-378.

Klevay, L.M., et al.: Hair analysis in clinical and experimental medicine. *Am. J. Clin. Nutr.* 1987; 46: 233-236.

Live Cell Analysis

Lowell JA. Live cell analysis: High-tech hokum. *Nutrition Forum* 1986, 3(11): 81-85.

Biochemical Biopsy

Fernandes JJ: Realistic expectations of laboratory testing. *JAOA* 1991; 91(12): 1223-1228.

Furda A: *Biochemical biopsy.* East Lansing, MI. Privately published, 1978.

Gottfried EL, Wagar ED: Laboratory testing: A practical guide. *Disease-A-Month* 1983; 29(11): 1-41.

Black ER, et al.: Characteristics of diagnostic tests and principles for their use in quantitative decision making. In: RJ Panzer, ER Black, PF Grinler (eds.): *Diagnostic strategies for common medical problems,* Philadelphia: American College Of Physicians, 1991: 1-16.

Optimal Laboratory Values

R Grasbeck, I Alstrom, T: *Reference Values in Laboratory Medicine,* New York: John Wiley and Sons, 1981.

Cytotoxic Testing for Food Allergies

Sawyer CE, Adams AH: The cytotoxic leukocyte test. *ACA J. Chiro.* 1987; 21 (2): 59-61.

Appendix References

Guidelines for Clinical Laboratory Investigation and Laboratory Protocols for Spinal Disorders

Deyo R. Early Diagnostic Evaluation of Low-back Pain. *J Gen Intern Med* 1986; 1: 328-338.

Deyo R, Diehl A. Cancer as a Cause of Back Pain: Frequency, Clinical Presentation, Diagnostic Strategies. *J Gen Intern Med* 1988; 3: 230-238.

Waddell G. An Approach to Backache. *Br J Hosp Med* 1982; Sept.: 187-219.

Focused Organ/Health Problem Profiles

Henry JB, Howanitz PJ. Organ Panels and the Relationship of the Laboratory to the Physician. In RJ Jones and RM Palulonis *Laboratory Tests in Medical Practice.* Chicago: American Medical Association, 1980: 25-45.

IX. MINORITY OPINIONS

None.

X. APPENDIX

A. Useful Guidelines for Clinical Laboratory Investigation of Spinal Disorders

1. Positive Health History for:

   Previous malignancy

   Striking weight loss

   Persistent pain, more than 50 years old

   Use of corticosteroids

   Drug or alcohol abuse

2. Positive Clinical Examination for:

   Systemic signs (i.e., fever)

3. Radiographic findings suggestive of pathology

4. Failure to improve with conservative care

   (See Chapter 8, Frequency of Care)

B. Laboratory Procedures Which May Be Useful for Spinal Disorders

Cause/Dysfunction		Tests
Mechanical	Compression fracture	Serum alkaline phosphatase, Total protein, Albumin, Serum total calcium, Inorganic PO4
Inflammatory	Infective: TB of the spine	ESR or CRP CBC, Urine and sputum cultures
	Other infectious agents	ESR or CRP CBC Blood culture Agglutination titers
	Noninfective rheumatoid arthritis	ESR, CRP, Serum viscosity Rheumatoid factor (anti-IgG)
	Ankylosing spondylitis	ESR or CRP CBC, Alkaline phosphatase, HLA-B27
Metabolic	Nutritional Osteoporosis	Alkaline phosphatase, Calcium, Inorganic PO4, Total protein, Albumin, BUN, Creatinine, sTSH or FT4
	Osteomalacia	CBC, BUN, Creatinine, Calcium, Inorganic PO4,

		Alkaline phosphatase, Total protein, Albumin, Vitamin D assay			Serum and urine amylase, Serum lipase, Serum trypsin
	Endocrine: Adrenal	Serum electrolytes, Urinary free cortisol		Chronic pancreatitis	Glucose, Serum amylase, Serum lipase, Stool fat, Serum bilirubin, Lundh test meal
	Parathyroid	Calcium, Inorganic PO4, Ionized calcium, PtH assay, Alkaline phosphatase, Serum chloride (C1/PO4 ratio)		Carcinoma of the pancreas	Glucose, AST, Alkaline phosphatase, T. bilirubin, GGT, Tumor marker assays, ESR
Other	Paget's disease	Alkaline phosphatase, Calcium, Inorganic PO4, Urinary hydroxproline		Cholecystitis	CBC, T. bilirubin, AST, Alkaline phosphatase, Serum amylase
Neoplastic	Multiple myeloma	Total protein, Albumin, CBC, Serum protein electrophoresis, Urinary protein electrophoresis, Uric acid, BUN, Creatinine, Immunoelectrophoresis, Urinary light chain typing		Pyelonephritis	Urinalysis, Urine culture, Colony count, BUN and creatinine, CBC, ESR
	Metastatic tumors	Alkaline phosphatase Calcium, Inorganic PO4, Uric acid, Acid phosphatase, Prostate specific antigen (PSA), LDH, Serum protein electrophoresis, ESR or CRP			
	Primary tumors	Same as metastatic tumors			
Visceral Referred Pain	Myocardial infarction	Total CK, CK and LD isoenzymes			
	Posterior peptic ulcer	CBC BUN Stool Occult blood test			
	Acute pancreatitis	Glucose Calcium			

C. Examples of Focused Organ/Health Problem Profiles

Utilization of these procedures requires clinical judgment and appropriateness.

Multisystem Involvement with Vague and Unexplained Physical Changes

Serum Alkaline Phosphatase	Serum Creatinine
Serum LDH	Serum Calcium
Serum Total Bilirubin	Serum Glucose
CBC	Serum Inorganic Phosphorous
Serum Urea Nitrogen	Serum Cholesterol
Serum HDL	Serum Total Protein
Serum AST	Serum Uric Acid
sTSH or Free T4 Index	Serum Albumin
Urinalysis	Serum Triglycerides

Urinary Tract Involvement

Serum Urea Nitrogen	Routine Urinalysis
Serum Creatinine	Urine Culture and Colony Count
Serum Uric Acid	

Hyperlipidemia and Lipid Transport Disorders

Serum Cholesterol	Serum LDL
Serum Triglycerides	Plasma Glucose
Serum HDL Cholesterol	Serum Uric Acid

Thyroid Involvement

T4	Thyroid Autoantibodies
Free T4 Index	(Anti-thyroglobulin antibody)
T3	(Anti-microsomal antibody)
sTSH	

Joint and Connective Tissue Involvement

ANA	RA Factor
ASO-T	Serum Uric Acid
CRP and/or ESR	CBC

Hepato-Biliary Involvement

Serum Alkaline Phosphatase	Serum ALT
Serum Total Bilirubin	Serum GGT
Serum Cholesterol	Serum Albumin
Serum LDH	Serum Protein Electrophoresis
Serum AST	

Anemia

CBC	Direct Coombs (Antiglobulin)
Reticulocyte Count	Serum B-12
Serum Iron	Serum Ferritin
Serum Iron Binding Capacity (IBC)	Hemoglobin Electrophoresis
RBC Folate	

Pregnancy

CBC	Indirect Coombs (Antiglobulin)
Blood Group (ABO)	Rubella
Blood Type (RH)	VDRL (RPR)

Hypertension

Serum Urea Nitrogen	Metanephrines 24-hour Urine
Serum Creatinine	Urinalysis
Serum Electrolytes	Urinary Free Cortisol
Plasma Aldosterone	

Cardiac Involvement (Chest Pain)

Serum CK	Serum CK Isoenzymes
Serum LDH	Serum LDH Isoenzymes

Metabolic Bone Involvement

Serum Total Protein	Serum Calcium
Serum Albumin	Serum Phosphorus
Serum Alkaline Phosphatase	Urinary Hydroxyproline

Skeletal Muscle

Serum CPK	Serum Calcium
Serum Aldolase	Electrolytes
Urine Myoglobin	

Pancreatic Involvement

Serum Amylase	Serum Calcium
Urinary Amylase	Serum Creatinine
Serum Lipase	Serum Trypsin

5

Record Keeping and Patient Consents

"If it isn't written down, it doesn't exist."
— *Anonymous and Ubiquitous*

Chapter Outline

I. OVERVIEW

The health care record serves many important functions and is one of the critical components of the health care delivery system. The most important function is in the immediate care and treatment of the patient. The record also permits different members of a health care team, or successive health care providers, to have access to relevant data concerning the patient to see what procedures have been performed and with what results. The health care record is important for documenting the specific services received by the patient so that the provider can be reimbursed for them. Records should be maintained in a manner that makes them suitable for utilization review. The health record is helpful in the evaluation of practitioners, provides data for public health purposes, and may be used for the purpose of teaching and research. It is critical in a variety of legal contexts, including litigation by patients and malpractice claims.

Construction of an adequate patient chart involves the accumulation of essential information from the patient by interview, use of questionnaires, examination and special studies. There should also be transfer of pertinent information where available from previous or other care given to the patient. This chapter describes the documents, internal and external, that are used to arrive at a diagnosis, to determine and document necessity of care, and to provide a foundation for the chiropractic treatment plan. The chapter also discusses appropriate patient consents and other legal disclosures.

Once the initial patient work-up has been completed, all record/chart entries should be made in a systematic, organized and contemporaneous manner. Recommendations on what constitutes necessary information to be contained in the day-to-day patient record are offered. The information contained in such records provides a foundation for writing accurate reports to other health care providers, insurance companies, attorneys and other interested parties. The practitioner is encouraged to use a charting system that is effective and complete, yet practical and efficient.

The organization of the patient chart may be enhanced by using preprinted forms and by having proper identifying information on each page. Minimum recommendations for legibility and clarity of chart entries are offered. The importance of confidentiality and professional courtesy with respect to patient records is emphasized and guidelines are offered.

Patient consent may be implied or expressed, depending upon the circumstances. Where it is expressed, it may be obtained either verbally or in writing. Often the process is facilitated by the use of preprinted forms completed and signed by involved parties then kept as part of the health record as evidence of the consent process. The practitioner is encouraged to consult with legal counsel for proper document design and application. Less common forms of consent are diagnosis waiver and consent to participate in research.

II. DEFINITIONS

A. General Definitions

Chart Notes: General term indicating notes made on the patient's work chart.

Health Record: All documents and recorded information relating to the clinical management of a patient.

Peer Review: Evaluation by peers or colleagues of the quality, quantity, and efficiency of services ordered or performed by a practitioner.

POMR - Problem Oriented Medical Records.

Progress Notes: Generally brief notations recorded in the patient's file for each office visit once management has commenced.

SOAP: Acronym for Subjective symptoms, Objective signs, Assessment and Plan.

SORE: Acronym for Subjective, Objective, Rx (treatment) and Exercise (ergonomics).

Work Chart: The form that the practitioner and/or staff uses to record patient's chart notes.

B. Legal Definitions

Consent to Treatment: Permission to treat from the patient or, where the patient is a minor or otherwise without legal capacity to consent, from the patient's guardian. Valid consent must be voluntary, informed, and related to a specific act or set of acts. It may be oral or written if expressly given, or may be implied.

Consent to Participate in Research: As above, but with the additional requirement that the subject has adequate information regarding the research and the power of free choice to participate in the research or decline participation.

Rule of Confidentiality: The rule which requires that all information about a patient that is gathered by a practitioner as part of the provider/patient relationship be kept confidential unless its release is authorized by the patient or, in exceptional circumstances, serves some other overriding purpose.

III. LIST OF SUBTOPICS

A. Internal Documentation

- Patient file
- Doctor/clinic identification
- Misc. assessment & outcome instruments
- Clinical impression

- Patient identification
- Patient demographics
- Health care coverage
- Patient history
- Examination findings
- Special studies

- Treatment plan
- Chart/progress notes
- Re-examination/ reassessment
- Financial records
- Internal memoranda

B. External Documentation

- Direct correspondence
- Health records

- Diagnostic imaging
- External reports

C. Chart/File Organization

- General considerations
- Use of pre-printed forms

- Legibility and clarity
- Use of abbreviations/ symbols

D. Maintenance of Records

- Confidentiality
- Records retention
- Administrative records

- Records transfer
- Clinic staff responsibilities

E. Patient Consents

- Informed consent
- Consent to treat minor child
- Authorization to release patient information

- Financial assignments
- Consent to participate in research
- Publication/photo/ video consent
- Authority to admit observers

IV. LITERATURE REVIEW

The literature search for this topic was accomplished through the use of CLIBCON indexing, referencing subject headings pertinent to the scope of the chapter. Other information was obtained through retrieval from personal libraries of committee members and advisors, especially with respect to recently published papers and monographs.

Much of the published literature on health record documentation and patient consents is either found in guidebooks, usually with significant contribution from the legal profession, or in popular publications containing sections dedicated to legal advice. Since 1979 there has been little information published on these topics in the chiropractic peer reviewed journals. A notable exception is the *Journal of the Canadian Chiropractic*

Association which is refereed but also serves as an important conduit of such information to association members.

In the general chiropractic literature, there are notable bound publications that have contributed to the knowledge-base. In 1973 Simmons[44] prepared a concise guide to assist the practitioner in maintaining daily records and recording elements of case history and consultation. Schafer[41,43] published procedural manuals through the American Chiropractic Association which underscored the importance of documenting necessity of chiropractic care through adequate record-keeping and the support of chiropractic paraprofessionals. In a publication of the International Chiropractors' Association Kranz[22] provides guidance for the practitioner in the hospital environment. There have been two recent publications promoting malpractice prevention or risk management strategies for practitioners. Campbell, Ladenheim, Sherman and Sportelli [5] identify many pitfalls of lax patient chart management and failure to obtain patient consents, and offer recommendations that can be implemented in office management systems. Harrison[18] crisply identifies shortcomings of patient records and the risks in the context of malpractice claims.

The Canadians lead the way in publishing contemporary articles in the chiropractic refereed journals relative to risk management, charting procedures and report writing. Authors such as Carey,[6] Cassidy,[7] Gotlib,[12,13] Nixdorf,[31] Vear and Vernon have contributed material that assists practitioners in management of patient records and obtaining appropriate consents. Elsewhere Reinke and Jahn[38] provide pointed commentary correlating the importance of the patient's health record and the practitioner's "legal well-being." Other direction has been offered by Turnbull[47] from New Zealand and Gledhill.[11] Bolton[4] adds to the published knowledge base on informed consent. Nyiendo and Haldeman[32] have analysed practice activities of student interns in a chiropractic college teaching clinic and summarize the need for standardized accountability in patient care.

Recently many monographs have been establishing guidelines for the management of chiropractic cases. These include a surge in efforts to publish standards of care in a number of state and provincial jurisdictions. Within these are position statements or "standards" on obtaining and documenting clinical information. Practitioners in Connecticut[36] were among the first to provide practice guidelines, noting that there must be adequate documentation of the necessity for chiropractic care. They established recommended formats for interval reporting. The workers' compensation guidelines produced by the Washington State Chiropractic Advisory Committee[16] adapted an outline proposed earlier by Vear, Haldeman and West citing six primary case management objectives supported by "standards." Vear[48] has subsequently republished these objectives and standards in a major text. Efforts by Olson,[34] LaBrot,[23] and state chiropractic organizations in Ohio,[33] Michigan[26] and Minnesota[27] have all produced practice guidelines that emphasize the need for better standards in record keeping. Similar efforts are underway in Oregon, Quebec, Manitoba, Oklahoma, Texas, South Carolina and other jurisdictions.

Chiropractic professional liability carriers have contributed to the information pool with monographs that are a part of their risk management program. Both the OUM Group and the National Chiropractic Mutual Insurance Company (NCMIC) have produced many articles through newsletters and booklets.[e.g., 42]

Chiropractic popular publications produced by the national and state associations periodically give guidance on efficient record keeping, risk management[e.g.,19,21] and report writing.[e.g., 7] Other popular publications that contribute articles include *The American Chiropractor,*[35] *Today's Chiropractic,*[28] *Digest of Chiropractic Economics*[e.g., 1-3] and *Dynamic Chiropractic.* Chiropractic specialty councils have contributed white papers[e.g., 14] on essential elements of the patient's case file, report composition and clinical workup. Popular publications outside the chiropractic field also contribute valuable knowledge that can be used in the development of guidelines.[e.g., 37, 40]

Probably the richest technical source of information relative to documentation and patient consents is found in legal publications.[e.g., 20, 25] The legal standard found in these publications is supported with citation of case law. Publications such as this are not easily accessed by the average practitioner in the field, nor are they available in all chiropractic college libraries. The profession must rely on its legal consultants to assist in review of such literature. Fortunately, publications such as *Legal Update* (formerly *Chiropractic Amicus)* edited by Ladenheim et al., and the *Chiropractic Report* edited by Chapman-Smith have emerged to fulfill this role and assist practitioners to understand legal ramifications of health care practice.

V. ASSESSMENT CRITERIA

Procedure Ratings (System II)

Necessary: Strong positive recommendation based on Class I evidence, or overwhelming Class II evidence when circumstances reflect compromise of patient safety.

Recommended: Positive recommendation based on consensus Class II and/or strong Class III evidence.

Discretionary: Positive recommendation based on strong consensus of Class III evidence.

Unnecessary: Negative recommendation based on inconclusive or conflicting Class II and Class III evidence.

Quality of Evidence

The following categories of evidence are used to support the ratings.

Class I:

A. Evidence of clinical utility from controlled studies published in refereed journals.

B. Binding or strongly persuasive legal authority such as legislation or case law.

Class II:

A. Evidence of clinical utility from the significant results of uncontrolled studies in refereed journals.

B. Evidence provided by recommendations from published expert legal opinion or persuasive case law.

Class III:

A. Evidence of clinical utility provided by opinions of experts, anecdote and/or by convention.

B. Expert legal opinion.

VI. RECOMMENDATIONS

Disclaimer — These guidelines may necessarily be superceded by statutory law in respective state or provincial jurisdictions. They do not purport to convey legal advice. It is recommended that each practitioner should obtain his/her own independent legal advice.

A. Internal Documentation

(Records generated within the chiropractor's office.)

1. The Patient File

When a new patient enters the office, a file is created which becomes the foundation of the patient's permanent record. Adequate systems may include personal patient data (e.g., name, address, phone numbers, age, sex, occupation); insurance and billing information; appropriate assignments and consent forms; case history; examination findings; imaging and laboratory findings; diagnosis; work chart for recording ongoing patient data obtained on each visit; the service rendered; health care plan; copies of insurance billings; reports; correspondence; case identification (e.g., by number) for easy storage and retrieval of patient's documents, etc.

5.1.1 **Rating:** Necessary
Evidence: Class I, II, III
Consensus Level: 1

A folder is used to house most of the patient's records. This may also be part of the record, if the practitioner writes patient data on the folder, such as patient personal information or x-ray/examination/treatment plan data. The practitioner may attach a patient work chart to the inside of the folder along with the other items in the patient's file. On periodic file review, outdated portions may be removed and stored in an archive file. A permanent note should be kept in the active file indicating that the patient has additional records.

5.1.2 **Rating:** Recommended
Evidence: Class II, III
Consensus Level: 1

2. Doctor/Clinic Identification

Basic information identifying the practitioner or facility should appear on documents used to establish the doctor-patient relationship. This can be preprinted on forms, affixed by rubber stamp or adhesive labels or typed or handwritten in ink. Basic information should include:

- practitioner's name/specialty
- specialty designation (if applicable)
- facility name (if different)
- legal trade name (if applicable)
- street address and mailing address (if different)
- telephone number(s)

5.1.3 **Rating:** Necessary
Evidence: Class I, II, III
Consensus Level: 1

3. Patient Identification

Clear identification of the patient with relevant demographic information (see item #4 below) is a necessary component of the chart. This information can be obtained with ease by using preprinted forms for completion by the patient. Identifying information may include:

- case/file number (if applicable)
- name (prior/other names)
- birthdate, age
- name of consenting parent or guardian (if patient is a minor or incapacitated)
- copy letter of guardianship (where appropriate)
- address(es)
- telephone number(s)
- social security number (if applicable)
- radiograph/lab identification (if applicable)
- contact in case of emergency (closest relationship name/ phone number)

5.1.4 **Rating:** Necessary
Evidence: Class I, II, III
Consensus Level: 1

4. Patient Demographics

- sex (M or F)
- occupation (special skills)

5.1.5 **Rating:** Necessary
Evidence: Class I, II, III
Consensus Level: 1

- marital status
- race
- number of dependents
- employer, address, phone number
- spouse's occupation

5.1.6 **Rating:** Discretionary
Evidence: Class I, II, III
Consensus Level: 1

5. Health Care Coverage

Health care coverage information is important for the business function of a health care facility, and such records are a part of the health care record. However, the information obtained and the format used are at the discretion of the practitioner.

- current incident result of accident or injury?
- insurance company or responsible party (auto/work comp/health/other)
- group and policy numbers, effective date
- spouse's insurance company and policy information (if applicable)

5.1.7 **Rating:** Discretionary
Evidence: Class III
Consensus Level: 1

6. Patient History

(See Chapter 1 of this document)

This is the foundation of the clinical database for each patient. The practitioner may choose to enter this data on a formatted or unformatted page. There should be an adequate picture of the patient's subjective perception of the history. Important elements of the history may include:

- date history taken
- present complaint/chief complaint
- description of accident/injurious event or other etiology
- past history, family history, social history (work history and recreational interests, hobbies as appropriate)
- review of systems (as appropriate)
- past and present medical/chiropractic treatment and attempts at self-care
- signature or initials of person eliciting history

5.1.8 **Rating:** Necessary
Evidence: Class I, II, III
Consensus Level: 1

When possible, history questionnaires, drawings and other information personally completed by the patient should be included in the initial documentation.

5.1.9 **Rating:** Recommended
Evidence: I, II, III
Consensus Level: 1

7. Examination Findings

(See Chapters 1, 3, & 4)

Objective information relative to the patient's history is obtained by physical assessment/examination of the area of complaint and related areas and/or systems. Gathering and recording this information may be facilitated by use of preprinted and formatted examination forms. If abbreviations are used, a legend should be available. Such documentation should include the date of the examination and name or initials of the examining practitioner. If persons other than the primary examining practitioner perform and/or record elements of the objective examination, their names and/or initials should appear on the exam/data form. Such evaluations may include:

- vital signs
- physical examination
- neuromusculoskeletal examination
- instrumentation
- other chiropractic examination procedures

5.1.10 **Rating:** Necessary
　　　　Evidence: Class I, II, III
　　　　Consensus Level: 1

8. Findings of Special Studies

(See Chapters 2, 3, & 4)

Documented results of special studies become a component part of the contemporaneous file. This documentation should include date of study, facility where performed, name of technician, name of interpreting practitioner, and relevant findings. Special studies ordered by practitioner may include:

- diagnostic imaging (e.g., plain film radiography; tomography or computed tomography; magnetic resonance imaging; diagnostic ultrasound; radionuclide bone scan)
- neurophysiologic/ electrodiagnostic testing (e.g., nerve conduction velocities; electromyography; somatosensory evoked responses)
- other laboratory tests

5.1.11 **Rating:** Recommended
　　　　Evidence: Class I, II, III
　　　　Consensus Level: 1

9. Miscellaneous Assessment and Outcome Instruments

(See Chapters 3 & 10)

Various assessment and outcome instruments can contribute to clinical management and become part of the case record. Many of these instruments are used in a repeated or serial fashion, which makes it essential for the record to identify the date(s) of completion and name(s) of scoring practitioner/technician. Measurement instruments currently in use include:

- visual analog scale
- pain diagrams
- pain questionnaires (e.g., McGill)

- pain disability instruments (e.g., Oswestry, Neck Disability Index)
- health status indices (e.g., SF-36, Sickness Impact Profile)
- patient satisfaction indices
- other outcome measures

5.1.12 **Rating:** Recommended
　　　　Evidence: Class I, II, III
　　　　Consensus Level: 1

10. Clinical Impression

(See Chapters 6, 9, & 12)

Upon completion of the subjective and objective data base, the practitioner formulates a clinical impression or diagnosis. This may be preliminary only, and may comprise more than one diagnosis. This clinical impression should be recorded within the file or in the contemporaneous visit record. As the clinical impression may change with new clinical information or in response to treatment, it is important that each clinical impression be dated. The record may include:

- primary, secondary and/or tertiary elements of diagnosis
- appropriate diagnostic coding (e.g., ICD-CM)

5.1.13 **Rating:** Necessary
　　　　Evidence: Class I, II, III
　　　　Consensus Level: 1

11. Treatment Plan

(See Chapters 6, 7, 8, 9 & 12)

This arises from the accumulation of clinical data and the formulation of the initial clinical impression. The plan may include further diagnostic work to monitor progress, or a therapeutic trial to test clinical impressions and assess appropriateness of treatment procedures selected. The treatment plan documents the approach to management by the practitioner and staff (e.g., spinal adjusting, therapy modalities, recommended exercise regime, lifestyle and dietary modifications). Any plan for referral to or consultation with other health care providers is appropriately listed in the record. The written treatment plan may appear on a form dedicated to the clinical work-up, or in the contemporaneous visit record, and may include:

- diagnostic/reassessment plan
- practitioner's treatment plan (modes and frequency of care)
- patient's education and self-care plan
- intra- or interdisciplinary referral or consultation

5.1.14 **Rating:** Recommended
　　　　Evidence: Class I, II, III
　　　　Consensus Level: 1

12. Chart/Progress Notes

Once the initial patient work-up has been completed, all record entries should be made in a systematic organized manner.

5.1.15 **Rating:** Necessary
Evidence: Class I, II, III
Consensus Level: 1

Clinical Information. The patient's records must be sufficiently complete to provide reasonable information requested by a subsequent health care provider, insurance company, and/or attorney (e.g., progress notes, SOAP notes, SORE notes). A dated record of what occurred on each visit, and any significant changes in the clinical picture or assessment or treatment plan need to be noted. The method in which chart notes are recorded is a matter of preference for each practitioner.

5.1.16 **Rating:** Necessary
Evidence: Class I, II, III
Consensus Level: 1

There are many different adjusting/manipulation/manual techniques. It is important to record what area was adjusted/manipulated/treated and the procedure used.

5.1.17 **Rating:** Necessary
Evidence: Class II, III
Consensus Level: 1

Anyone other than the attending practitioner who enters data into the contemporaneous chart must initial the entry.

5.1.18 **Rating:** Necessary
Evidence: Class I, II, III
Consensus Level: 1

13. Re-examination/Reassessment:
(See Chapter 9)
All relevant information from every reassessment and re-examination must be recorded in the patient file.

5.1.19 **Rating:** Necessary
Evidence: Class I, II, III
Consensus Level: 1

14. Financial Records
Financial records are important for the business function of a health care facility, and such data are part of the health care record:

- patient account ledgers
- billing statements
- explanation of benefits (EOB) from payers, proof of payment

5.1.20 **Rating:** Necessary
Evidence: Class I, III
Consensus Level: 1

The precise information obtained and the means of storage and retrieval are at the discretion of the chiropractor.

5.1.21 **Rating:** Discretionary
Evidence: Class III
Consensus Level: 1

15. Internal Memoranda Regarding Patient

- patient sign-in sheets
- staff messages (intra-office)
- phone messages and summaries/transcription of phone conversations

5.1.22 **Rating:** Discretionary
Evidence: Class I, III
Consensus Level: 1

B. External Documentation

External documentation includes all records arising from outside the practitioner's office, but also includes any communication with third parties.

1. Direct Correspondence
Correspondence in the form of letters or memoranda that leave the office should have information identifying the practitioner and/or clinic, address, and telephone number and be contemporaneously dated. A copy must always be kept on file.

- introductory letter(s) to or from referring practitioner (DC, MD, etc.)
- general correspondence to or from other practitioners
- general correspondence to or from attorney(s)
- general correspondence to or from patient
- general correspondence to or from various payer groups

5.2.1 **Rating:** Recommended
Evidence: Class II, III
Consensus Level: 1

2. Health Records

- pertinent copies of health records from previous or concurrent health care providers
- special consultative reports
- reports of special diagnostic studies

5.2.2 **Rating:** Recommended
Evidence: Class II, III
Consensus Level: 1

3. Diagnostic Imaging
(See Chapter 2)

- When indicated, a reasonable attempt should be made to obtain recent x-rays (or copies) relevant to the presenting problem of the patient, and summarize and record pertinent information.
- Copies of external radiology reports.

5.2.3 **Rating:** Recommended
Evidence: Class II, III
Consensus Level: 1

4. External Reports

Frequently a practitioner will be required to write various reports. The information for these reports comes from patient records. Adequate reporting usually requires the practitioner to review the patient's history, examination findings, diagnosis, treatment procedures, progress notes/work chart and other reports that may have been written together with records from other health care providers that have treated or evaluated the patient. There are many types of reports that serve various needs. There are many acceptable styles and formats.

> 5.2.4 **Rating:** Recommended
> Evidence: Class II, III
> **Consensus Level: 1**

C. Chart/File Organization

1. General Considerations

Records should be kept in chronological order and entered as contemporaneously as possible. They should not be backdated or altered. Corrections or additions should be dated and initialled. The chart or file should be fully documented and contain all relevant, objective information; extraneous information should not be included. The record must be complete enough to provide the practitioner with information required for subsequent patient care or reporting to outside parties.

> 5.3.1 **Rating:** Necessary
> Evidence: Class I, II, III
> **Consensus Level: 1**

2. Use of Pre-printed Forms

The use of forms can assist in tasks such as obtaining case history, noting examination findings and charting case progress. Use of forms is at the discretion of the individual practitioner but should favor comprehensiveness and completeness rather than brevity.

> 5.3.2 **Rating:** Discretionary
> Evidence: Class II, III
> **Consensus Level: 1**

3. Legibility and Clarity

Health records should be neat, organized and complete. Entries in charts should be written legibly in ink. Entries must not be erased or altered with correction fluid (whiteout) or tape or adhesive labels, etc. If the contents of any document are changed, the practitioner should initial and date such changes in the corresponding margin.

> 5.3.3 **Rating:** Necessary
> Evidence: Class I, II
> **Consensus Level: 1**

4. Use of Abbreviations/Symbols

Use of abbreviations or coding can save record space and time. A legend of the codes or abbreviations should appear on the form or be available in the office in order that another prac-titioner or interested person can interpret and use the information. The legend can also be used for intra-office communications and as a dictation aid.

> 5.3.4 **Rating:** Recommended
> Evidence: Class II, III
> **Consensus Level: 1**

D. Maintenance of Records

1. Confidentiality

The rule of confidentiality requires that all information about a patient gathered by a practitioner as any part of the doctor-patient relationship be kept confidential unless its release is authorized by the patient or is compelled by law. The rule is an ethical responsibility as well as a legal one. Assurance of confidentiality is necessary if individuals are to be open and forthright with the practitioner. Patients rightly expect that such information as their health will remain private and secure from public scrutiny. Thus the principle that all doctor-patient communications are privileged and confidential.

> 5.4.1 **Rating:** Necessary
> Evidence: Class I, II
> **Consensus Level: 1**

2. Records Retention and Retrieval

Health records should be retained, and in a way that facilitates retrieval. To the extent possible, they should be kept in a centralized location. In most circumstances, recent records are maintained on premises either as hard copy or electronically, and after a period of time can be archived, microfilmed or microfiched and placed in storage. The length of time that records, in whatever form, must be kept varies. Many states/provinces have legislated minimum periods of time for retention of health records, usually between five to fifteen years. When the decision is made to dispose of health records, the manner of disposal must protect patient confidentiality. If a chiropractic office closes or changes ownership, secure retention of the health care record must be ensured.

> 5.4.2 **Rating:** Necessary
> Evidence: Class I, II
> **Consensus Level: 1**

Even when legal time limits have elapsed, it is advisable to continue to retain records because of the valuable information they contain.

> 5.4.3 **Rating:** Discretionary
> Evidence: Class III
> **Consensus Level: 1**

3. Administrative Records

Administrative records are primarily those relating to the non-clinical side of practice, but there is some overlap into the doctor/patient relationship. Examples of administrative records may include: telephone logs, schedule and record of appointments, patient personal data information, insurance forms and billing, collection and patient billing, routine correspondence, a record filing system that makes for accurate retrieval of patient data. These records must be maintained in a legible and retrievable format.

5.4.4 **Rating:** Necessary
Evidence: Class I, II, III
Consensus Level: 1

4. Records Transfer

It is mandatory that health care data (excluding data and reports from outside sources) requested by another provider currently treating a present or former patient be forwarded upon receipt of an appropriate request and patient consent. In some jurisdictions, this duty to forward information to another treating health professional is imposed by statute also. However, even in the absence of a statutory requirement a practitioner has a responsibility to comply with such a request, and as expeditiously as possible.

5.4.5 **Rating:** Necessary
Evidence: Class I, II, III
Consensus Level: 1

5. Clinic Staff Responsibilities

The practitioner is responsible for staff actions regarding record keeping and consent forms, and for assuring that administrative tasks are handled correctly and promptly. Any employee involved in the preparation, organization, or filing of records should fully understand professional and legal requirements, including the rules of confidentiality.

5.4.6 **Rating:** Necessary
Evidence: Class I, II, III
Consensus Level: 1

E. Patient Consents

1. Informed Consent/Consent to Treatment - Generally

(See also Chapter 12)

Patient consent to treatment is always necessary. It is often implied rather than expressed. However, where there is risk of significant harm from the treatment proposed, this risk must be disclosed, understood, and accepted by the patient. Such informed consent is required for ethical and legal reasons. The best record of consent is one that is objectively documented (e.g., a witnessed written consent or videotape).

5.5.1 **Rating:** Necessary
Evidence: Class I, II, III
Consensus Level: 1

2. Consent to Treatment - Competence

A patient must be competent to give consent to treatment. The treatment of minors (age of majority varies from 14 to 21 according to jurisdiction) and mentally incompetent adults requires the prior consent of a guardian in most circumstances.

5.5.2 **Rating:** Necessary
Evidence: I, II, III
Consensus Level: 1

3. Authorization to Release Patient Information

With the consent of a competent patient or guardian, records may, and in most situations must, be provided to third parties with a legitimate need for access. The patient consent should not be more than 90 days old, or as provided by law. Whenever health care information is released pursuant to authorization from a patient, documentation of the authorization should be requested and retained (except in some emergencies). If the request is for all or part of the health care record, the original record should never be released, unless compelled by law, only copies. Before the copy chart or other records are sent out, they should be reviewed to make certain they are complete.

5.5.3 **Rating:** Necessary
Evidence: Class I, II, III
Consensus Level: 1

4. Financial Assignments

While financial data is important for the business function of a health care facility, and such records are indeed part of the health care record, the information obtained and the method of acquiring such information is at the discretion of the practitioner. Any alteration of standard fees charged necessitates documentation (e.g, in cases of financial hardship).

5.5.4 **Rating:** Discretionary
Evidence: Class III
Consensus Level: 1

5. Consent to Participate in Research

When a practitioner engages in research, the ethical basis of the doctor-patient relationship changes to an investigator-subject interaction. The new relationship must meet a new set of criteria different from clinical practice.

If a patient is requested to participate in a research study or project the request must be accompanied by informed consent that meets the minimum request for the protection of human subjects as established by competent authorities (e.g., NIH/ NSF or state/provincial law).

5.5.5 **Rating:** Necessary
Evidence: Class I, II, III
Consensus Level: 1

6. Publication/Photo/Video Consent

All records from which a patient may be identified (e.g., photographs, videotapes, audiotapes) should only be created once consent has been obtained. Such consents should identify the purposes of the record and the circumstances under which it will be released.

a. records for clinical management

5.5.6 **Rating:** Recommended
Evidence: Class I, II III
Consensus Level: 1

b. records for all other purposes (e.g., research, training, distribution)

5.5.7 **Rating:** Necessary
Evidence: Class I, II, III
Consensus Level: 1

7. Authority to Admit Observers

Persons not participating in the treatment of the patient should not be permitted to watch examinations or procedures without authorization from the patient. This principle is subject to some exceptions where the patient is a minor.

5.5.8 **Rating:** Necessary
Evidence: Class I, II, III
Consensus Level: 1

VII. COMMENTS, SUMMARY OR CONCLUSION

This chapter presents guidelines for the chiropractic profession in North America with regard to creation and maintenance of a patient chart/file. It is suggested in chiropractic literature [38] that the development of keener clinical awareness and improved patient care are the most important reasons to maintain competent records. Fundamental training of the practitioner in charting skills exists in the educational process, but reinforcement of the need for quality records must come through published literature, postgraduate seminars and risk management efforts.

However, there are additional administrative requirements in health care practice that underline the necessity for sound records maintenance. Today there is a heightened awareness of the need for good records because of accountability of all practitioners in managed care, intraprofessional peer review, and interactive claims management used by public and private sector purchasers. This rapid expansion of clinician accountability underscores the need for mature systems, and dissemination of information on recordkeeping throughout the chiropractic profession. It will be important for the sponsoring organizations of this consensus meeting on standards of practice to take the lead in the dissemination process.

VIII. REFERENCES

1. Baird R: Health record documentation: Charting guidelines. *Dig Chir Econ* 1981; 32-33, July/Aug.

2. Baird R: Confidentiality statements. *Dig Chir Econ* 1986; July/Aug: 60.

3. Baird R: Obtaining health record information. *Dig Chir Econ* 1981; Nov/Dec:137.

4. Bolton SP: Informed consent revisited. *J Aust Chir Assoc* 1990; 20 (4): 135-38.

5. Campbell LK, Ladenheim CJ, Sherman RP, Sportelli L: *Risk Management in Chiropractic*. Virginia Health Services Publications, Ltd. 1990.

6. Carey P: Informed consent - the new reality. *J Can Chir Assoc.* 1998; 32(2): 91-94.

7. Cassidy JD et al.: Medical-chiropractic correspondence-when and how to write effectively. *J Can Chir Assoc* 1985; 29 (1): 29-31.

8. Coulehan JL, Block MR: *The Medical Interview: A Primer for Students of the Art*. F.A. Davis Co., Philadelphia, 1987.

9. Gatterman MI: *Chiropractic Management of Spine Related Disorders*. Baltimore, MD. Williams & Wilkins 1990.

10. Gatterman MI: Standards of practice relative to complications of and contraindications to spinal manipulative therapy. *J Can Chir Assoc* 1991; 35 (4): 232-236.

11. Gledhil SJ: Expert opinion and legal basis of standards of care determination. *J Chir Technique* 1990; 2 (3):94-97.

12. Gotlib AC: The nature of the informed consent doctrine and the chiropractor.*J Can Chir Assoc* 1984; 28(2):272-274.

13. Gotlib AC: The chiropractor and third party access to confidential patient health records. *J Can Chir Assoc* 1984; 28(3):327.

14. Gunderson BV: *The Case History. Orthopedic Brief*. Council on Chiropractic Orthopedics of the American Chiropractic Association. 1989.

15. Haldeman S: Importance of record keeping in the evaluation of chiropractic results. *J Chir* 1975.

16. Hansen DT (ed): *Chiropractic standards and utilization guidelines in the care and treatment of injured workers*. Chiropractic Advisory Committee, Department of Labor & Industries. State of Washington 1988.

17. Hansen DT, Sollecito PC: Standard chart abbreviations in chiropractic practice. *J Chir Technique* 1991; 3(2):96-103.

18. Harrison JD: *Chiropractic Practice Liability: A Practical Guide to Successful Risk Management*. International Chiropractors Association. Arlington, VA. 1991.

19. Harrison JD: Standards of practice. *ICA Review* 1989; (Nov/Dec);45(6):11-13.

20. Huffman EK: *Medical Record Management*. Physician's Record Company. Berwyn, IL. 1972.

21. Hug PR: General consideration of "consent." *J Chiro* (Dec) 1985; 22(12):52-53.

22. Kranz KC: *Chiropractic and Hospital Privileges Protocol*. International Chiropractors Association. Arlington, Virginia 1987.

23. LaBrot TM: *A Standard of Care for the Chiropractic Practice*. Self-published. Phoenix, Arizona. 1990.

24. Lewkovich GN: Progress notes made easier. *Calif Chir J* 1989; July:32-35.

25. MacDonald MG, Meyer DC, Essig B: *Health Care Law: A practical guide*. New York, Matthew Bender & Co. 1986.

26. Michigan Chiropractic Society. *Chiropractic Care and Utilization Review Guidelines*. Lansing, Michigan. 1991.

27. Minnesota Chiropractic Association. *Standard of Practice*. Roseville, MN. 1991.

28. Mootz RD: Chiropractic clinical management and record-keeping. *ICA Review* 1988; 3:56-59.

29. Mootz RD: Interprofessional referral protocol. *Today's Chir* 1989; 16(4):37-39.

30. Murkowski K, Semlow DG: *Doctor's Guidebook to Risk Management*. Self-published. Associated Practice Liability Consultants. Jackson, Michigan 1986.

31. Nixdorf D: Current standards of material risk. *J Can Chir Assoc.* 1990; 34(2):87-89.

32. Nyiendo JA, Haldeman S: A critical study of the student interns' practice activities in a chiropractic college teaching clinic. *J Manip Physiol Ther* 1986; 9(3):197-207.

33. Ohio State Chiropractic Association. *The Chiropractic Manual for Insurance Claims Personnel*. Columbus, OH. 1990.

34. Olson RE: *Chiropractic/Physical Therapy Treatment Standards: A Reference Guide.* Data Management Ventures, Inc. Atlanta, GA. 1987.

35. Oxford G: Progress notes: Keeping track of patients. *Am Chir* 1988; March:26-33.

36. Peyser MD (ed): *Chiropractic and the HMO environment in Connecticut.* Connecticut Chiropractic Association. 1985.

37. Polit DF, Hungler BP: *Nursing Research Principles and Methods.* J.B. Lippincott, Philadelphia.

38. Reinke T, Jahn W: Commentary: Preventing legal suicide with medical records. *J Manip Physiol Ther* 1988; 11(6):511-513.

39. Rothman EH: *Manual of Narrative Report Writing. Chiropractic on paper: recordkeeping and the narrative report.* Self-published. Western States Chiropractic College. Portland, OR.

40. St. Paul Fire and Marine Ins. Co. Defensible Documentation. *Physical Therapy Today* 1991; Spring:62-63.

41. Schafer RC (ed): *Basic Chiropractic Procedural Manual.* American Chiropractic Association. Des Moines, IA. 1978: V4-10.

42. Schafer RC: *Chiropractic Physicians Guide: Clinical Malpractice.* National Chiropractic Mutual Insurance Company, Des Moines, IA. 1983.

43. Schafer RC: *Chiropractic Paraprofessional Manual.* American Chiropractic Association. Des Moines, Iowa. 1978.

44. Simmons DF: *The Chiropracto-Legal Story.* Self-published. Tacoma, WA. 1973.

45. Strachan G: Chiropractic physician records: Essential for defense and new practice areas. *DC TRACTS* 1990; 2(6):315-321.

46. Thomas MM: Chiropractic research and the I.R.B. *J Chiropractic* 1987; 6:60-63.

47. Turnbull G: Peer Review: an outline. NZ *Chir J.*

IX. MINORITY OPINIONS

None

Clinical Impression

Chapter Outline

I. OVERVIEW

This chapter will consider the use of the concepts of a "clinical impression," "diagnosis," and "analysis" in the practice of chiropractic.

The concept of diagnosis has been a matter of significant historical debate. The application of diagnosis in chiropractic practice, the perspective of the practitioner relative to diagnosis, and the diagnostic responsibility of the practitioner have varied with respect to state laws, board regulations, and court rulings.

While the exact language may vary, it is clear, however, that the practitioner is dealing with the process of conveying the salient findings of his or her examination relative to the patient in question. The consequence of the diagnosis, clinical impression, or analysis impacts directly on the management of the patient.

Guidelines for quality assurance and standards of practice are expressed and understood within historical, legal and professional perspectives of the profession. In addition, standards must be developed to reflect the advancement in the quality of chiropractic care, the protection of the patient and the continuing process of assessment of effectiveness.

II. DEFINITIONS

Diagnosis: A decision regarding the nature of the patient's complaint; the art or act of identifying a disease or condition from its signs and symptoms.

Clinical Impression: A working hypothesis formulated from significant items in the history and the physical findings; a tentative diagnosis; or a working diagnosis.

Differential Diagnosis: The determination of which one of two or more complaints or conditions a patient is suffering from by systematically comparing and contrasting their clinical findings.

Analysis: The act of separating into component parts the clinical evaluation of a condition or disease in order to identify the clinical impression or determine the diagnosis.

Utility: Significant benefit to both the patient and clinician resulting from a reduction in uncertainty of the diagnosis, clinical impression, or analysis.

Portal of Entry: First level of contact with and intake into the health delivery system.

III. LIST OF SUBTOPICS

A. **Necessity**
B. **Initial Responsibility**
C. **Subsequent Responsibility**
D. **Terminology**
E. **Content**
F. **Process**
G. **Dynamics**
H. **Communication**

IV. LITERATURE REVIEW

Information regarding the evolution of concepts of diagnosis, clinical impression, or analysis has been available from the writings of early chiropractic pioneers [Palmer, D.D.;[2] Palmer, B.J.;[3] Firth[4]] through to current chiropractic experts.[1,8-23] It has also been described in a legislative framework.[23-30]

Chiropractic Analysis

The concept of chiropractic analysis as something unique and distinct from a diagnosis was expressed as early as 1910 by Palmer[2] and 1916 by Firth.[4] The term has continued to be used in this way by various members of the profession.[7,31] The commonality in its use is based on the concept that structure, primarily the spine, affects function.[3,4,5,6,7,9]

Chiropractic analysis can also be viewed in more general terms as the process of reaching a clinical impression or diagnosis. This incorporates the complete art of clinical decision-making.[1,34]

Diagnosis

Like chiropractic analysis, the term diagnosis has been defined in differing ways in chiropractic practice. As with many practitioners today, D.D. Palmer accepted the importance and necessity of making a diagnosis. His definition of diagnosis was not so dissimilar to that presented above, namely, "determining the character of disease; also the decision arrived at, is diagnosis."[2]

In earlier years, when legislation was not enacted, members of the chiropractic profession were accused of practicing medicine without a license when they treated patients after arriving at a diagnosis. Thus "diagnosis" was replaced with the term "analysis." This alteration may have been made for the following reasons: 1) to avoid prosecution; and 2) to make chiropractic a separate and distinct profession with no allegiance to medicine.[16]

As a portal of entry provider, the chiropractic practitioner is charged with certain responsibilities, legal and professional, and possesses certain rights and privileges shared by all doctors. The courts have not concerned themselves with which words a practitioner elects to use to describe a diagnostic situation but rather have strived to protect the public.[24,25] Therefore, the issue of diagnosis, clinical impression, or analysis is paramount for the reason that it is necessary prior to the implementation of an appropriate plan of care.

The purpose of a diagnosis as described in legislative acts, government commission hearings and the literature is two-fold: 1) to identify the problem to determine if it is amenable to chiropractic care, and 2) to determine if the patient should be referred. [1,13,18,20,21,24,25]

The process of arriving at a diagnosis depends upon logic and reasoning,[1,14] and includes the evaluation of information obtained from the interview, examination and diagnostic procedures. The methods used in the gathering and analysis of information are beyond the scope of this review but can be found in many sources among them are Jamison[1] and Weinstein and Fineberg.[37] (See also Chapter 5 of these guidelines.) This culminates in a clinical decision making process from which a diagnosis, clinical impression, or analysis is made concerning the disease or condition affecting the patient. Gitelman presents the concept of a double diagnosis. This double diagnosis takes into consideration firstly the articular dysfunction, secondly its influence upon the patient's general well-being and broader symptom complex.[15,36]

Regardless of the variety of views, the state of the art with respect to diagnosis is that which is currently described in the literature. This includes case reports published in reputable scientific journals, as an avenue by which chiropractic establishes the spectrum of conditions that its members are responsible for diagnosing.[33]

In perusing the standardized channels of literature review for the application of the concepts of diagnosis, it is important to note that case studies abound in chiropractic literature. In JMPT alone, over the last 14 years there have been 90 case reports. Although subluxation is mentioned in some of those reports as a portion of the diagnosis, additional diagnoses are used to describe the patients or conditions.

The significance of diagnostic responsibility is emphasized in statements contained within the Clinical Quality Assurance Guidelines of the CCE,[19] the Policy Guidelines of the International Chiropractors' Association,[40] the Consensus Report of the American Chiropractic Association Council on Technique[32] and the guidelines of the Canadian Chiropractic Protective Association, an agency of the Canadian Chiropractic Association.[35]

Application of Diagnostic or Analytical Concepts

Williams,[11] Slosberg,[10] Winterstein,[12] and Masarsky and Weber [38] have all attempted to address the question of the role of diagnosis from the point of view of the practicing chiropractor. Harrison[27] and Sportelli, et. al.,[28] have addressed the issue from the perspective of legal necessity as a component of legal defense. Herfert [39] has addressed the question from the perspective of the relationship with third party payers.

It is clear that all of these authors advocate acceptance of the diagnostic responsibility of the chiropractic profession.

The concern remains for the appropriate use of language and the context of a diagnostic statement. Choice of language — diagnosis, clinical impression, analyses or assessment — reflects the clinician's philosophical constructs. There is, however, uniformity regarding the need for appropriate, responsible steps to be taken on the patients' behalf, regardless of the paradigm, to establish the clinical findings of each individual practitioner. It is the right of the patient to receive an appropriate evaluation and statement of their problem as a prerequisite for delivery of care.

The ethical, moral, legal and professional responsibility of a chiropractic practitioner does not change with the terminology used to express his or her clinical findings. The practitioner is required to assess the patient on presentation and respond to the clinical situation in a manner consistent with the best interests of the patient and the practitioner's clinical judgment.

V. ASSESSMENT CRITERIA

Procedure Ratings (System II)

Necessary: Strong positive recommendations based on Class I evidence, or overwhelming Class II evidence when circumstances reflect compromise of patient safety.

Recommended: Positive recommendation, based on consensus Class II and/or strong Class III evidence.

Discretionary: Positive recommendation, based on consensus of Class III evidence.

Unnecessary: Negative recommendation, based on inconclusive or conflicting Class II, III evidence.

Quality of Evidence

The following categories of evidence are used to support the ratings:

Class I:

  A. Evidence of clinical utility from controlled studies published in refereed journals.
  B. Binding or strongly persuasive legal authority such as legislation or case law.

Class II:

  A. Evidence of clinical utility from the significant results of uncontrolled studies in refereed journals.
  B. Evidence provided by recommendations from published expert legal opinion or persuasive case law.

Class III:

  A. Evidence of clinical utility provided by opinions of experts, anecdote and/or convention.
  B. Expert legal opinion.

VI. RECOMMENDATIONS

A. Necessity

Arrival at a clinical impression or diagnosis, or diagnostic conclusion or analysis, is a necessary outcome of the patient encounter.

Comment: The responsibility of a chiropractic practitioner does not change with the terminology used to describe clinical findings. The practitioner is required to assess the patient upon presentation and respond to the clinical situation in a manner consistent with the best interests of the patient, the practitioner's clinical judgment, and the law of the jurisdiction in question.

6.1.1 **Rating:** Necessary
Evidence: Class I, II, III
Consensus Level: 1

B. Initial Responsibility

The initial level of responsibility of the practitioner involves the immediate discernment as to the nature and status of the patient on initial presentation. A practitioner should be expected to recognize and respond to life-threatening situations in a manner consistent with the patient's best interest.

6.2.1 **Rating:** Necessary
Evidence: Class I, II, III
Consensus Level: 1

C. Subsequent Responsibility

After the initial evaluation has been completed the practitioner begins a series of differentiations that result in many clinical decisions being implemented. This process is not an end in itself, but merely designates suspected conditions that become the focus for prognostic judgments, further assessment and patient management. Initiation of chiropractic care, additional studies, referral with or without continuing chiropractic care and cessation of chiropractic care are possible.

6.3.1 **Rating:** Necessary
Evidence: Class I, II, III
Consensus Level: 1

D. Terminology

The terminology utilized to describe a clinical impression, diagnosis, diagnostic conclusion, or analysis should be consistent with appropriate usage in chiropractic (e.g., subluxation complex/fixation/misalignment) and related health care communities. If a practitioner is required to use specific terminology, or is prohibited from the use of such terminology by law, then that legal requirement is the guiding factor.

6.4.1 **Rating:** Recommended
Evidence: Class II, III
Consensus Level: 1

E. Content

1. Patients may have various conditions/symptoms/findings that result in a number of unrelated clinical impressions. The primary clinical impression, diagnosis, diagnostic conclusion, or analysis should address the chief complaint expressed by the patient. Secondary diagnoses should be prioritized and addressed as needed and may be of greater clinical consequence to the patient.

6.5.1 **Rating:** Recommended
Evidence: Class II, III
Consensus Level: 1

2. The clinical impression, diagnosis, diagnostic conclusion, or analysis should reflect a classification scheme that consists of statements reflective of severity, region, and organ/tissue involvement.

6.5.2 **Rating:** Recommended
Evidence: Class II, III
Consensus Level: 1

3. The clinical impression, diagnosis, diagnostic conclusion or analysis should be related to the subjective and/or objective findings of the patient, and be consistent with evidence-based criteria.

6.5.3 **Rating:** Established
Evidence: Class I, II, III
Consensus Level: 1

F. Process

1. When additional confirmatory tests are required to establish the clinical impression, diagnosis, diagnostic conclusion, or analysis it is the practitioner's responsibility to ensure that these studies are completed in as timely and efficient a manner as possible. Practitioners may perform such procedures consistent with their qualifications and the law, or they may seek to have such procedures performed by other qualified parties.

6.6.1 **Rating:** Necessary
Evidence: Class I, II, III
Consensus Level: 1

2. Where procedures relevant to a diagnosis, clinical impression, diagnostic conclusion, or analysis are not within the qualifications or competence of a practitioner, the practitioner should make appropriate consultations with others.

6.6.2 **Rating:** Recommended
Evidence: Class II, III
Consensus Level: 1

3. The clinical impression, diagnosis, diagnostic conclusion, or analysis should be recorded in the patient's record and qualified as to its certainty.

6.6.3 **Rating**: Necessary
Evidence: Class I, II, III
Consensus Level: 1

G. Dynamics

The clinical impression, diagnosis, diagnostic conclusion, or analysis should be a working hypothesis that may change over time, given additional information and/or changes in the condition of the patient.

6.7.1 **Rating**: Necessary
Evidence: Class I, II, III
Consensus Level: 1

H. Communication

The practitioner should communicate the diagnosis or clinical impression or diagnostic conclusion or analysis, and its significance, to the patient in understandable terms, and convey such findings to other providers or agencies as the patient requests and consents to, or as the law requires.

6.8.1 **Rating**: Necessary
Evidence: Class I, II, III
Consensus Level: 1

VII. COMMENTS, SUMMARY OR CONCLUSION

None.

VIII. REFERENCES

1. Jamison JR: Diagnostic Decision Making in Clinical Practice, *Seminars in Chiropractic* 1991, 2: 1-128, 2.

2. Palmer DD: *The Science, Art, and Philosophy of Chiropractic*, Portland, published by the author, 1910.

3. Palmer BJ: *The Science of Chiropractic*, 1920, Davenport, Iowa, Palmer School of Chiropractic.

4. Firth JN: *Chiropractic Symptomology*, Indianapolis, published by the author, 1919.

5. Firth JN: *Chiropractic Diagnosis*, Indianapolis, published by author, 1929.

6. Firth JN: *A Textbook of Chiropractic Diagnosis*, Indianapolis, published by the author, 1948.

7. Dinetenfass J: A Question of Diagnosis: The Acceptance of Chiropractic Analysis in New York State, 1963, *Chiropractic History*,1989; 9 (2).

8. Schafer RC: *Physical Diagnosis*, Arlington, VA, The American Chiropractic Association, 1988.

9. Smallie P: *Chiropractic Diagnosis*, Stockton, World Wide Books, 1980.

10. Slosberg M: Understanding the role of diagnosis within the scope of chiropractic. *The Digest of Chiropractic Economics*, January/February, 1984.

11. Williams S: *Chiropractic Science and Practice in the United States*, Arlington, The International Chiropractors Association, 1991.

12. Winterstein, JF. Options. *Outreach: National College of Chiropractic*, 1990 March; VI (3): 1.

13. Maxwell TD: Our diagnostic responsibility as a primary contact profession. *J Can Chirop Assoc* June 16-17, 1975.

14. Engel GL, Morgan WL: *Interviewing the Patient*. Philadelphia; WB Saunders, 1973.

15. Gitelman R: A chiropractic approach to biomechanical disorders of the lumbar spine and pelvis, in Haldeman, S (ed) *Modern Developments in the Principles and Practice of Chiropractic*. New York, Appleton-Century-Crofts, 1980.

16. Beech RA: Some thoughts about diagnosis. *Swiss Annals* 196 iv: 27-31.

17. Janse J: *Principles and Practice of Chiropractic: an Anthology*. Hildebrandt, RW (ed) Lombard, National College of Chiropractic, 1976.

18. Chiropractic in New Zealand, *Report of the Commission of Inquiry*. Government Printer, Wellington, 1979.

19. Council on Chiropractic Education, *Clinical Competency Document*. Clinical Quality Assurance Panel, Oct. 1, 1989.

20. Jaquet P: The importance of laboratory methods in chiropractic diagnosis. *Swiss Annals* 1971; V: 215-229.

21. Jaquet P: *An Introduction to Clinical Chiropractic*, 2nd ed., Geneva,Jaquet and Grounauer, 1974.

22. Jamison JR: Science in chiropractic clinical practice: identifying a need. *J Manip Physiol Ther*, June 1991; 14(5): 298-304.

23. MacDonald B, Cordry D: Development of a grand rounds program. *Journal of Chiropractic Education*, March 1991; 4(4): 115-121.

24. Gledhill SJ: Expert opinion and legal basis of standards of care determination. *Chiropractic Technique* 1990; 2(3): 94-97.

25. Hirtle RL: Chiropractic Jurisprudence and Malpractice Considerations, in Vear (ed), *Chiropractic Standards of Practice and Quality of Care*, Gaithersburg, Aspen 1991: 239-252.

26. Foreman SM, Stahl MJ: Medico-Legal Issues in Chiropractic, in *Seminars in Chiropractic*. Lawrence DJ, Foreman SM (eds), Summer 1990 1 (3); Baltimore: Williams and Wilkins.

27. Harrison J: *Chiropractic practice liability*. Arlington, The International Chiropractors Association, 1990.

28. Sportelli L, et al.: *Risk Management in Chiropractic*, Fincastle, VA, Health Services Publications, Ltd., 1990.

29. Attorney General vs. Beno: Docket No. 72852, Argued October 3, 1984 (Calendar No. 8) Decided August 27, 1985.

30. Lamm, Lester C: Chiropractic Scope of Practice: What the Law Allows. *American Journal of Chiropractic Medicine*, December 1989; 2(4): S-14 - S-15.

31. Levine M: Chiropractic analysis vs. medical diagnosis. *ACA Journal of Chiropractic*, February, 1967.

32. Panel of Advisors, ACA Council on Technique, Chiropractic Terminology: A Report, *ACA Journal of Chiropractic*, 1988, 46-57.

33. Lawrence DJ: Fourteen years of case reports, editorial, *J Manip Physiol Ther*, 1991; 14: 447-449.

34. Hansen DT: Quality of Care and Chiropractic Necessities, in *Chiropractic Standards of Practice and Quality of Care*, Vear, HT (ed) Gaithersburg, Aspen, 1991; 85-113.

35. Janse, Joseph, *Chiropractic Principles and Technic: for use by students and practitioners*, National College of Chiropractic, 1947.

36. Gatterman MI: *Chiropractic Management of Spine Related Disorders*. Baltimore, Williams and Wilkins, 1990.

37. Weinstein MC, Fineberg HV. *Clinical decision analysis.* Philadelphia, Saunders, 1980.

38. Masarsky, Charles, Weber, Marion: Stop paradigm erosion. *J Manip Physiol Ther*, June 1991; 14 (5): 323-326.

39. Herfert R: *Communicating the Vertebral Subluxation Complex*, published by the author, 1986.

40. *Policy Handbook and Code of Ethics.* International Chiropractors Association, Arlington, Virginia, April, 1991.

41. *Information/Risk Managment Manual.* Canadian Chiropractic Protective Association, Toronto, Canada, 1991.

IX. MINORITY OPINIONS

None.

7

Modes of Care

Chapter Outline

I. OVERVIEW

This chapter provides a generic topical summary of typical chiropractic procedures in current use. Most chiropractic named technique procedures consist of a combination of various analytic and treatment components. This chapter does not serve to review and pass judgment on any particular named technique system as a whole. Rather, generic procedures are presented and ratings are made based on current available information and expert opinion. Clinical practice and scientific investigation are ongoing processes and it is understood that this document is a dynamic entity that will require modification as new knowledge becomes available.

Although this chapter does not include every possible chiropractic technique or procedure, an overall categorization of chiropractic approaches is presented. Chiropractic procedures are categorized according to the Bartol algorithm that has been recommended by the American Chiropractic Association's Council on Technique and has been adopted as a template for consensus development by the Consortium for Chiropractic Research. In addition, a more elaborate classification system is presented here for the non-manual chiropractic procedures.

II. DEFINITIONS

A. Chiropractic Adjustment

Chiropractic Adjustment: This term refers to a wide variety of manual and mechanical interventions that may be high or low velocity; short or long lever; high or low amplitude; with or without recoil. Procedures are usually directed at specific joints or anatomic regions. An adjustment may or may not involve the cavitation or gapping of a joint (opening of a joint within its paraphysiologic zone usually producing a characteristic audible "click" or "pop"). The common denominator for the various adjustive interventions is the concept of removing structural dysfunctions of joints and muscles that are associated with neurologic alterations. The chiropractic profession refers to this concept as a "subluxation." This use of the word subluxation should not be confused with the term's precise anatomic usage which considers only the anatomical relationships.

B. Manipulation and Mobilization

During joint motion, three barriers or end ranges to movement can be identified. The first is the active end range which occurs when the patient has maximally contracted muscles controlling a joint in a particular directional vector. At this point, the clinician can passively move the joint toward a second barrier called the passive end range. Movement up to this barrier is termed physiologic joint space. Beyond this point, the practitioner can move the joint into its paraphysiologic space. The third barrier encountered is the anatomic end range. Movement beyond this will result in rupture of the joint's ligaments.

Manipulation: Passive movement of short amplitude and high-velocity which moves the joint into the paraphysiologic range. This is accompanied by cavitation or gapping of the joint which results in an intrasynovial vacuum phenomenon thought to involve gas separating from fluid. Usually accompanied by an audible pop or click, manipulation has been shown to result in increased joint motion compared to mobilization alone. This increase in motion lasts for a 20-30 minute refractory period during which an additional cavitation of the same joint will not occur. Manipulation is a passive dynamic thrust that causes cavitation and attempts to increase the manipulated joint's range of motion.

Mobilization: Passive movement within the physiologic joint space administered by a clinician for the purpose of increasing overall range of joint motion.

C. Descriptors of Adjustment, Manipulation, Mobilization

Amplitude: Amplitude refers to the depth of, or distance traveled by, the practitioner's thrust. Most adjustment/manipulation is of low amplitude, minimizing total force applied to the patient. When placing a joint in position prior to treatment the practitioner pre-stresses the joint in the appropriate direction to take up soft-tissue slack (joint play). When joints are less accessible and/or involve a longer lever contact, or when inadequate pre-stress is obtained, amplitude will necessarily increase.

Dynamic Thrust (Thrust): The therapeutic force or maneuver delivered by the practitioner during manipulation and most adjustment techniques. It is typically a high-velocity, low-amplitude movement applied to a joint when all joint play has been passively removed. It may be applied with follow through, which means that the end amplitude of the thrust is briefly maintained, or it may be applied with recoil. This means that once the end amplitude is reached the thrust is immediately withdrawn. There are low-velocity thrust techniques, but all thrusts involve some element of rapid acceleration.

Force: The product of the amplitude and velocity applied during a thrust. An adjustment or manipulation may be very fast (high velocity) but of extremely low-amplitude, and in these circumstances the force will be relatively low.

Joint Play (Accessory Movement): The small, precise joint movements, not under the control of the voluntary muscles or patient, that are necessary to permit normal voluntary joint movement. Joint play may include spin, glide and roll of the articulation. The full range of active movement of a joint without practitioner assistance is a combination of voluntary movement (voluntary muscles) and joint play.

Lever: During manual joint manipulation there are a variety of mechanical factors considered including the practitioner's contact points, stabilization points, fulcrums of movement, specific features of the joint to be manipulated, particular vectors, etc. Depending on which joint or motion segment is addressed, the stabilization and contact points selected, and a patient's position, biomechanical leverage considerations can become quite complex. For the sake of simplification and communication, descriptors of leverage can be defined as follows.

Long-lever Contacts: those in which joints and structures not primarily involved in the procedure are positioned between the practitioner's contact point and the adjusted or manipulated joint. For example, an adjustment of the right sacroiliac (SI) joint with a contact on the ischium is considered short-lever because there are no articulations between the contact point and the SI joint. However, an adjustment of the L5/SI facet using the same contact is long-lever because the SI joint is located between the contact and the L5/SI facet joint.

Short-lever Contacts: those which involve contacts and stabilizations on osseous structures directly involved in the joint being manipulated.

Line of Drive (Vector): The direction of thrust, usually described in terms of the three cardinal planes of skeletal motion: 1. Flexion/Extension, 2. Right/Left Rotation, 3. Right/Left Lateral Flexion. As manipulation of a joint may be both difficult and uncomfortable when a joint is in a compressed or close-packed position, nearly all adjustive or manipulative maneuvers include axial distraction as part of the pre-stress. For this reason, this vector is usually omitted but implied in descriptions of thrust.

Pre-Stress: The process in which, prior to manipulation, a joint is moved passively to its end range, controlling joint play. The joint is near the limit of its passive end range.

Velocity (Acceleration): The speed with which a thrust is delivered. This term is strictly incorrect because a thrust does not maintain a constant velocity but rather changes speed constantly. However, thrusts are commonly described as "high-velocity" or "low-velocity" and these relative terms are useful.

D. Soft Tissue Procedures

There are a variety of techniques for manual soft tissue procedures, some unique to chiropractic practitioners. As muscles and non-contractile structures lose function and elasticity, they have an effect on joint function. Most soft tissues are richly innervated with a variety of proprioceptive mechanisms, and often chiropractic application of soft tissue procedures will follow a traditional chiropractic rationale of at-tempting to improve a clinically identifiable aberrant neurologic reflex or pain pattern. Such work may be used in conjunction with other adjustive or manipulative approaches. Some chiropractors use a variety of soft tissue procedures for non-articular purposes as well. For example, abdominal pressure points may be stimulated in a constipated patient.

E. Descriptors of Some Common Soft Tissue Procedures

Contract-Relax: Application of a combination of active and passive muscle tightening and stretching.

Ischemic Compression (Acupressure, Shiatzu, Myotherapy)**:** Application of a progressively increasing pressure on a pressure point, trigger point, or tight muscle. This typically reduces the point's tenderness and produces a flushing and a relaxation of tightness.

Massage: Application of pressure to a tight muscle in an attempt to relax it. Similar procedures may be used in other soft tissues. There are many specific procedures such as effluerage, petrissage, cross-friction, and J-stroking, along with certain techniques that may be used.

Passive Stretch (Spray and Stretch)**:** Application of a lengthening force along a muscle by passive movement of the associated joint(s). Sometimes used with a distractor such as a coolant spray or ice prior to applying the stretch.

F. Neuromusculoskeletal Conditions:

For the purposes of this document, conditions which display symptoms and/or signs related to two or more of the nervous, muscular and skeletal body systems. Such conditions may be contrasted with those which produce advanced pathologic states (e.g., neurofibromatosis). Neuromusculoskeletal conditions are sometimes referred to as "type M disorders," and distinguished from "type O disorders," which refer to internal organ disorders.

III. LIST OF SUBTOPICS

A. Manual, Articular Manipulative and Adjustive Procedures
   1. Specific Contact Thrust Procedures
   2. Nonspecific Contact Thrust Procedures
   3. Manual Force, Mechanically Assisted Procedures
   4. Mechanical Force, Manually Assisted Procedures

B. Manual, Nonarticular Manipulative and Adjustive Procedures
   1. Manual Reflex and Muscle Relaxation Procedures
   2. Miscellaneous Procedures

C. Nonmanual Procedures
1. Exercise and Rehabilitation
2. Education Procedures
3. Electrical Modalities
4. Thermal Modalities
5. Ultraviolet
6. Ultrasound and Phonophoresis
7. Bracing, Casts, and Supports
8. Traction

D. Special Interest Areas
1. Manipulation under Sedation/Anesthesia
2. Acupuncture
3. Homeopathic Remedies

IV. LITERATURE REVIEW

Specific literature on named chiropractic techniques has traditionally been proprietary and procedurally oriented. In addition, it has rarely been peer reviewed or indexed, which makes access difficult. This problem has been addressed in recent years by the chiropractic profession primarily through three vehicles.

Firstly, the *Journal of Chiropractic Technique* was established to provide a forum for articles relevant to chiropractic procedures. Secondly, a number of discussions, position papers and round tables have been sponsored by professional associations. The Consortium for Chiropractic Research, in collaboration with the Council on Technique and others, held a series of consensus conferences attended by technique teachers, academicians, chiropractic researchers, and private practitioners. See, for example, the proceedings of the 1990 Seattle Consensus Conference (Bergman 1990). Thirdly, a sophisticated standards of care project has been undertaken jointly by the RAND Corporation, the Consortium for Chiropractic Research, and the Foundation for Chiropractic Education and Research (Shekelle, et al., 1991a, Shekelle et al., 1991b).

These efforts have resulted in a number of helpful developments. At the state level, one of the first methodical publications attempting to describe chiropractic management in some detail was a set of standards of practice guidelines developed in Washington (Hansen, 1988). This provides a variety of recommended guidelines and practices for the delivery of chiropractic care in the management of industrial injuries in Washington state. Of particular note are the definitions regarding types of care, abstracts of literature relevant to manipulation, and clinical practice objectives.

Kaminski (1987) proposed an algorithm for the classification of chiropractic procedures, using the classifications "fully accepted," "provisionally accepted" and "unsubstantiated." This algorithm provides general guidelines for the review of procedures based on the reasonableness of the models, utility in practice and scientific investigation. This algorithm was adopted at subsequent consensus conferences and, in modified form, serves as the template for the rating of techniques in this chapter.

The organizational scheme for the classification of chiropractic techniques that is used here is based on Bartol's model (1991a, 1991b), which has been adopted by the ACA Council on Technique. The classification for nonmanual chiropractic approaches is expanded. There are some differences in specific categorization methods as well.

The reader is directed to Greenman (1989), Cox (1990), White & Anderson (1991), Schafer (1984), Haldeman (1992), and Grieve (1989) for in-depth discussions of particular manipulative approaches and more comprehensive references. With respect to information on ancillary procedures, Schafer (1984) provides a review of protocols adopted by the American Chiropractic Association.

Manipulative and adjustive procedures are currently in growing and widespread use, with the chiropractic profession having the most comprehensive training and practice in this field. Manipulative care has been shown to have value for a variety of ailments, but studies of patients seeking chiropractic care suggest that painful conditions of the spine and extremities are by far the leading symptoms presented (Nyiendo, 1989, Phillips, in press). Exact mechanisms of action in spinal adjustment and manipulation remain uncertain but result in mechanical, neurological, trophic and psychosocial effects (Mootz, 1992, Stonebrink, 1990).

There are over 30 randomized trials in the literature comparing manipulation and mobilization to other forms of treatment for low-back pain (Shekelle, et al. 1991a, Anderson, et al., 1992). The majority show manipulation to be more effective than the many interventions to which it has been compared. A few of the studies found no significant differences. In no studies has manipulation been shown to be less effective than other comparison approaches or a control group. There have also been a small number of trials on manipulation for other musculoskeletal conditions such as headache, neck pain, and thoracic pain, which have shown promising outcomes (Parker, 1978, see review by Meeker, 1990). The recent recommendations of the North American Spine Society's Ad Hoc Committee on Diagnostic and Therapeutic Procedures has rated chiropractic adjustment as an established procedure for mechanical low back pain (NASS, 1991).

Some studies have demonstrated the utility of thoracic manipulation in relieving pain associated with angina pectoris (Rogers, 1976, Rinzler, 1948, see review by Mootz, 1992). However, it was not clear whether patients had true angina or suffered from a referred costo-thoracic syndrome that mimicked the pain of angina. There are published case studies suggesting successful management of enuresis with spinal adjustment. However, a recent study, which confirmed some positive response rate, did not find a success rate that matched other behavioral medicine regimens (Leboeuf, 1991).

Another comparative study evaluated chiropractic dynamic thrust adjustment with typical medical management of asthma patients (Bronfort, 1989). This study, which employed a crossover design, showed that patients in both treatment groups obtained a beneficial initial response. However, long-term success rates were better in the medically managed group, even after crossover into the alternative treatment group.

There is evidence that adjustment stimulates certain metabolic activity within some types of white blood cells (Brennen, 1990). There is also preliminary evidence suggesting a relationship between adjustment and serum beta-endorphin levels and other circulating pituitary hormones (Vernon, 1989). A randomized controlled study on a small number of patients with elevated blood pressure demonstrated a significant reduction in posttreatment blood pressure for subjects adjusted in the thoracic spine employing an Activator adjusting instrument (Yates, 1988).

There is a paucity of information in the literature comparing one manual approach to another. Even in the area of low-back pain, where there are now over thirty trials, only a few authors have clearly defined the specific manipulative intervention employed. Usually it is unclear whether adjustment, manipulation, mobilization or a combination of these has been used. Hence it is beyond the scope of this chapter, and capabilities of the contributors, to consider individual conditions and interventions and exact appropriateness. Rather, procedures are presented on a basis of generic categorizations, with discussion regarding utility for specific conditions only where this is possible and appropriate.

The exact number of named chiropractic techniques is thought to be about 200. However, there is a great deal of overlap, and a number of techniques involve only minor modifications of others. Additionally, many named techniques have both analytical and therapeutic components. Only the treatment portions of technique procedures are presented here. Analysis and other diagnostic considerations are discussed in other chapters (see History and Physical Examination, Diagnostic Imaging, Clinical Laboratory, Clinical Impression, Frequency of Care, and Outcomes Assessment).

Exercise has been the subject of a number of clinical trials and was recently the subject of meta-analysis which showed most exercise regimens to be far less consistent in beneficial effects than studies on manipulation (Koes, et al., 1991; Anderson, 1992). However, many exercise and education protocols are in widespread use and considered standard approaches within the medical community (White and Anderson, 1991, Mayer and Gatchell, 1987). Physiotherapeutic modalities are relatively standardized (Schaefer, 1984, Stonebrink, 1990) and are generally used as ancillary procedures in chiropractic practice.

Manipulation under anesthesia or sedation (MUA) has been traditionally performed by allopathic and osteopathic practitioners. With inclusion in hospitals in recent years, some chiropractic practitioners are now trained to perform these procedures in the hospital setting. There is one randomized controlled trial (Siehl, 1971) and at least six clinical reports (Francis, 1989; Krumhansl, 1986; Morey, 1976; Morey, 1973; Rumney, 1968; Siehl, 1963) in the literature describing the results of MUA and suggesting it can be an effective procedure upon carefully selected patients. These patients usually have specific neuromusculoskeletal disorders and fail to respond to conservative treatments, including manipulation, in the hospital or office setting. Force required during MUA is usually less than during adjustment or manipulation without anesthesia. Both high-velocity and low-velocity maneuvers are used. There is, however, less patient feedback and control.

V. ASSESSMENT CRITERIA

Note: The Kaminski algorithm (1987) was proposed for the purpose of allowing technique developers and colleges to determine the current state of development of chiropractic procedures. Kaminski's categories have been revised and an expanded scale is used here to allow for greater consensus and expert input.

Procedure Ratings (System I)

Established: Accepted as appropriate by the practicing chiropractic community for the given indication in the specified patient population.

Promising: Given current knowledge, this appears to be appropriate for the given indication in the specified patient population. As more evidence and experience accumulates, this interim rating will change. This connotes provisional acceptance, but permits a greater role for the current level of clinical use.

Equivocal: Current knowledge exists to support a given indication in a specified patient population, though its value can neither be confirmed nor denied. As more evidence and experience accumulates this interim rating will change. Expert opinion recognizes a need for caution in general application.

Investigational: Evidence is insufficient to determine appropriateness. Further study is warranted. Use for a given indication in a specified patient population should be confined to research protocols. As more evidence and experience accumulates this interim rating will change.

Doubtful: Given current knowledge, this appears to be inappropriate for the given indication in the specified patient population. As more evidence and experience accumulates this interim rating will change.

Inappropriate: Regarded by the practicing chiropractic community as unacceptable for the given indication in a specified patient population.

Quality of Evidence:

The following categories of evidence are used to support the ratings.

Class I:

Evidence provided by one or more well-designed controlled clinical trials; or well-designed experimental studies that address reliability, validity, positive predictive value, discriminability, sensitivity, and specificity.

Class II:

Evidence provided by one or more well-designed uncontrolled, observational clinical studies, such as case-control, cohort studies, etc.; or clinically relevant basic science studies that address reliability, validity, positive predictive value, discriminability, sensitivity, and specificity; and published in refereed journals.

Class III:

Evidence provided by expert legal opinion, descriptive studies or case reports.

Suggested Strength of Recommendations Ratings

Type A. Strong positive recommendation. Based on Class I evidence or overwhelming Class II evidence when circumstances preclude randomized clinical trials.

Type B. Positive recommendation based on Class II evidence.

Type C. Positive recommendation based on strong consensus of Class III evidence.

Type D. Negative recommendation based on inconclusive or conflicting Class II evidence.

Type E. Negative recommendation based on evidence of ineffectiveness or lack of efficacy based on Class I or Class II evidence.

Safety and Effectiveness

Safety: a judgment of the acceptability of risk in a specified situation, e.g., for a given health problem, by a provider with specified training (at a specific stage of the disorder, etc.).

Effectiveness: producing a desired effect under conditions of actual use.

VI. RECOMMENDATIONS

A. Manual, Articular Manipulative and Adjustive Procedures

1. Specific Contact Thrust Procedures

a. **High Velocity Thrust:** High-velocity thrust procedures (also referred to as osseous adjusting proce-

dures) are probably the most commonly recognized, most widely taught, and most widely used of the adjustive and manipulative techniques within the chiropractic profession.

7.1.1 **Rating:** Established for the care of patients with mechanical low-back problems.
Evidence: Class I, II, III
Consensus Level: 1

7.1.2 **Rating:** Established for the care of patients with many other neuromusculoskeletal problems.
Evidence: Class II, III
Consensus Level: 1

7.1.3 **Rating:** Equivocal for other purposes.
Evidence: Class II, III
Consensus Level: 1

Comments: These procedures must be considered in light of their intended application, types of patients and conditions independently managed, and the nature of the thrust.

b. **High Velocity Thrust with Recoil:** There is little evidence in the literature specifically evaluating the effectiveness of thrust with recoil as compared to non-recoil thrust. Although distinct in application due to the recoil, typical joint cavitation and movement occurs with this procedure as it does with dynamic thrust without recoil. It is reasonable to assume that similar physiologic responses occur with both forms of thrust. Although comparative trials are needed, this modification is not controversial and it is reasonable to assume that studies evaluating thrust with or without recoil would have similar outcomes.

7.1.4 **Rating:** Promising to established for the care of patients with neuromusculoskeletal problems.
Evidence: Class II, III
Consensus Level: 1

7.1.5 **Rating:** Equivocal for other purposes.
Evidence: Class II, III
Consensus Level: 1

Comments: These procedures must be considered in light of their intended application, types of patients and conditions independently managed, and the nature of the thrust.

c. **Low-Velocity Thrust:** Low-velocity thrust may or may not result in joint gapping, depending on degree of pre-stress and amplitude. In the absence of specific comparative studies on low-velocity thrust, it is reasonable that any low-velocity thrust that results in joint gap is likely to have effects similar to high velocity thrusts from a mechanical point of view. For low-velocity thrust that does not cause cavitation, the literature on mobilization is thought to be representative if substantial range of motion to joints and soft tissues is induced. Reflex and global (widespread) effects of such procedures have not been well studied and are addressed in the section on reflex procedures.

7.1.6 **Rating**: Equivocal to promising for the care of patients with neuromusculoskeletal problems.
Evidence: Class II, III
Consensus Level: 1

7.1.7 **Rating:** Investigational to equivocal for the care of patients with some organic conditions.
Evidence: Class II, III
Consensus Level: 1

Comments: These procedures must be considered in light of their intended application, types of patients and conditions independently managed, and the nature of the thrust.

2. Non-Specific Contact Thrust Procedures

Mobilization: Mobilization (passive movement through the physiologic joint range) does not exceed the passive end range and therefore involves no cavitation of the joint and hence is distinct from manipulation. The purpose of mobilization is to increase range of motion within a restricted joint. Much of the clinical outcome literature on mobilization is blended with the manipulation literature.

7.2.1 **Rating:** Established
Evidence: Class I, II, III
Consensus Level: 1

3. Manual Force, Mechanically Assisted Procedures

a. **Drop Tables and Terminal Point Adjustive Thrust:** This procedure is a dynamic thrust with or without recoil that is in widespread use within the profession. The thrust involves positioning and pre-stress of joints in similar and modified fashion to other dynamic thrust procedures but involves small translational movement of a section of the adjusting table beneath the patient and the segment to which the thrust is applied.

7.3.1 **Rating:** Promising to established for the care of patients with neuromusculoskeletal problems.
Evidence: Class III
Consensus Level: 1

7.3.2 **Rating:** Investigational to equivocal for other purposes.
Evidence: Class III, with probable applicability of Class II studies involving high velocity thrust without mechanical assistance.
Consensus Level: 3

Comments: These procedures must be considered in light of their intended application, types of patients and conditions independently managed, and the nature of the thrust.

b. **Flexion-Distraction Tables:** These devices allow for manually assisted mechanical distraction to be applied primarily to the lumbar and thoracic spine along

with other ranges of motion. This approach of flexion-distraction is a standard, widely taught procedure. There is a great deal of supportable and reasonable mechanical and physiologic rationale in the literature for the appropriate use of these procedures for the care of patients with neuromusculoskeletal problems.

7.3.3 **Rating:** Established
Evidence: Class II, III
Consensus Level: 2

c. **Pelvic Blocks:** These paired wedges are used primarily for positioning the lumbosacral and sacroiliac joints to produce a sustained stretch. This procedure is in fairly common use, and there is reasonable rationale and expert opinion on its utility in certain situations.

7.3.4 **Rating:** Promising for the care of patients with neuromusculoskeletal problems.
Evidence: Class III
Consensus Level: 1

4. Mechanical Force, Manually Assisted Procedures

a. **Fixed Stylus, Compression Wave Instruments:** These devices are typically used in the upper cervical spine. A non-moving stylus is positioned against a pre-stressed motion segment. A moving piston strikes the stylus producing a compression wave along the stylus. It is speculated that a force is transmitted to the adjacent tissue and transmitted to the osseous and articular structures. With minimal tissue deformation and no amplitude change, the pliability and elasticity of the intermediate soft tissue is likely to absorb and disperse some or all of the force transmitted.

7.4.1 **Rating:** Equivocal
Evidence: Class III
Consensus Level: 1

Comments: Rationale for procedure is poorly substantiated and good efficacy studies are lacking. There are no direct safety concerns with proper application. These sorts of instruments suffer from the same limitations as low-force thrusts and will require significant investigation over time. Although use is not widespread, such instruments and protocols are taught in the curriculum of a few institutions and are not known to be restricted by regulatory agencies. There is clinical opinion and some case study information suggesting utility.

b. **Moving Stylus Instruments:** Spring loaded and piston activated adjusting instruments can be adjusted by amplitude, position and/or acceleration. One instrument known as an "Activator" has an adjustable amplitude with a spring loaded cocking mechanism that permits an adjustable range of reproducible accelerations. This instrument has been tested in animal models using pressure transducers and accelerometers and has demonstrated small but reproducible oscillation of bony vertebrae. Other devices employing similar mechanisms (such as the Pettibon instrument) may have similar effects.

These instruments when applied by and for rationales similar to dynamic thrust are likely to produce effects similar to some low-amplitude manual thrusting or mobilization procedures. They are also likely to stimulate cutaneous nerve endings and produce reflex effects. However, more investigation is required regarding rationales for application for several of these instruments.

7.4.2 **Rating:** Promising to established.
Evidence: Class I, II, III
Consensus Level: 1

B. Manual, Nonarticular Manipulative and Adjustive Procedures

1. Manual Reflex and Muscle Relaxation Procedures

a. **Muscle Energy Techniques:** A variety of procedures fall under this classification including post-facilitation stretch, post-isometric relaxation, and reciprocal inhibition, among others. In addition, there are several chiropractic techniques that use procedures mechanically and physiologically similar to these as part of their therapeutic armamentarium. The rationale for such procedures is based on the concept of reciprocal innervation and inhibition between agonist and antagonist muscles. Treatment is directed at finding such sites and having the patient do movements and muscle contractions, typically against some kind of active resistance in order to cause a relaxation of a hypertonic muscle. These techniques are commonly in use and are the subject of much investigation.

7.5.1 **Rating:** Promising
Evidence: Class II, III
Consensus Level: 1

b. **Neurologic Reflex Techniques:** These are a variety of techniques that attempt to stimulate proprioceptive and other sensory nerve endings by application of light touch or sustained pressure on various soft tissue or bony structures.

7.5.2 **Rating:** Equivocal for muscle relaxation.
Evidence: Class III
Consensus Level: 1

7.5.3 **Rating:** Investigational for other purposes.
Evidence: Class III
Consensus Level: 1

Comments: There is evidence that demonstrates that mechanical stimulation may influence muscle relaxation, sudomotor activity, vasoconstriction/dilation, gastric secretions.

Some practitioners use varieties of passive spring tension "plunger" devices for this purpose. Persuasive clinical studies only exist for somatic conditions. Procedures that result in only slight temporary soft tissue deformation or none at all (such as brief or sustained touch-like pressure to the skin) are not presently represented in the literature, and no well-articulated or substantiated physiologic rationales exist for effectiveness. These procedures would benefit from detailed investigation.

c. **Myofascial Ischemic Compression Procedures:** Ischemic compression involves placing a sustained compressive force on a tight or contracted muscle. This is thought to relax the muscle and thereby reduce stress to any joints to which the muscle is attached. The chiropractic profession has employed myofascial ischemic compression procedures and other soft tissue procedures as part of a care regimen for a long time (e.g., Receptor-tonus Technique, myofascial trigger point therapy).

7.5.4 **Rating:** Established for muscle relaxation.
Evidence: Class II, III
Consensus Level: 1

d. **Miscellaneous Soft Tissue Techniques:** There are many different kinds of muscle work in widespread use. They involve applying manual pressure in order to relieve muscle spasm. Some common techniques of muscle work include: massage (superficial, effleurage, petrissage, percussion), pressure point work (acupressure and shiatsu), and deep tissue techniques (Rolfing). There is little controversy regarding the clinical utility of such procedures for relaxation and uncomplicated musculoskeletal dysfunction. However, comparative clinical investigations are sparse. Light massage has occasionally been used as a placebo control in manipulation studies.

7.5.5 **Rating:** Established
Evidence: Class II, III
Consensus Level: 1

2. Miscellaneous Procedures

a. **Neural Retraining Techniques:** A variety of procedures aimed at developing neuromuscular coordination exist within the chiropractic profession. Such procedures constitute portions of some popular techniques. Primarily, these approaches involve repeated active movements under a variety of mechanical conditions in order to "pattern" the motor system for particular activities. There is rationale and support in the exercise physiology, kinesiology, and neurologic rehabilitation literature for many of these practices. There is overlap with other reflex procedures including muscle energy techniques. In terms of training for developing coordination and conditioning there is little controversy due to the plausibility of rationale, but a minimum of outcome investigations. Examples of these approaches include Janda, Feldenkrais, Alexander, cross crawl, etc.

7.6.1 **Rating**: Equivocal to promising in some conditioning and neuromuscular coordination contexts.
Evidence: Class II, III
Consensus Level: 1

7.6.2 **Rating:** Investigational for other purposes.
Evidence: Class II, III
Consensus Level: 1

Comment: There are proponents of other neural "organization" or "reeducation" procedures that claim a variety of clinical applications including the treatment of visceral, psychologic, and genetic conditions. There are poorly described rationales that may offer a starting point for model development, but no truly scholarly efforts are available to date. There is little or no literature available which documents effectiveness and such protocols are rarely taught as core material at accredited institutions. At best these procedures should be considered investigational, and, depending on the plausibility of certain applications, may be considered inappropriate to doubtful.

b. **Conceptual Mind-Body Approaches:** These approaches are based on the idea that mental thought (by the clinician) can influence physiological function of the patient. However, there is no information that suggests that a given doctor can directly influence a patient's physiology or disease process in specific situations. Although interesting, application to chiropractic care is speculative.

7.6.3 **Rating:** Inappropriate
Evidence: Class III
Consensus Level: 1

Comment: There is widespread acceptance of the importance of the doctor-patient relationship in the healing process. There is also burgeoning popular support for the mind-body relationship in the healing process. Facilitating this process in all types of therapeutic encounters is likely to be of benefit for patients' mental and social states. However, there is no justification for the substitution of metaphysical modalities for standard mechanical and chiropractic interventions. These issues are important fields in and of themselves (psychology, psychoneuroimmunology). It should be noted that one well-designed prospective, randomized, controlled trial of intercessory prayer on 393 hospitalized cardiac patients did demonstrate beneficial therapeutic effects (Byrd, 1988).

c. **Surrogate Approaches:** All chiropractic treatment approaches that utilize another person or a device as a mediator for receiving treatment on behalf of the patient have no defensible rationale or documentation of effectiveness and are therefore unacceptable in chiropractic practice.

7.6.4 **Rating:** Inappropriate
Evidence: Class III
Consensus Level: 1

C. Nonmanual Procedures

1. Exercise and Rehabilitation

a. **Mobility and Stretching Exercise:** Active mobility maintenance and stretching by the patient are traditionally encouraged in chiropractic practice. Training, counseling and advice in stretching and mobility exercises are common, and various descriptions of chiropractic programs exist in the literature. Trials on exercise in chiropractic settings have not been published, but there is function and performance information available in exercise physiology and sports medicine literature.

7.7.1 **Rating:** Promising to established.
Evidence: Class I, II, III
Consensus Level: 1

b. **Strengthening, Conditioning and Rehabilitation:** Active conditioning exercise is thought to be helpful for both healing and prevention of many mechanical back and neck problems. Conditioning and spinal stabilization programs are becoming more common for chiropractic management of low-back conditions. In addition, numerous programs are in place that involve job simulation and work hardening protocols that are directed at chiropractic management and conditioning for specific tasks.

7.7.2 **Rating:** Promising to established.
Evidence: Class I, II, III
Consensus Level: 1

c. **Passive Stretch:** Passive stretch is gentle sustained muscle lengthening applied by the practitioner or therapist. Its use is common within the chiropractic profession. There are a number of variations of application including several modalities to distract the patient from potential discomfort such as 1. cryotherapy (ice, coolant sprays, etc.) and 2. analgesic balms. These distractors are usually applied just before or simultaneous with the passive stretch and are for the purpose of distracting the patient from the possible discomfort of sustained stretch on the muscles and tissues. Practitioners, especially within the field of sports chiropractic, teach and use these procedures frequently.

7.7.3 **Rating:** Established
Evidence: Class I, II, III
Consensus Level: 1

2. Educational Programs

a. **Back School/Spinal Care Courses:** Knowledge about how to take care of one's health problems and how to modify behavior or lifestyle is likely to be beneficial for most patients. Back school programs and patient education have traditionally been an integral part of chiropractic case management. It is supportable when used as an appropriate teaching aid.

7.8.1 **Rating:** Promising to established.
Evidence: Class I, II, III
Consensus Level: 1

b. **Wellness Care/Disease Prevention/Health Promotion:** A relatively new area of interest in chiropractic as a distinct service, prevention has long been a primary consideration of the chiropractic profession's approach to health care. Typical disease prevention programs, smoking cessation, weight reduction efforts and the like fit well within chiropractic practice scopes. Organizations such as the American Chiropractic Association, International Chiropractors' Association and the Chiropractic Forum of the American Public Health Association have adopted policies or expressed support for such programs and practitioners with a particular expertise and interest in this area are increasing in number.

7.8.2 **Rating:** Promising to established.
Evidence: Class II, III
Consensus Level: 1

c. **Nutritional Counselling:** Nutritional training is included in the chiropractic curriculum. As a general issue concerning scope of practice, there is little disagreement regarding the capability or qualifications of practitioners to counsel patients concerning nutritional matters.

7.8.3 **Rating:** Established
Evidence: Class I, II, III
Consensus Level: 1

Comment: Specific nutritional therapy is an extensive field that requires a great deal of delineation. This should be addressed in the future.

d. **Biofeedback:** Some practitioners have begun to use biofeedback training as a means of teaching patients to control stress and other conditions. Its utility has been fairly well documented and its clinical application in chiropractic case management may be beneficial.

7.8.4 **Rating:** Promising to established.
Evidence: Class II, III
Consensus Level: 1

3. Electrical Modalities

Electrical modalities (e.g., muscle stimulating, electro-chemical, electro-acupuncture) have long been a part of chiropractic education and they are specifically included in scope of practice regulations in most jurisdictions. Standard electrical modalities are often used as ancillary to chiropractic manual procedures, and although there has been historical and political controversy regarding the clinical utility of all physiotherapeutic modalities in chiropractic practice, their inclusion in chiropractic scope of practice is not a significant area of debate. Protocols are well delineated. Muscle stimulation, galvanic current, microcurrent, iontophoresis, and TENS among others are representative modalities within this grouping. There is good evidence that many of these procedures produce therapeutic changes in muscle tone. There is some conflicting evidence for the effectiveness of electroanalgesia. Iontophoresis of some compounds may be regulated specifically in some jurisdictions.

7.9.1 **Rating:** Promising to established.
Evidence: Class I, II, III
Consensus Level: 1

4. Thermal Modalities

These include cryotherapy, infrared, hydrotherapy, hydrocollator, diathermy and others. These are standard within the chiropractic scope of practice in most jurisdictions. Protocols are documented and standardized. Cooling modalities are well established in the control of inflammation whereas heating modalities tend to promote palliation and general relaxation.

7.10.1 **Rating:** Established
Evidence: Class I, II, III
Consensus Level: 1

5. Ultraviolet

Ultraviolet radiation is a conservative procedure used in the treatment of superficial cutaneous and mucosal conditions. It is typically included as a physiotherapeutic modality in most chiropractic jurisdictions.

7.11.1 **Rating:** Established
Evidence: Class II, III
Consensus Level: 1

6. Ultrasound and Phonophoresis

Ultrasound is thought to be beneficial in increasing metabolic activity through deep heating and micromassage. Standard ultrasound and phonophoresis are typically included as standard ancillary procedures in chiropractic care. However, limitations may exist regarding phonophoresis of regulated compounds. Protocols are documented and standardized but may vary between jurisdictions.

7.12.1 **Rating:** Established
Evidence: Class I, II, III
Consensus Level: 1

7. Bracing, Casting, and Supports

Supports, braces, casting, orthotics and the like are often useful components of chiropractic care. Practitioners are trained for the application of many such appliances. However, more specialized training is required for scoliosis appliance prescription and other complex procedures.

7.13.1 **Rating:** Promising to established.
　　　Evidence: Class II, III
　　　Consensus Level: 2

8. Traction

Mechanical traction is frequently employed to stretch muscles, joints, and intervertebral discs. Its use is typically included in chiropractic education and is considered as a viable mechanical modality.

7.14.1 **Rating:** Promising to established.
　　　Evidence: Class I, II, III
　　　Consensus Level: 1

D. Special Interest Areas

1. Manipulation Under Sedation/Anesthesia (MUS/MUA)

Manipulation under sedation has been included in medical and osteopathic practice for some time. Chiropractic practitioners, because of their expertise in manual methods, have begun participating in the application of these procedures in the hospital setting in conjunction with anesthesiologists. These programs are subject to strict protocols as well as state and federal regulations.

7.15.1 **Rating:** Equivocal
　　　Evidence: Class II, III
　　　Consensus Level: 1

Comment: Although MUS/MUA is considered potentially useful, chiropractic involvement in such programs is a new area of special interest that requires further exploration.

2. Acupuncture

Acupuncture is a healing art that has been utilized for over 5,000 years. It is taught at some chiropractic colleges and is utilized by some practitioners. Its primary clinical use is for pain control.

7.16.1 **Rating:** Promising
　　　Evidence: Class I, II, III
　　　Consensus Level: 1

Comment: This is a complex field that warrants special training. A thorough discussion is beyond the scope of this document. Use may be regulated in some jurisdictions.

3. Homeopathic Remedies

Homeopathic remedies are thought to be of therapeutic value in some circumstances. Many homeopathic preparations are in use by some practitioners. Typically used for the relief of immediate symptoms and pain, homeopathic preparations are usually non-toxic to the patient and protocols for their usage are standardized and documented.

7.17.1 **Rating:** Equivocal
　　　Evidence: Class II, III
　　　Consensus Level: 1

Comment: This is a complex field that warrants special training. A thorough discussion is beyond the scope of this document. Use may be regulated in some jurisdictions.

VII. COMMENTS, SUMMARY OR CONCLUSIONS

Chiropractic modes of care encompass a wide variety of approaches. As chiropractic addresses health care from a perspective involving the role that body structure plays in overall physiologic function, many procedures emphasize manual care procedures such as adjusting, manipulation, soft tissue work, and physiotherapeutic modalities. However, the profession has traditionally maintained a strong interest in wellness care and disease prevention, as well as lifestyle and ergonomic issues. Therefore education, conditioning, nutrition, counseling and other approaches are often used by many practitioners. Although some specialty certification programs exist within the profession, these are not yet fully standardized.

The literature on the effectiveness of manual interventions has shown great promise for manipulation and to a lesser degree mobilization for care of various mechanical problems, especially certain low-back and neck conditions. There is an absence of good comparative studies to help clarify differences between technique approaches. The recommendations in this section are based on reasoning from biologic models, clinical experience, and expert opinion derived from both Delphi and Nominal Group consensus methodology.

It should be emphasized that chiropractic practitioners are typically well trained in a variety of standard assessment procedures, as well as specialized neuromusculoskeletal evaluation protocols. There has traditionally been an emphasis in chiropractic practice on lifestyle, wellness, prevention, and other natural approaches to health care.

Many practitioners have training and experience in a variety of alternative procedures such as acupuncture or homeopathy. It is beyond the scope of this chapter to cover these and other procedures (e.g., psychosocial, lifestyle and nutrition) to the level of detail they deserve. It is recommended that future guidelines on modes of chiropractic care give the detail for these procedures that is found for manual procedures in this chapter.

VIII. REFERENCES

Anderson R, Meeker W, et al.: Meta-analysis of randomized clinical trials on manipulation for low-back pain. *J Manip Physiol Ther* 1992, 15(3): 181-194.

Bartol KM: A model for categorization of chiropractic treatment procedures. *J Chiropractic Technique* 1991, 3(2):78-80.

Bergman T (ed): Special Issue on Seattle Consensus Conference. *J Chiropractic Technique* 1990, 2(3).

Brennan PC, Kokjohn K, Kaltinger CJ, et al.: Enhanced phagocytic cell respiratory burst induced by spinal manipulation: potential role of substance p. *J Manip Physiol Ther* 1991, 14(7).

Bronfort G, Nielsen N, Bendixt B, Madsen F, Weeks B: Chiropractic treatment of asthma: a controlled clinical trial. *Proceedings of International Conference on Spinal Manipulation FCER*, Arlington, Va.,1989.

Byrd RC: Positive therapeutic effect of intercessory prayer in a coronary care unit population. *Southern Med J* 1988, 81(7):826-829.

Cleveland C, Luttges M: Spinal correction effects on motor and sensory functions. In Mazzerelli J (ed): *Chiropractic Interprofessional Research*, Edizioni Minerva Medica, Torino Italy: 1985, 21-32.

Cox JM: *Low-Back Pain, Mechanism, Diagnosis and Treatment, 4th ed.* Williams & Wilkins, 1985.

Francis R. Spinal manipulation under general anesthesia: a chiropractic approach in a hospital setting. *ACA J Chiropractic* 1989, 12:39-41.

Frost EAM, Hsu C, Saadonski D: Acupuncture therapy: comparative values in acute and chronic pain. *NY State J Med* 1976, 76:695-697.

Fuhr AW, Smith DB: Accuracy of piezoelectric accelerometer measuring displacement of a spinal adjusting instrument. *J Manip Physiol Ther* 1986, 9(2):15-21.

Greenman P: *Principles of Manual Medicine.* Baltimore, Williams & Wilkins, 1989.

Grieve G: *Modern Manual Therapy.* Edinburgh, Churchill Livingstone, Edinburgh, 1986.

Hansen D, Jansen RD, et al. (eds): Emphasis on Consensus: *Proceedings of the 6th Annual Conference on Research and Education.* Consortium for Chiropractic Research, Belmont, CA, 1991.

Hansen D (ed): *Chiropractic Standards of Practice and Utilization Guidelines in the Care and Treatment of Injured Workers.* Washington State Department of Labor and Industry, 1988.

Haldeman S (ed): *Modern Developments in the Principles and Practice of Chiropractic, 2nd ed.* Appleton-Lange, 1992.

Kaminski M: Validation of chiropractic methods. *J Manip Physiol Ther* 1987, 10(2):61-64.

Kirk CR, Lawrence DJ, Valvo NL: *States Manual of Spinal, Pelvic, and Extravertebral Technique, 2nd ed.,* Lombard, National College of Chiropractic, Lombard, II, 1985.

Koes BW, Bouter LM, Beckerman H, van der Heijden G, Knipschild PG: Physiotherapy exercises and back pain: a blinded review. *Brit Med J* 1991, 302:1572-76.

Krumhansl BR, Nowacek CJ. Manipulation under anesthesia. In: Grieve GP. (ed.) *Modern Manual Therapy of the Vertebral Column.* Edinburgh, Churchill Livingston, 1986, 777-786.

Leach RA: *The Chiropractic Theories: a Synopsis of Chiropractic Research, 2nd ed.,* Baltimore, Williams & Wilkins, 1986.

Leboeuf C, Brown P, Herman A, et.al.: Chiropractic care of children with nocturnal enuresis: a prospective outcome study. *J Manip Physiol Ther* 1991, 14(2):110-115.

Liebenson C: Active muscular relaxation techniques. Part I: basic principles and methods. J *Manip Physiol Ther* 1989, 12(6): 446-454.

Liebenson C: Active muscular relaxation techniques. Part II: clinical application. *J Manip Physiol Ther* 1990, 13(1):2-6.

Maitland GD: *Vertebral Manipulation, 4th ed.* London, Butterworths, 1977.

Mayer TG, Gatchel RJ, et al.: A prospective two-year study of functional restoration in industrial low-back pain. *J Am Med Assoc* 1987, 258:1763-1767.

Meeker WC: Chiropractic manipulation: techniques and rationale for the cervical spine. In White A (ed): *Cervical Spine and Upper Extremity in Sports and Industry.* Daly City, San Francisco Spine Institute, 1990.

Morey LW. Osteopathic manipulation under general anesthesia. *J Amer Osteopathic Assoc* 1973, 73:116-127.

Morey LW. Manipulation under general anesthesia. *Osteopathic Annals* 1976, 3:127-132.

Mootz RD: Chiropractic Models: Current understanding of vertebral subluxation and manipulable spinal lesions. In Sweere J (ed): *Chiropractic Family Practice.* Gaithersburg, Aspen Publishers, (in press due 1992).

New Zealand Commission of Inquiry: *Chiropractic in New Zealand,* PD Hasselberg, Wellington, 1979.

North American Spine Society's ad hoc committee on diagnostic and therapeutic procedures: Common diagnostic and therapeutic procedures of the lumbosacral spine. *Spine* 1991, 16(10):1161-1167.

Nyiendo J, Phillips RB, Meeker WC, et al.: A comparison of patients and patient complaints at six chiropractic colleges. *J Manip Physiol Ther* 1989, 12(2):79-85.

Parker G, Tupling H, Pryor D: A controlled trial of cervical manipulation for migraine. *Aust NZ J Med* 1978, 8(6):589-593.

Phillips RB, Mootz RD, Nyiendo J, et al.: *A comparison of patients and patient complaints presenting to private chiropractic practioner's offices.* (in press).

Quebec Task Force on Spinal Disorders: Scientific Approach to the Assessment and Management of Activity-related Spinal Disorders. *Spine Supplement* 1987, 12(7s).

Rinzler SH, Travell J: Therapy directed at the somatic component of cardiac pain. *Am Heart J* 1948, 35:248.

Rogers JT, Rogers JC: The role of osteopathic manipulative therapy in the treatment of coronary heart disease. *J Am Osteop Assoc* 1976, 76:71-81.

Rumney IC. Manipulation of the spine and appendages under anesthesia: an evaluation. *J Amer Osteopathic Assoc* 1986, 68:235-245.

Schaefer RC (ed): *Basic Chiropractic Procedural Manual, 4th ed.* Arlington, American Chiropractic Association, 1984.

Shekelle PG, Adams AH, et.al.: *The Appropriateness of Spinal Manipulation for Low-Back Pain: Project Overview and Literature Review* (R-4025/1-CCR/FCER). Santa Monica, RAND: 1991a.

Shekelle PG, Adams AH, et.al.: *The Appropriateness of Spinal Manipulation for Low-Back Pain: Indications and Ratings by a Multidisciplinary Expert Panel* (R-4025/2-CCR/FCER). Santa Monica, RAND, 1991b.

Siehl D. Manipulation of the spine under general anesthesia. *J Amer Osteopathic Assoc* 1963, 62: 881-887.

Siehl D. Olson DR, Ross HE, Rockwood EE. Manipulation of the lumbar spine with the patient under general anesthesia: evaluation by electromyography and clinical-neurologic examination of its use for lumbar nerve root compression syndrome. *J Amer Osteopathic Assoc* 1971, 70:433-440.

Smith DB, Fuhr AW, Davis BP: Skin accelerometer displacement and relative bone movement of adjacent vertebrae in response to chiropractic percussion thrusts. *J Manip Physiol Ther* 1989, 12(1):26-37.

Stonebrink RD: *Evaluation and Manipulative Management of Common Musculoskeletal Disorders.* Portland, Stonebrink, 1990.

Travell JG, Simons D: *Myofacial Pain and Dysfunction. The Trigger Point Manual.* Baltimore, Williams & Wilkins 1983.

Ulman D: *Homeopathy: Medicine for the 21st Century.* Berkeley, North Atlantic Books, 1988.

Vernon H, Dhami M, Howley TP, Annett R: Spinal manipulation and beta-endorphin: a controlled study of the effect of a spinal manipulation on beta-endorphin levels in normal males. *J Manip Physiol Ther* 1986, 9(2):115-124.

White AH, Anderson R (eds): *Conservative Care of Low-Back Pain.* Baltimore,Williams & Wilkins, 1991.

Yates RG, Lamping DL, et.al.: Effects of chiropractic treatment on blood pressure and anxiety: a randomized controlled trial. J *Manip Physiol Ther* 1988, 11(6):484-488.

IX. MINORITY OPINIONS

None

Frequency and Duration of Care

Chapter Outline

I. OVERVIEW

Guidelines concerning the treatment plan should be tempered with a balance of scientific information and systematic observation derived from clinical experience.[1] Further, in order to be practical, they must be periodically upgraded to reflect advances in the ever-changing knowledge database. Their purpose is to assist the clinician in decision making based on the expectation of outcome for the **uncomplicated case.** They are NOT designed as a prescriptive or cookbook procedure for determining the absolute frequency and duration of treatment/care for any specific case.

The review and recommendations made in this section have been drawn from clinical experience and clinical/scientific data on the response of patients receiving chiropractic health care services. No attempt has been made to select for individual conditions by region of complaint or by diagnosis. Most data reported in the clinical literature does not make these kinds of distinctions.

The majority of quantitative information available addresses the management of low-back and leg pain complaints. This is not surprising since these conditions currently account for most of the complaints seen by all health care providers who work with musculoskeletal disorders. The references to low-back disorders in this section are used only as examples. There is no intent to imply that these conditions constitute the totality of chiropractic expertise or practice. Rather, since these recommendations were born from experience and from data on multivariate clinical circumstances, they may be extrapolated with appropriate case-specific modifications to most of the common complaints for which chiropractic care is sought.

Virtually all chiropractic providers who submit claims for payment from third party payers receive disbursements based on contractual language. Commonly this requires that "treatment/care" be documented as having "therapeutic necessity." For that reason this chapter will refer to provider services under the rubric of "treatment/care" as a pragmatic representation of the business actually conducted by the chiropractic profession on a daily basis. There is no intent to engage in or to settle any philosophical debate on appropriate language.

Reducing Variations in Practice

The endurance of robust treatment variations in common practice [2] results from an absence of tested theory. Treatment diversity, or uncertainty, exists because of the differences among practitioners in their clinical evaluation of patients (diagnosis), or in their belief in the value of a procedure for meeting their patient's needs (therapy).[3] Some scattered efforts have been made to categorize treatment outcomes by condition (Connecticut,[4] Georgia,[5] Oregon,[6] Minnesota,[7] Ohio,[8] Washington.[9]) Each has struggled with competing priorities and with quality of evidence. This review is based

upon a formal consideration of the available database and seeks to draw appropriate conclusions seasoned by the cumulative years of practical experience of the panel members.

Clinical expectation regarding treatment outcome must be based upon more than personal opinion. The approach to the development of guidelines for chiropractic quality assurance and standards of practice pertaining to the frequency and duration of treatment focuses on the uncomplicated case and logically includes the following considerations:

1. The natural history of common spinal disorders
2. The characteristics and stages of tissue repair processes
3. Reasonable treatment/care outcome classified into short and long range goals

Classifications of Patients

The care of common spinal complaints does not fit well into any diagnostic classification system because of a dual uncertainty surrounding the diagnosis and the efficacy of treatment.[10] Theoretically, complaints can be formulated into structural, neurophysiologic, and biomechanical diagnostic subsets.[11] Yet, these categorizations are not always helpful in setting realistic short and long term treatment/care goals. For example, a disc herniation may be discovered fortuitously in an asymptomatic patient and not require care. On the other hand, in an anatomically small spinal canal it may become quite disabling and defy conservative management.

Clinical descriptors such as those proposed by the Quebec Task Force[12] are useful in helping predict the course of the condition. More concrete treatment/care protocols, then, may be based on the clinical impressions rather than on knowledge of the lesion mechanics or treatment efficacy.[13, 14, 15]

Principles of Case Management

The primary missions of health care delivery are to provide sufficient care to restore health, maintain it, and prevent the recurrence of injury and illness. To meet these objectives, the practitioner uses a myriad of procedures and skills that collectively can be grouped into three categories—passive intervention, active intervention, and patient education. The practical boundaries on what will constitute necessary and sufficient treatment/care are situational. However, guidelines framing expectations of treatment outcome can be drawn from the literature and adapted by practical experience on a case-by-case basis.

The first principle of case management is that early return to activity is associated with reduced disability and symptoms.[16, 17, 18] A second principle is based upon the experience gained from monitoring the response of patients having no treatment,[19, 20] and those with treatment. The lesson learned is that there is a natural history of recovery for uncomplicated cases[21] that can serve as a time frame from which to evaluate and shape a successful treatment plan. A third principle is that chronicity should be prevented wherever possible. Patients who are at risk for becoming chronic show characteristic patterns involving their illness and life situation.[22] Warning signs include:

1. Somatic complaints that remain static longer than 2-3 weeks
2. Anxiety or depression
3. Functional or emotional disability
4. Family turmoil
5. Drug dependence: recreational, non-prescription or prescription

A fourth guiding principle is that repeated use of acute care measures alone generally fosters chronicity, physician dependence and over-utilization.[23] Finally, therapeutic motivation, goals and fiscal responsibility are different for elective care than for therapeutically necessary care.

II. DEFINITIONS

Active Rest: The resting of a tissue or body part only to the point of restriction of deforming and pathological forces during the healing period, while at the same time allowing normal physiological stresses. Also called relative rest.

Adequate Trial of Treatment/Care: A course of two weeks each of two different types of manual procedures (four weeks total), after which, in the absence of documented improvement, manual procedures are no longer indicated.

Chronicity: Stages of progress of a disorder that are related both to severity and duration: acute, subacute, chronic, and recurrent.

Complicated Case: A case where the patient, because of one or more identifiable factors, exhibits regression or retarded recovery in comparison with expectations from the natural history.

Elective Care: Treatment/care requested by the patient designed to promote optimum function to alleviate subjective symptomatology in cases having reached maximum therapeutic benefit.

Manual Procedures: For purposes of this chapter this term includes adjustive or manipulative procedures, and other manual techniques.

MaximumTherapeutic Benefit (Maximum Medical or Chiropractic Improvement): Return to pre-injury/illness status or failure to improve beyond a certain level of symptomatology or disability, whatever the treatment/care approach.

Natural History: The anticipated clinical course of recovery for uncomplicated disorders either without treatment/care, or with conservative treatment/care.

Preventative/Maintenance Care: Care given to reduce the incidence or prevalence of illness, impairment, and risk factors, and to promote optimal function.

Stages of Treatment/Care: (sequential or concurrent)

1. **Acute Intervention:** Initial therapeutic intervention to assist and promote anatomical rest, reduce muscle spasm and inflammatory reaction, and alleviate pain.
2. **Remobilization:** Continuing intervention to increase the pain-free ranges of motion and to minimize de-conditioning.
3. **Rehabilitation:** Efforts to restore strength and endurance in the pain-free range, and increase physical work capacity. Rehabilitation is treatment/care applied for more chronic or complex problems in patients with impaired capabilities. It may be used sequentially or concomitantly with other care depending on the specific characteristics of a problem.
4. **Life Style Modification:** Adaptations of life style necessary to modify social and recreational activity, diminish work environment risk factors, and adapt to psychological elements affecting, or altered by, the disorder.

Supportive Care: Treatment/care for patients having reached maximum therapeutic benefit, in whom periodic trials of therapeutic withdrawal fail to sustain previous therapeutic gains that would otherwise progressively deteriorate. Supportive care follows appropriate application of active and passive care including lifestyle modifications. It is appropriate when rehabilitative and/or functional restorative and alternative care options, including home-based self-care and lifestyle modifications, have been considered and attempted. Supportive care may be inappropriate when it interferes with other appropriate primary care, or when the risk of supportive care outweighs its benefits, i.e, physician dependence, somatization, illness behavior, or secondary gain.

Therapeutic Necessity: Exists in the presence of an impairment (illness/injury) evidenced by recognized signs and symptoms, and likely to respond favorably to the treatment/care planned.

Treatment/Care Dynamics-Manual Procedures:

1. **Threshold:** The minimum rate and magnitude of joint load needed to bring about a change.
2. **Dosage:** The frequency of care necessary and sufficient to maintain effects while healing occurs.
3. **Duration:** The minimum treatment/care interval to obtain a stable response.
4. **Combination:** The potentiation or competition of response by simultaneous treatment/care applications.

Treatment/Care Goals: Written short term and long range expectations of patient response to the treatment plan.

Treatment/Care Type:

1. **Passive Care:** Application of treatment/care modalities by the care-giver to a patient, who "passively" receives care.

2. **Active Care:** Modes of treatment/care requiring "active" involvement, participation, and responsibility on the part of the patient.

Treatment Plan: A written description of intended therapeutic actions divided according to relevant treatment/care goals and prognosis.

Uncomplicated Case: A case where the patient exhibits progressive recovery from an illness or injury at a rate greater than, or equal to, the expectation from the natural history.

III. LIST OF SUBTOPICS

A. Short and Long Range Treatment Planning
B. Treatment/Care Frequency
C. Patient Cooperation
D. Failure to Meet Treatment/Care/Objectives
E. Uncomplicated Cases
F. Complicated Cases
G. Elective Care

IV. LITERATURE REVIEW

Natural History

Earlier schools of thought in chiropractic placed less emphasis on diagnosis and more on the response to therapeutic trial—a descriptive analysis. When combined into groups as is done in the DRG or Quebec schemes of classification, patterns emerge in the course of treated and untreated conditions.[24,25,26,27,28] These observations provide a natural history that can serve as a reference point for treatment/care expectations. The most meaningful outcome measures available are the rate of return to work, continued use of health care services, and recurrence of back-related injuries.[29]

Regardless of how a patient is categorized diagnostically, clinical decision-making can be rationally organized for most back pain sufferers. The natural history of back pain and other conditions for uncomplicated episodes gives a defensible basis from which a measurable plan of action can be made.

Clearly, the duration and intensity of in-office treatment/care for an uncomplicated case should not extend beyond the time frame observed in reports of the natural untreated course. As a set of minimal standards, attention to how the patient is progressing in comparison with the natural history helps to set an upper limit on the time during which a case should be fol-

lowed without modification of the treatment plan. Figure 8-1 (page 128) shows the progress believed to characterize most back pain patients who require intervention.

Each episode of the condition can be perceived in the context of its own time course and described as acute, subacute, chronic, or recurrent. Some controversy exists about definitions for each category. They appear to be loosely based upon the duration of absence from work or upon an assessment of relative clinical improvement.

Episode Time-Course

Table I lists the aggressive, intermediate, and conservative time limits for each category. Recurrent episodes of back pain are not listed separately, since they are treated similarly to acute cases. Differences in the cutoffs chosen in each study reflect the relative values each group places upon intervention to avert chronicity. There is universal agreement that of those whose symptoms persist for more than 3 to 4 months, more than half will still be disabled at the end of a year.[30]

Table 1 Staging the Episode: Time-Course

	Quebec Study (1987)	Frymoyer (1988)	Mayer & Gatchel (1988)
Acute	0-7 days	0-6 weeks	0-8 weeks
Subacute	7 days-7 weeks	6-12 weeks	8-16 weeks
Chronic	7 weeks +	> 12 weeks	> 16 weeks

Standards in patient management require close attention to three elements of the treatment plan. They are: 1) criteria for selecting treatment/care procedures; 2) close monitoring of the therapeutic response in comparison with the expected outcome of natural history; and 3) flexibility of the treatment/care protocol when less favorable or unexpected responses are encountered.

As with any other form of therapy, it is likely that manual procedures follow dynamic principles. That is, treatment/care response will depend upon threshold effect, dosage, duration of administration, and additive effects from combination with other agents.[31]

Scientific study of the relative efficacy and mechanism for different procedures and combined efforts has only begun recently.[32] For example, the mechanical response of a motion segment may be influenced by many modifiers. Local muscle tone and the patterning of recruitment during voluntary movement affect the distribution of stresses that are transmitted through the spinal tissues. The passive mechanical properties of disc, ligaments, and muscle may be altered by inflammatory or degenerative processes. Pathologic barriers imposed by intra-articular adhesions or meniscoid entrapments may be present and are thought by some to be potential mechanisms for disrupting normal mechanics. Finally, the occupational hazards of prolonged static postures or high peak spinal loads can inhibit responses. For example, the body's healing processes must proceed and inflammation subside before the effects of prolonged antalgic loading of the spine can be mitigated.

Treatment Plans

The treatment plan for therapeutically necessary care can be divided into four phases (Table II), each having distinct objectives that allow for passive and active benefits. When the patient exhibits acute distress, efforts to reduce soft tissue and joint stresses are applied to diminish inflammation and swelling. A short term of reduced mobility to limit the joint loading effects of gravity may be warranted. Passive forms of treatment/care, including manual and palliative procedures, may be used with deference to the type of mechanical lesion present. When pain and discomfort have abated, the area can be remobilized with low speed and minimal load exercises directed to improve flexibility without incurring mechanical stress. As the range of pain free motion is improved, a gradual increase in exertion can be introduced. Lastly, when a maximal range of motion is achieved, rehabilitation for strength and endurance can begin.

Table II Stages of Treatment/Care: Goals and Objectives

Passive Care
1. **Acute Intervention** (including manual procedures)
   A. To promote anatomical rest
   B. To diminish muscular spasm
   C. To reduce inflammation
   D. To alleviate pain

Active Care
1. **Remobilization**
   A. To increase the range of pain free motion
   B. To minimize deconditioning
2. **Rehabilitation**
   A. To restore strength and endurance
   B. To increase physical work capacity
3. **Life Style Adaptations**
   A. To modify social and recreational activity
   B. To diminish work environment risk factors
   C. To adapt psychological factors affecting or altered by the spinal disorder.

It is beneficial to proceed to the rehabilitation phase (if warranted) as rapidly as possible, and to minimize dependency upon passive forms of treatment/care. Studies have shown a clear relationship between prolonged restricted activity and the risk of failure in returning to pre-injury status. Often a complete resolution of pain is not possible until patients begin to focus on increasing the number and kind of activities in which they participate. Return to work usually can be commenced at 80-90% level of pre-injury status.[33] Even then, some residual pain can be expected, although usually it will be offset by the benefits of increased productive functioning.

Predictions from the Case History

Most back pain studies have found that the duration of symptoms is a predictor of response to treatment/care with manual procedures. The duration of symptoms is inversely related to the likelihood of positive clinical response. Bronfort[34] reported that patients with a shorter duration of symptoms were more likely to respond to manipulation (85% cured within six months for patients with less than seven days of initial pain, only 35% with more than 28 days of initial pain.) Similar results are shown by Maitland,[35] Glover,[36] Evans,[37] and Potter.[38]

Singer et al.[39] describe a relationship between three descriptive factors in the episode history noted at the time of patient consultation, and the duration of conservative care. Pain intensity and duration prior to the consultation, and the number of prior episodes were observed to affect the time necessary to return the patient to preinjury activity and recovery at least to a point of mild pain. In general, more severe pain at treatment/care onset was associated with longer treatment/care times. In like manner, patients suffering with pain longer than eight days before commencing therapy took a mean of 21 days to recover. With less duration of pain, only 13 days were required. Similarly, patients with up to three prior episodes required 12 days, while more than eight episodes extended recovery to 27 days.

Passive Care

The scientific literature is not helpful in deciding when manual treatment/care should be stopped, either with respect to improvement or worsening of symptoms. Controlled trials or case series have been reported with ranges between 1 and 19 sessions of manipulation lasting anywhere from a single day to two months. Triano[40] has suggested an algorithm of decision-review points triggered by the individual patient's response in contrast to the natural history. Hansen[41] recommends a second opinion if there is no objective or subjective sign of improvement (or worsening of the condition) in two weeks, or treatment of three times per week that exceeds four weeks. The 1990 RAND Consensus Panel unanimously agreed to a definition of adequate therapeutic trial for spinal manipulation. They recommended a trial course of two weeks each using alternative manipulative procedures before considering treatment/care to have failed. Without evidence of improvement over this time frame, spinal manipulation is no longer indicated.

Several observational or retrospective studies have compiled information on the number of treatments that have been given to patients. Varying experimental methodologies were used. Reporting on case records of 3,943 patients from multiple private offices, Phillips and Butler[42] found a mean of 12.5 treatments (SD, 13.1). Separately, Phillips[43] reported a mean of 9.0 treatments in 871 cases. Patients fit all categories from acute, subacute to chronic. Symptoms had been present for less than 30 days in 57%, for 60 to 180 days in 11% and for longer than 180 days in 22%. The mean length of case management was 11.4 days. Twenty-four percent were attended for a week or less while 56% received care for up to 30 days. One hundred and three patients[44] with lumbosacral pain were treated with up to four sessions of manipulation. They were followed for one to three years. Recurrence of symptoms appeared in only 11.7% during that time. In another study examining workers' compensation case data, Jarvis et al.[45] calculated a mean of 12.9 treatments over an average of 54.5 days.

Manipulative services on patients with work-related back disorders in Florida averaged 29 office-based procedures per patient.[46] In another office based prospective observation of 100 consecutive low back pain cases, Cox et al.[47] found a 50% pain reduction within a mean of 10 treatment sessions over 16 days. Maximum relief was gained at 41 days and after 16 treatment sessions.

Nyiendo and Haldeman[48] reported a range for the number of patient visits across all complaints as 1-81, with a mean of 4.4. In a prospective study controlled for volunteer bias, Triano et al. reported a range of 1-22 sessions.[49] Moreover, the results of this study appear more representative of private practice experience than other published profiles. Several conclusions from this study are helpful in judging the frequency and duration of care for symptomatic episodes:

1. Patients with chronic disorders may require more treatment/care to resolve symptomatic episodes than do other categories of complaint.
2. Lordotic areas of the spine, on average, required twice the care of complaints involving the thoracic and transitional regions.
3. Most cases studied resolved well within six weeks of intervention consistent with the expectations from natural history (Figure 8-1, Page 128).
4. Patients for whom care is necessary beyond six weeks may require up to 11 (mean = 3.8) additional sessions before reaching resolution.

Statistics describing clinical experience with manipulation fit well within guidelines based upon natural history outcomes. More aggressive in-office intervention early during treatment/care may ultimately result in reducing the amount of disabling injury and the necessity to engage in more extensive inpatient procedures. These conclusions closely resemble determinations derived from functional rehabilitation and from the recommendations of the Ontario study for an earlier aggressive treatment approach.

It is possible that the presence of pathologic or anomalous structures may impede clinical progression.[50] Re-injury and exacerbation from unexpected events also may alter treatment/care goals. Likewise, biomechanical and psychosocial stress may be important deterrents to recovery. Bronfort[51] showed that the presence of psychological overlay (defined by the hysteria and hypochondriasis scores on the MMPI), and

the presence of ergonomic influences was associated with poorer response to chiropractic manipulation. Circumstances such as these require the artful practice of patient management. The ability of the attending clinician to identify the primary problem is a major factor in minimizing the time of patient suffering.[52] A decision algorithm simplifies the sorting out process in these cases (Figure 8-2, Page 129). Its value lies in helping clarify and discriminate practitioner and patient responsibilities in working toward case resolution. The overriding concern is a focus upon the patient's rate of improvement in comparison with that predicted by the natural history.

The patient who experiences sufficient severity or duration of back discomfort may wish to seek consultation. From that time forward, treatment/care is divided into the four stages of intent described above. Case management includes decisions about timing in the implementation of each stage. Some small variation can be expected from case to case as this derives from circumstances in the patient's habits, life style, or occupation, and accidental encounter. These circumstances should be sought whenever the progress of treatment/care approximates or intersects the estimated time line of Figure 8-1. A systematic interview with the patient, sometimes including members of the family, will often reveal influences competing with treatment/care objectives. After correcting these factors, trial therapy should be reimplemented.

If extenuating circumstances are not evident, or if a renewal of trial therapy fails to bring about an adequate rate of improvement, it is wise to reconsider the initial diagnosis. Special testing or imaging may be warranted depending upon the practitioner's level of suspicion and the results of monitoring the renewed treatment plan. Whether or not the diagnostic impression is upheld, a change in the therapeutic plan needs to be instituted. Failure to achieve a satisfactory response after working through the scenario laid out in the algorithm should result in an assessment for maximum therapeutic improvement or referral for a second opinion. Patients who progress into a state of chronicity can be identified and aggressively rehabilitated at an earlier stage.

Active Care

While only 4 percent of back pain patients fail to return to pre-injury status after six months, these patients are responsible for most back related health care costs. The preponderance of evidence from studies of medication treatment, manipulation, back school, and physical therapy shows that when any of these conservative treatments cease,[53] the natural course of on-going disability reasserts itself for these cases. Clearly, new treatment/care options are needed to improve upon these long range clinical outcome statistics.

The chiropractic profession has responded to this need in managing cases at risk for becoming chronic. Advanced understanding for the progression of acute pain to chronic,[54] deconditioning syndromes,[55] illness behavior,[56] and the risk of physician dependence has resulted in more providers actively specializing in preventive and rehabilitative practice.[57] Their primary purpose is to provide a vehicle for successful transition of patient care from relying upon passive treatment/care intervention to active patient participation. The factors that enter into consideration of appropriateness include:

1. Duration of the painful episode
2. The number of previous episodes
3. Response to acute intervention
4. Anticipated future physical activity
5. Patient motivation
6. Training of the practitioner and staff

Once therapeutic necessity has been determined, success of the rehabilitation plan will be determined primarily by the latter three elements.

Some anti-inflammatory approaches might be applicable at this phase, i.e., relative rest or active rest.[58] Other forms of passive treatment/care, including manual and palliative procedures, are used with deference to the type of mechanical lesion present, and are discussed under the section above on passive care. Pain-free isometric contraction signals the appropriate timing for expanding the range of motion. Once pain and discomfort are controlled, the area is remobilized with low speed, minimal load exercises directed to improve flexibility without being mechanically stressful. As range of pain-free motion is improved, a gradual increase in exertion can be introduced. Finally, rehabilitation for strength and endurance can begin.

Should the patient fail to progress through the stages proportional to the natural history, a search for complication, somatization, non-compliance, or reinjury should be made. After correcting these factors, trial therapy should be implemented again. Cases persisting without substantial improvement and that have no underlying complications warrant consideration for rehabilitation.

Patients at risk for becoming chronic generally present common warning signs.[59] They include: 1) stationary symptoms of somatic pain for two or three weeks; 2) functional impairment; 3) chemical dependency used recreationally or for pain control; and 4) emotional distress that may include family disruption. The presence of such indicators should signal the practitioner to move quickly away from passive care as the primary emphasis.

Reaching the rehabilitation phase as rapidly as possible and minimizing dependence upon passive forms of treatment/care usually lead to the optimal result. Prolonged limited activity is related to risk of failure in returning to preinjury status. Often complete resolution of pain is not possible until the patient begins to focus on increasing the number and kind of activities in which they participate. Even then, some residual pain can be expected, but it may be offset by the benefits of increasingly productive function. While optimization of physical performance may be desirable, continuation of care past the treatment/care goal is considered elective care.

Treatment/Care Protocols

There are nearly as many preferences in exercise programs available as there are health care providers using them. What is more important, however, is the recognition that care should not focus selectively on the injured areas alone but should involve associated areas that support the injury. Program design should have balanced components based on the needs of the patient. Elements that should be addressed include:

1. The dissuasion of pain related behavior
2. Education on body biomechanics
3. Supervised training for flexibility with stability, strength, coordination, and endurance

For patients already demonstrating signs of deconditioning or chronicity, this will require more than handing out a simple list of exercises to be performed at home.

Pain Behavior

Pain behavior and illness conviction are best managed with a conceptual shift in thinking about pain. The care giver must switch focus from injury and attention to the patient's level of discomfort to what the patient is able to do.[60] An understanding that movement is safe and helpful, even if not completely comfortable, needs to be emphasized. Where psychosocial factors predominate in the assessment, referral for counseling should be made. However, lesser psychosocial effects arise from ongoing pain itself. Focus upon rehabilitation as a means to improve the quality of life and to reduce suffering can result in a significant reduction on secondary somatization.

Patient Education

Educational instructions are to be given to promote safe habits. Job and biomechanical analyses help steer topics toward specific activities and conditions in which the person is likely to find himself or herself. However, a general comprehension of function and stressors should be attempted using terms familiar to the patient. Topics including the classical bending, lifting, pushing and pulling, entry and exit from vehicles, sitting, yard work, recreation, personal care, and sexual activity all should be included.[61,62] Emphasis should be placed on personalizing the activities commonly experienced by the patient.

Exercise Training

Flexibility and Stability: The long term goal of rehabilitation is to restore the patient to preinjury function and reduce the chances of recurrent episodes. Repetitive microtrauma superimposed on previous injury can lead to advanced degeneration.[63] Spinal stabilization is designed to teach trunk muscle recruitment as an effort to control and reduce flexion and torsional stresses on the joint segments. Through the use of voluntary muscles, pain-free regional postures can be maintained while the patient carries out normal daily activities. The necessary posture and combination of muscle actions determined experimentally are specific for each case. Once the comfortable position is found, the patient is assisted while rehearsing progressively more complex tasks, keeping the body part in its neutral, pain-free position.

Strength and Endurance: Early on, during recovery, isometric exercises and stretching within the pain-free range of motion may be used to limit the effects of deconditioning.[64] Once the case has successfully passed the remobilization phase, progressively increasing loads throughout the full range of motion are initiated. These may be accomplished through use of free weights, weight stack machines, or the same computerized isokinetic or isoinertial machines that aid in assessment of function.

The usual exercise training plan begins with direct supervision, three to five times per week, of assigned exercise tasks intermixed with rest periods. Many progressive-resistance protocols are available. These are summarized by Christensen[65] and Saal and Saal.[66] The combination of multiple sets of repetitions with increasing or decreasing increments of weight results in benefits for both strength and endurance. The maximum exertion is increased weekly over a course of four to six weeks for the typical case. Computerized instruments may be used in analogous fashion. They offer immediate feedback and may help maintain user interest, but their use is not essential to a good clinical outcome.

Persons who fail to comply with the treatment/care schedule or who are insincere in their efforts should be discontinued and discharged from care. The remaining patients are reassessed near the completion of the treatment plan to determine the outcome.

V. ASSESSMENT CRITERIA

Procedure Ratings (System I)

Established: Accepted as appropriate by the practicing chiropractic community for the given indication in the specified patient population.

Promising: Given current knowledge, this technology appears to be appropriate for the given indication in the specified patient population. As more evidence and experience accumulate this interim rating will change. This connotes provisional acceptance, but permits a greater role for the current level of clinical use.

Equivocal: Current knowledge exists to support a given indication in a specified patient population, though value can neither be confirmed nor denied. As more evidence and experience accumulates this interim rating will change. Expert opinion recognizes a need for caution in general application.

Investigational: Evidence is insufficient to determine appropriateness. Further study is warranted. Use for a given indication in a specified patient population should be confined largely to research protocols. As more evidence and experience accumulates, this interim rating will change.

Doubtful: Given current knowledge, this appears to be inappropriate for the given indication in the specified patient population. As more evidence and experience accumulate this interim rating will change.

Inappropriate: Regarded by the practicing chiropractic community as unacceptable for the given indication in the specified patient population.

Quality Of Evidence

The following categories of evidence are used to support the ratings.

Class I:
Evidence provided by one or more well-designed controlled clinical trials; or well-designed experimental studies that address reliability, validity, positive predictive value, discriminability, sensitivity, and specificity.

Class II:
Evidence provided by one or more well-designed, uncontrolled, observational clinical studies such as case control, cohort studies, etc.; or clinically relevant basic science studies that address reliability, validity, positive predictive value, discriminability, sensitivity, and specificity; and published in refereed journals.

Class III:
Evidence provided by expert opinion, descriptive studies or case reports.

Suggested Strengths of Recommendation Ratings

Type A. Strong positive recommendation based on Class I evidence, or overwhelming Class II evidence when circumstances preclude randomized clinical trials.

Type B. Positive recommendation based on Class II evidence.

Type C. Positive recommendation based on strong consensus of Class III evidence.

Type D. Negative recommendation based on inconclusive or conflicting Class II evidence.

Type E. Negative recommendation based on evidence of ineffectiveness or lack of efficacy based on Class I or Class II evidence.

Safety and Effectiveness

Safety: a judgment of the acceptability of risk, in a specified situation, e.g., for a given health problem, by a provider with specified training (at a specific stage of the disorder etc.).

Effectiveness: producing a desired effect under conditions of actual use.

VI. RECOMMENDATIONS

Note: Statistical descriptors of treatment frequency, such as mean/median/mode, should NOT be used as a standard to judge care administered to an INDIVIDUAL patient. The particular factors of each case will govern the course of recovery and need to be a part of the considerations in assessing clinical progress.

A. Short and Long Range Treatment Planning:

At the outset of treatment/care, a written estimated time frame for reaching intermediate functional milestones (short term goals, e.g., the ability to move the affected part, exert force, walk, etc.) and treatment/care outcomes (long term goals, e.g., return to work, renew sports, full activity, etc.) should be made. The length of time to reach these objectives can be affected by specific historical factors.
NOTE: These factors, when combined (two or more), do not necessarily imply combined delay in recovery, but must be evaluated on a case-by-case basis.

1. **Preconsultation Duration of Symptoms.** Pain less than eight days: No anticipated delay in recovery. Pain more than eight days: Recovery may take 1.5 times longer.
2. **Typical Severity of Symptoms.** Mild pain: No anticipated delay in recovery. Severe pain: Recovery may take up to two times longer.
3. **Number of Previous Episodes.** 0-3: No anticipated delay in recovery. 4-7: Recovery may take up to two times longer.
4. **Injury Superimposed on Preexisting Condition(s).** Skeletal anomaly: May increase recovery time by 1.5-2 times. Structural pathology: May increase recovery time by 1.5-2 times.

8.1.1 **Rating:** These recommendations are **safe** and have **limited effectiveness** in predicting recovery rate. They have a rating of **promising** based on Class II and III evidence.
Consensus Level: 1
Strength of Recommendation: Type B

B. Treatment/Care Frequency:

Specific recommendations related to acute, subacute and chronic presentations are given below. In general, more aggressive in-office intervention (three to five sessions per week for one to two weeks) may be necessary early. Progressively declining frequency is expected to discharge of the patient, or conversion to elective care.

8.2.1 **Rating:** The general approach to frequency is **safe** and **effective** provided it is carried out within the guidelines of natural history. The rating is **established** and is supported by Class II and III evidence.
Consensus Level: 1
Strength of Recommendation: Type B

C. Patient Cooperation:

The nature of the patient's disorder and the purpose and strategy of the treatment plan should be adequately explained to the patient. Patients who prove to be insincere or non-compliant to treatment/care recommendations should be discharged from care, with referral when appropriate.

8.3.1 **Rating:** This recommendation is **safe** and **effective**. The rating of **promising** is given when used in an effort to avoid physician dependence and overuse of services based on Class II and III evidence.
Consensus Level: 1
Strength of Recommendation: Type B

D. Failure to Meet Treatment/Care Objectives :

1. **Acute Disorders:** After a maximum of two trial therapy series of manual procedures lasting up to two weeks each (four weeks total) without significant documented improvement, manual procedures may no longer be appropriate and alternative care should be considered.

2. **Unresponsive Acute, Subacute, or Chronic Disorders:** Repeated use of passive treatment/care normally designed to manage acute conditions should be avoided as it tends to promote physician dependence and chronicity.

3. Systematic interview of the patient and immediate family should be carried out in search for complicating or extenuating factors responsible for prolonged recovery.

4. Specific treatment/care goals should be written to address each issue.

5. Continued failure should result in patient discharge as inappropriate for chiropractic care, or having achieved maximum therapeutic benefit.

8.4.1 **Rating: Safe** and **effective** procedures that are **established** and supported by Class I, II, and III evidence.
Consensus Level: 1
Strength of Recommendation: Type A

E. Uncomplicated Cases: (acute episode)

Observing the consistency of practice experience defined by the studies listed in the review of literature for passive care, *only* acute episodes can truly be considered uncomplicated. Acute episode (first occurrence, recurrent, or exacerbation of a chronic condition).

1. Symptom Response: Significant improvement within 10-14 days; three to five treatments per week.
2. Activities-of-Daily-Living (ADL): The promotion of rest, elevation, active rest, and remobilization, as needed, are expected to improve ADL followed by a favorable response in symptoms.
3. Return to Pre-episode Status: six to eight weeks; up to three treatments per week.
4. Supportive Care: Inappropriate.

8.5.1 **Rating:** These recommendations are **safe** and **effective** in meeting the desired objectives. It has an **established** rating based upon the relationship to natural history. It is supported by Class I, II, and III evidence.
Consensus Level: 1
Strength of Recommendation: Type A.

F. Complicated Cases:

Implementation of up to two independent treatment plans relying on repeated use of passive care is generally acceptable in the management of cases undergoing prolonged recovery.

1. Signs of Chronicity: All episodes of symptoms that remain unchanged for two to three weeks should be evaluated for risk factors of pending chronicity.

Patients at risk for becoming chronic should have treatment plans altered to de-emphasize passive care and refocus on active care approaches.

8.6.1 **Rating:** Criteria for chronicity are **established, safe** and **effective** with Class I, II, and III evidence.
Consensus Level: 1
Strength of Recommendation: Type A

2. Subacute Episode:
   a. Symptom Response: Symptoms have been prolonged beyond six weeks, and passive care in this phase is as necessary, not generally to exceed two treatments per week, to avoid promoting chronicity or physician dependence.

   b. Activities of Daily Living (ADL): Management emphasis shifts to active care, dissuasion of pain behavior, patient education, flexibility and stabilization exercises. Rehabilitation may be appropriate.
   c. Return to Pre-episode Status: 6-16 weeks.
   d. Supportive Care: Inappropriate.

8.6.2 **Rating:** These recommendations are **safe** and **effective** in reaching the desired objective. They have a **promising** rating based upon the relationship to natural history and are supported by Class II and III evidence.
Consensus Level: 1
Strength of Recommendation: Type B

3. Chronic Episode
   a. Symptom Response: Symptoms have been prolonged beyond 16 weeks, and passive care is for acute exacerbation only.
   b. Activities of Daily Living (ADL): Supervised rehabilitation and life style changes are appropriate.
   c. Return to Preinjury Status: May not return. Maximum therapeutic benefit and declaration should be considered.
   d. Supportive Care: Supportive care using passive therapy may be necessary if repeated efforts to withdraw treatment/care result in significant deterioration of clinical status.

8.6.3 **Rating:** These chronic episode recommendations are **safe** and **effective** in reaching the desired objectives of sustaining the optimal health status under the circumstances. The rating is **promising**. Chronic disorder treatment/care is supported by Class II and III evidence.
Consensus Level: 1
Strength of Recommendation: Type B.

G. Elective Care:

Under specific circumstances for individual cases, elective care may be safe and effective. Elective care must be designed to avoid physician dependence and chronicity. Therapeutic necessity is absent by definition.

8.7.1 **Rating:** Unrated
Consensus Level: 1

VII. COMMENTS, SUMMARY, OR CONCLUSION

There are many unknown features that obscure our understanding of the nature of most musculoskeletal disorders. Manipulative/ adjustive procedures are an important option in the initial management. While efforts continue to be made to understand more completely the pathoanatomical and functional features, a systematic method for adopting outcome expectations is available, and even perplexing cases can be managed within a time frame that avoids or reduces the risk of chronicity or the development of physician dependence. Treatment/care established upon documented therapeutic need can be more rationally based when elements of natural history and modifying factors from the patient's lifestyle and environment are considered.

VIII. REFERENCES

1. Kapp MB: "Cookbook" medicine—a legal perspective. *Arch Intern Med.*, 150:496-500, 1990.

2. Mulley AG, Eagel KA: What is inappropriate care? *JAMA*, 260:540-1, 1988.

3. Wennberg JE, Barnes BA, Zubkoff M: Professional uncertainty and the problem of supplier-induced demand. *Soc Sci Med.*, 16:811-24, 1982.

4. Peyson MD (ed): *Chiropractic and the HMO environment in Connecticut.* Connecticut Chiropractic Association, 1985.

5. Olson RE: *Chiropractic/physical therapy treatment standards: a reference guide.* Data Management Ventures, Inc., Atlanta, GA., 1987.

6. Lang MG (chm) et al.: *Oregon chiropractic practices and utilization guidelines for neuromusculoskeletal conditions,* Oregon Chiropractic Practice and Utilization Guidelines Committee.

7. Minnesota Chiropractic Association: *Standards of practice.* Roseville, MN., 1991.

8. Ohio State Chiropractic Association. *The chiropractic manual for insurance personnel,* Columbus, Ohio, 1988,1990.

9. Hansen DT (ed): *Chiropractic standards and utilization guidelines in the care and treatment of injured workers. Chiropractic Advisory Committee*, Department of Labor and Industries, State of Washington, 1988.

10. Wennberg J, et al.: Ibid, 1982.

11. Saal J: Diagnostic studies of industrial low-back injuries. Top Acute Care Trauma. *Rehabil,* 2:31-49, 1988.

12. Leblanc F (ed): Scientific approach to the assessment and management of activity-related spinal disorders. *Spine,* 12:16-21, 1987.

13. Furberg CD: The impact of clinical trials on clinical practice. *Drug Res.*, 39:986-8, 1989.

14. Haldeman S: Presidential address, North American Spine Society: Failure of the pathology model to predict back pain. *Spine,* 15:718-24, 1990.

15. Mulley A, Eagle K: Ibid, 1988.

16. Deyo RA, Diehl AK, Rosenthal M: How many days of bed rest for acute low-back pain? A randomized clinical trial. *New Eng J Med.*, 315:1064-70, 1986.

17. Frymoyer J: Back pain and sciatica. *N Engl J Med.*, 318:291-300, 1988.

18. Mayer T, Gatchel R: *Functional Restoration for Spinal Disorders: A Sports Medicine Approach.* Philadelphia, Lea & Febiger, 1988.

19. Roland M, Morris R: A study of the natural history of back pain, part I. Development of a reliable and sensitive measure of disability in low-back pain. *Spine,* 8:141-4, 1983.

20. Roland M, Morris R: A study of the natural history of back pain, part II. Development of guidelines for trials of treatment in primary care. *Spine,* 8:145-50, 1983.

21. Waddell G: A new clinical model for the treatment of low-back pain. *Spine,* 2:632-44, 1984.

22. Cailliet R: *Rehabilitation Forum,* 1987.

23. Riley JF, Ahern DK, Follick MJ: Chronic pain and functional impairment: assessing beliefs about their relationship. *Arch Phys Med Rehabil,* 69:579-82, 1988.

24. Roland M, Morris R: Ibid, 1983.

25. Roland M. Morris R: Ibid, 1983 B.

26. Vallfors B: Acute, subacute and chronic low-back pain: clinical symptoms, absenteeism and working environment. *Scand J Rehab Med.*, (Suppl) 11:1-90, 1985.

27. Frymoyer J: Ibid, 1988.

28. Mayer T, Gatchel R: Ibid, pp 3-14, 1988.

29. Mayer TG, Gatchel RJ, Mayer H, Kishino ND, Keeley J, Mooney V: A prospective two-year study of functional restoration in industrial low-back injury. An objective assessment procedure. *JAMA,* 258:1763-7, 1987.

30. Mayer T, Gatchel R: Ibid, pp 5-6, 1988.

31. Triano JJ: Studies on the biomechanical effect of a spinal adjustment. Invited paper: World Federation of Chiropractic, Toronto, Ontario. May 1991. In press: publication of proceedings by *J Manip Physiol Ther.*, January 1992.

32. Ongley M, Klein R, Dorman T, Eek B, Hubert L: A new approach to the treatment of chronic low-back pain. *Lancet,* 2:143-6, 1987.

33. Beimborn DS, Morrissey MC: A review of the literature related to trunk muscle performance. *Spine,* 13:655-60, 1988.

34. Bronfort G: Chiropractic treatment of low-back pain: a prospective survey. *J Manip Physiol Ther.*, 9:99-113, 1986.

35. Maitland GD: Low-back pain and allied symptoms, and their treatment results. *Med J Aust.*, 44:851-4, 1957.

36. Glover JR, Morris JG, Khosla T: Back pain: randomized clinical trial of rotational manipulation of the trunk. *Br J Med.*, 31:59-64, 1974.

37. Evans DP, Burke MS, Lloyd KN, Roberts EE, Roberts GM: Lumbar spinal manipulation on trial: part I, clinical assessment. *Rheumatol Rehabil.*, 17:46-53, 1978.

38. Potter GE: A study of 744 cases of neck and back pain treated with spinal manipulation. *J Can Chiropr Assoc.*, December, pp 154-5, 1977.

39. Singer, et al.: Outcome predictions: acute low-back/leg pain. *Can Fam Phys.*, 33:655-9, 1987.

40. Triano J: Standards of Care: Manipulation Procedures In: White A, and Anderson R (eds): *Conservative Care of Low-Back Pain.* Williams & Wilkins, Baltimore, pp 159-68, 1991.

41. Hansen DT: Ibid, 1988.

42. Phllips RB, Butler R: Survey of chiropractic in Dade County, Florida. *J Manip Physiol Ther.*, 5:83-9, 1982.

43. Phillips R: A survey of Utah chiropractic patients. *ACA J Chiro,* 18:113-28, 1981.

44. Guifu C, Zongmin L, Zhenzhong Y, Jianghua W: Lateral rotatory manipulative maneuver in the treatment of subluxation and synovial entrapment of lumbar facet joints. *J Trad Chin Med.*, 4:211-12, 1984.

45. Jarvis KB, Phillips RB, Morris EK: Cost per case comparison of back injury claims of chiropractic versus medical management for conditions with identical diagnostic codes. *J Occup Med.*, 33:847-52, 1991.

46. Wolk S: An analysis of Florida workers' compensation medical claims for back-related injuries. *Proc Amer Pub Health Assoc,* Boston, 1988.

47. Cox JM, Fromelt KA, Shreiner S: Chiropractic statistical survey of 100 consecutive low-back pain patients. *J Manip Physiol Ther.*, 6:117-28, 1983.

48. Nyiendo J, Haldeman S: A prospective study of 2,000 patients attending a chiropractic college teaching clinic. *Med Care,* 25:516-27, 1987.

49. Triano JJ, Hondras M, McGregor M: Differences in treatment history with manipulation for acute, subacute, chronic and recurrent spine pain. Proceedings: World Federation of Chiropractic, Toronto, 1991. In press: publication of proceedings by *J Manip Physiol Ther.*, January 1992.

50. Herrin G, Chaffin G, Mach R: Criteria for research on the hazards of manual materials handling. *NTIS* PB83-151902, 1974.

51. Bronfort G: Ibid, 1986.

52. Mayer T, Gatchel R: Ibid, 1988.

53. Haldeman S: Ibid, 1990.

54. Sullivan MD, Turner JA, Romano J: Chronic pain in primary care identification and management of psychosocial factors. *J Fam Pract.,* 32:193-199, 1991.

55. Mayer T, Gatchel R: Ibid, pp 1988.

56. Waddell G, Main CJ, Morris EW, DiPaola M, Gray L: Chronic low back pain, psychologic distress and illness behavior. *Spine,* 9:209-13, 1984.

57. Triano JJ: Chiropractic rehabilitation practice. In: Hochschuler S, Guyer R, Cotler H, Carranza C. (eds): *Rehabilitation of the spine: science and practice.* (in press: Springer-Verlag, 1992).

58. Peterson L, Renstrom P: *Sports injuries, their prevention and treatment.* Year Book Medical Publishers, Chicago, 1983.

59. Vallfors B: Ibid, 1985.

60. Sullivan MD, et al.: Ibid, 1991.

61. Triano J, Cramer G: Patient Information: Anatomy and Biomechanics. In White A, Anderson R. (eds): *Conservative Care of Low-Back Pain.* Williams & Wilkins, Baltimore, pp 45-57, 1991.

62. White AW: *Back school and other conservative approaches to low back pain.* St. Louis, Mosby, pp 48-9, 1983.

63. Saal JA, Saal JS: Rehabilitation of the patient. In White A, Anderson R (eds.): *Conservative Care of Low-Back Pain.* Williams & Wilkins, Baltimore, pp 25-29, 1991.

64. Campbell MK: Rehabilitation of Soft Tissue Injuries, In Hammer WI (ed.): *Functional Soft Tissue Examination and Treatment by Manual Methods: The Extremities.* Aspen, Gaithersburg, pp 277-291, 1991.

65. Christensen KD: *Chiropractic Rehabilitation Volume 1: Protocols.* Publication Division, CRA Ridgefield, pp 45, 1991.

66. Saal JS, Saal JA: Strength training and flexibility. In White A, Anderson R (eds.): *Conservative care of low-back pain.* Williams and Wilkins, Baltimore, pp 65-77, 1991.

67. Shekelle P: *The appropriateness of spinal manipulation for low back pain.* CCR Conference on Research and Education, The RAND Corporation, Monterey, California, June 21, 1991.

IX. MINORITY OPINIONS

None.

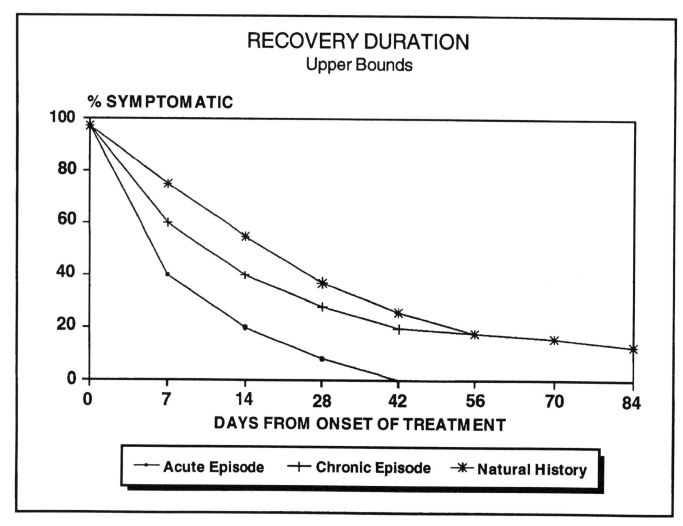

Figure 8-1 Patient's progression in comparison with the natural history (From Triano, 1991).

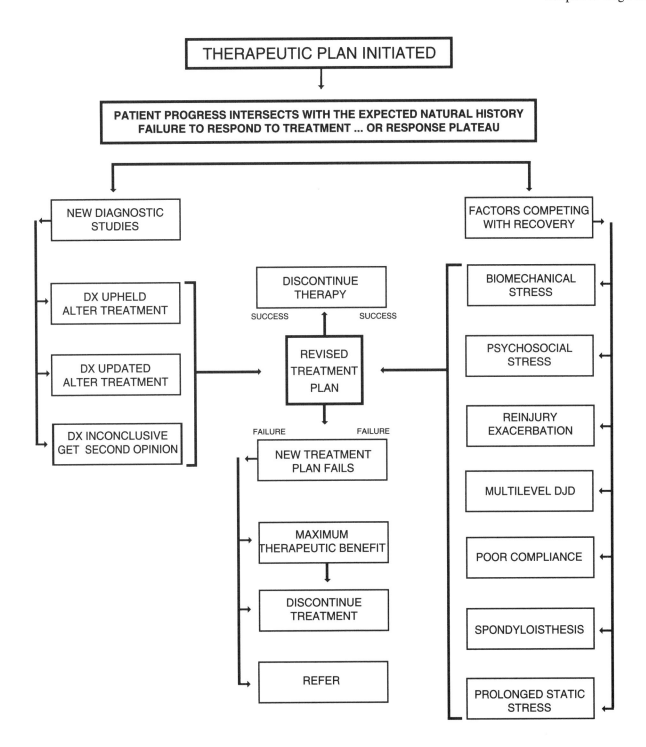

Figure 8-2

9

Reassessment

Chapter Outline

I. OVERVIEW

Reassessment refers to patient evaluations performed after the initiation of patient care. Reassessment is essential for monitoring the patient's progress and is also termed "outcomes assessment." Clinical research addresses the development and application of reassessment instruments and procedures. Appropriate application of these to clinical practice is of great importance.

The primary reason for reassessment is to evaluate the patient's clinical state. From this and a knowledge of prior condition, rate of progress and specific interventions utilized to manage the patient's condition, more informed decisions can be made regarding the appropriateness of care, efficiency of care rendered, need for continued care, and the need to modify care. A number of questions have been raised with regard to reassessment such as: Why should patients be reassessed, what specifically should be reassessed, when should reassessment be performed, and how should reassessment be conducted? In considering these topics, it is important to keep in mind the distinctive qualities of chiropractic as a manual healing art.

For the purposes of this paper, three temporal patterns of reassessment are identified: interactive, periodic, and follow-up. Since the practice of chiropractic inherently involves continual reassessment by virtue of the "hands-on" nature of the therapies, an ongoing evaluation is required with each visit. This is done in order to arrive at an ongoing clinical impression and determine the immediate need for chiropractic intervention. This is referred to here as "interactive" reassessment. Periodic reassessment is utilized in situations where changes are likely to be seen over a more extended period of weeks or months. The dynamic nature of the recuperative process requires that periodic reassessment be performed to track the patient's progress and determine the need for continued care or the need to modify the management program. Follow-up reassessment is performed at the end of the management program or when the patient has attained maximal clinical improvement. Such an assessment is often performed to ascertain the degree of residual deficit, such as disability ratings, or the degree of recovery.

II. DEFINITIONS

Assessment: An examination performed with the intent of arriving at a qualitative or quantitative description of a patient's condition. The term suggests any evaluation procedure performed for the purpose of obtaining information regarding the patient's state or condition.

Evaluation: Synonymous with assessment.

Initial Patient Evaluation: Represents the assessment procedures that are performed on a patient upon initial contact, and are used to arrive at a clinical impression and a plan for patient management. (Also: preliminary assessment, preliminary evaluation, clinical workup, preliminary workup.) Initial evaluation may include a series of diagnostic or evaluative sessions separated by days or weeks when the express purpose of these sessions is to evaluate the patient's state prior to the initiation of care (i.e., obtain a baseline).

Diagnosis: A specific decision regarding the nature of the patient's complaints.

Nominative: Pertaining to decisions based mainly on subjective or "soft" information (e.g., palpation, most ROM, reflex challenges, etc.).

Substantive: Pertaining to decisions based on mainly objective or "hard" information (such as x-ray, MRI, precise ROM).

Baseline: The temporal course of a patient's condition prior to the initiation of care, determined by a series of clinical evaluations performed during separate diagnostic sessions over a period of time.

Reassessment: Evaluation for the purpose of following the progress of a patient under clinical management. The term does not include multiple assessment sessions employed for baseline evaluation and carries the express connotation of assessment performed after the initiation of patient care.

Progress: Any change in the patient's condition. It does not necessarily mean improvement.

Interactive Reassessment: Evaluation of a patient by procedures utilized on each visit to assess the immediate need for manual intervention.

Periodic Reassessment: Evaluation of a patient at intervals of weeks or months, for the purpose of assessing the need for continued care, modified care, cessation of care or referral.

Follow-up Reassessment: Evaluation of a patient at the end of a course of therapy or management program for the purpose of assessing the status of the patient at maximal clinical improvement.

Vertebral Subluxation Complex (VSC): An aberration of normal spinal biomechanics, usually involving a restriction or loss of normal movement of a motion segment, and associated aberrations in the tissues which support articular motion (e.g., nerve, muscle, connective and vascular).

Subluxation Syndrome: The clinical signs and symptoms thought to relate to pathophysiology or dysfunction of spinal motion segments or to peripheral joints that may be amenable to manipulative/adjustive procedures.

III. LIST OF SUBTOPICS

    A. Reassessments—General Principles
    B. Interactive Reassessment
    C. Periodic Assessment

IV. LITERATURE REVIEW

Texts with chapters on diagnosis do not specifically deal with the issue of reassessment and are content to describe the procedures from a largely mechanical perspective. Therefore the frequency of reassessment is left implicitly to the judgment of the treating practitioner. Currently, justification for any particular pattern of reassessment must be culled from the clinical research literature and expert opinion. A representative selection of the literature is referenced at the end of this chapter.

In clinical practice there is typically a single assessment in the initial patient evaluation, but it is not uncommon for several consecutive assessments to be conducted to create a baseline for the patient's progress. The approach taken may depend upon the patient's condition. For example, a patient with severe, acute pain due to an apparent lumbar disc herniation will have little tolerance for multiple session evaluations to establish a baseline for management. By contrast, the establishment of a baseline for juvenile scoliosis patients typically requires evaluations over a period of several months.

Patients are reassessed for a number of reasons. Primary among them is the ongoing need for the practitioner to determine the necessity and appropriateness of further care. Reassessment gives the practitioner an opportunity to assess the effectiveness or success of the chosen treatment plan by providing a monitor of patient progress, either improvement or deterioration. It is important to determine whether improvement is occurring at an appropriate rate. If not, appropriate changes in the treatment plan can be made, including possible referral.

A reassessment is often performed to satisfy the requirements of third-party payers. Their concerns are often the justification of continued care, determination of patient progress, and determination of disability rating.

As a general rule, reassessment will focus on those areas in which positive findings were obtained during the initial clinical evaluation. Exceptions to this occur when additional signs or symptoms develop during the course of treatment which mandate re-evaluation of previously negative tests or the use of procedures not previously employed. When the natural history of a condition is known, reassessment can provide valuable insight into the effectiveness of the treatment program in altering its course.

It is unreasonable to adopt the approach that every known test is performed on the initial examination and subsequently repeated with each reassessment. Good clinical judgment combined with careful observation will direct the practitioner to those areas and procedures which will provide the most valuable information. The clinical tests used during reassessment will depend on the nature of the condition being evaluated.

"Interactive assessment" includes procedures which direct treatment for that patient visit. These typically include procedures which provide indications for manipulation/adjustment, such as palpation and other spinal motion assessment.

Periodic reassessment includes: 1) repetition of actions or clinical procedures which upon prior examination provided information about the chief complaint and which led to the clinical impression. Examples include range of motion, tenderness and positive pain provocation signs; 2) repetition of tests wherein abnormalities were detected on initial examination (e.g., deep tendon reflexes); 3) new procedures not previously performed but indicated by the patient's clinical condition; 4) special studies (e.g., C.T. scan) which may impact the course of therapy when there has been failure to improve or deterioration in the patient's condition.

Spinal radiography is used widely as a reassessment tool but definitive studies on level of appropriateness are lacking. There is also little scientific evidence to validate many of the commonly used procedures and tests in neuromuscular diagnosis. There is even less documentation of validity and reliability with respect to procedures specific to the manual arts. Existing criteria and practice appear to have evolved empirically from clinical experience and convention. However, such procedures are widely used. As in all health care, if we depend entirely upon scientific method to determine the inclusion or exclusion of evaluation procedures, we would be left with a paucity of procedures with which to arrive at a working clinical impression.

The way in which reassessments are made needs considerable clarification. Interactive procedures should be simple and allow for assessment in an ongoing practice. Analog pain scales provide a tool for regular pain assessment, whereas pain questionnaires are more cumbersome and difficult to administer on an ongoing basis. Periodic evaluations may have more formal structure and detail. They may include more extensive questionnaires regarding pain, patient satisfaction and activities of daily living, functional disability assessment, and more extensive physical examination procedures. The evaluative procedures selected will depend upon the nature and role of reassessment.

Frequency of periodic reassessment is determined by several factors such as the severity or urgency of the condition or the likelihood of progression and degeneration. Scoliosis is an excellent example of a condition in which the frequency of reassessment varies with the severity and location of the condition, the age of the patient and history of prior progression. Truly life-threatening conditions requiring continuous monitoring, or even daily monitoring, are rarely found in chiropractic practice, and if they are the patient should be referred to an appropriate facility. Severe acute conditions should be assessed frequently. A patient's need for reassessment may also change during the course of care, depending upon progress. If the patient's condition demonstrates marked improvement, then reassessment should become less frequent. Conversely, if the patient deteriorates, reassessment should be performed as soon as possible to determine an appropriate course of action.

The practitioner's role in integrating information from diverse sources and prescribing or administering treatment can be assisted by reassessment information contributed by a variety of individuals. Some aspects of reassessment may involve appropriately trained and qualified employees of the attending practitioner. Others may require the assistance of specialized facilities, such as advanced imaging centers. The chiropractic practitioner assumes the role of team captain, coordinating the efforts of a health care team in the evaluation, diagnosis and management of the patient.

V. ASSESSMENT CRITERIA

Procedure Ratings (System II)

Necessary: Strong positive recommendation, based on Class I evidence, or overwhelming Class II evidence when circumstances reflect compromise of patient safety.

Recommended: Positive recommendation, based on consensus of Class II and/or strong Class III evidence.

Discretionary: Positive recommendation, based on strong consensus of Class III evidence.

Unnecessary: Negative recommendation, based on inconclusive or conflicting Class II, III evidence.

Quality of Evidence:

The following categories of evidence are used to support the ratings.

Class I:

A. Evidence of clinical utility from controlled studies published in refereed journals.

B. Binding or strongly persuasive legal authority such as legislated or case law.

Class II:

A. Evidence of clinical utility from the significant results of uncontrolled studies in refereed journals.

B. Evidence provided by recommendations from published expert legal opinion or persuasive case law.

Class III:

A. Evidence of clinical utility provided by opinions of experts, anecdote and/or by convention.

B. Expert legal opinion.

VI. RECOMMENDATIONS

A. Reassessments - General Principles

Reassessments are an integral component of case management and should be made following an appropriate period of care.

9.1.1 **Rating:** Necessary
Evidence: Class II, III
Consensus Level: 1

The necessity for and the content of reassessments are determined by the patient's response. Patients responding as expected might be reassessed later and with fewer tests; those not responding or responding more slowly should be re-evaluated sooner and possibly more thoroughly. A knowledge of the natural history of the condition greatly facilitates decisions concerning the timing of reassessment.

9.2.1 **Rating:** Necessary
Evidence: Class II, III
Consensus Level: 1

Appropriate reassessment shall be made as soon as possible if the patient demonstrates a marked worsening of clinical status.

9.3.1 **Rating:** Necessary
Evidence: Class III
Consensus Level: 1

Appropriate reassessment shall be made if the patient begins to manifest clinical signs or symptoms in areas not previously evaluated.

9.4.1 **Rating:** Necessary
Evidence: Class II, III
Consensus Level: 1

Reassessment should be performed by persons appropriately trained and qualified in the specific procedures.

9.5.1 **Rating:** Necessary
Evidence: Class II, III
Consensus Level: 1

Reassessment should be performed, as closely as possible, in the same manner as the initial assessment.

9.6.1 **Rating:** Recommended
Evidence: Class I, II, III
Consensus Level: 1

Reassessments performed solely to satisfy third party interests should be performed with due regard for all the recommendations presented in this chapter.

9.7.1 **Rating:** Recommended
Evidence: Class III
Consensus Level: 1

Interactive reassessment should be performed during each patient encounter for the purpose of confirming or modifying a clinical impression.

B. Interactive Reassessment

9.8.1 **Rating:** Necessary
Evidence: Class III
Consensus Level: 1

C. Periodic Reassessment

Periodic reassessment should be performed only after it would be reasonably expected that some measurable change in the patient's clinical condition would have occurred.

9.9.1 **Rating:** Necessary
Evidence: Class III
Consensus Level: 1

Periodic reassessment should be made in all areas in which there were prior positive clinical findings.

9.10.1 **Rating:** Necessary
Evidence: Class III
Consensus Level: 1

VII. COMMENTS, SUMMARY OR CONCLUSION

None.

VIII. REFERENCES

Adams AH: Methodological considerations in the selection of outcome measures for chiropractic practice. *ICSM Proceedings*, April 1991.

Arnold L: *Chiropractic Procedures Examination.* Seminole Printing, Inc. Seminole, Florida 1978.

Banks RJ, LeBoeuf C, Webb MN: Recently graduated chiropractors in Australia, Part 3: interprofessional referrals. *J Aust Chiro Assoc* 1988; 18(1):14-16.

Bolton SP: When to re-x-ray? A case report. J *Aust Chiro Assoc* 1989:19(1):2-4.

Burns K, Johnson P: *Health Assessment in Clinical Practice.* Prentice-Hall, Inc., Englewood Cliffs, New Jersey, 1980.

Burton AK: Sciatic syndromes; a preliminary report of a search for criteria for identification and assessment. *Brit Osteopathic J* 1983;15:87-94.

Christensen K: *Clinical Chiropractic Orthopedics.* Foot Levelers, Inc., Dubuque, Iowa, 1984.

Cox JM: *Low-Back Pain.* Williams and Wilkins, 1987, Baltimore.

Cox JM, Aspergren DD: Scoliosis: diagnosis, detection, and treatment. *ACA Journal of Chiropractic* 1986; 20(1); 46-52.

Daniel M, Long C, Murphy W, Kores R, Hutcherson W: Therapists' and chronic pain patients' perceptions of treatment outcome. *J Nervous Mental Di* 1983;171(12):729-733.

DeGiacoma F: *Chiropractic analysis through palpation.* New York Chiropractic College, Glenhead, New York , 1979.

DeGowin EL, DeGowin RL: *Diagnostic Examination.* Macmillan Publishing Company, Inc., 1981.

Donelson R, Grant W et al.: Pain response to repeated end-range sagittal spinal motion. *Spine* (Sup 1991); 16(65):5206-5212.

Drummond D, Ranallo F, Lonstein J, Brooks HL, Cameron J: Radiation hazards in scoliosis management. *Spine* 1983;8(7) 741-748.

Evans JH, Kagan A: The development of a functional rating scale to measure the treatment outcome of chronic spinal patients. *Spine* 1986;11(3):277-281.

Gatterman M: *Chiropractic Management of Spine Related Disorders.* Williams & Wilkins Baltimore, Maryland, 1990.

Gehlbach SH: *Interpreting the Medical Literature.* Macmillian Publishing Company, 1988.

Greenstein G, Hsieh C-Y, Danielson C, Phillips RB, Lueder R: Intra-examiner reliability using the flexcurve to determine lumbar lordosis, sagittal mobility and a range of motion index. *Proc ICSM.* 1990, FCER 1701 Clarendon Blvd., Arlington, VA.

Haney PL, Mootz RD: A case report on nonresolving conservative care of low-back pain and sciatic radicular syndrome. *J Manip Physiol Ther* 1985; 8(2):109-114.

Hansen DT, Ayres JR: Chiropractic Outcome Measure. *Chiropractic Technique.* Williams & Wilkins 1991.

Hildebrandt RW: The chiropractic spinography issue (letter). *J Manip Physiol Therap* 1981; 4(4):171-172.

Hsieh C-Y, Phillips RB: Reliability of manual muscle testing with a computerized dynamometer. *J Manip Physiol Ther* 1990; 13(2):72-82.

Hsieh C-Y, Phillips RB, Adams AH, Pope MH: Functional outcomes of low-back pain: comparison of four treatment groups in a randomized controlled trial. *J Manip Physiol Ther* 1992; 15(1):4-9. Chiropractic.

Inglis B, Faser B, Penfold B: Chiropractic in New Zealand. *Report of the Commission of Inquiry.* Government Printer, Wellington, New Zealand 1979.

Jackson R, Schafer R: *Basic Chiropractic Paraprofessional Manual.* American Chiropractic Association , Arlington, Virginia, 1978.

Jamison JR: Chiropractic's functional integration into conventional health care: some implications. *J Manip Physiol Ther* 1987; 10(1):5-10.

LeBoeuf C, Gardner V: Chronic low-back pain: orthopaedic and chiropractic test results. *Aust Chiro Assoc* 1989;19(1):9-16.

Marback N: Complications in a low-back case. *ACA Journal of Chiropractic* 1980;14:131-134.

Mayer TG: Using physical measurements to assess low-back pain. *J of Musculoskeletal Med.* June 1985:44-59.

Meade TW, Dyer S, Browne W, Townsend J, Frank AO: Low-back pain of mechanical origin: randomized comparison of chiropractic and hospital outpatient treatment. *Brit Med J* 1990;300:1431-1437.

Mellin G: Physical therapy for chronic low-back pain: correlations between spinal mobility and treatment outcome. *Scand J Rehabil Med* 1985; 17(4):163-166.

Mennell JM: The validation of the diagnosis "joint dysfunction" in the synovial joints of the cervical spine. *J Manip Physiol Ther* 1990; 13(1):7-12.

Nash CL, Gregg EC, Brown RH, Pillai K: Risks of exposure to x-rays in patients undergoing long-term treatment for scoliosis. *J Bone Joint Surg* 1979; 61A:371-374.

Palmer M, Epler M: *Clinical Assessment Procedures in Physical Therapy.* Lippincott Company, Philadelphia, Pennylvania, 1990.

Pressman A, Adams A: *Clinical Assessment of Nutritional Status: A Working Manual.* Management Enterprises New York City, New York, 1982.

Quebec Task Force on Spinal Disorders. *Spine Supplement 1* - Harper & Row Publishers, 1987;12.

Rae PS, Waddell G, Venner RM: A simple technique for measuring lumbar spinal flexion. *Journal of the Royal College of Surgeons of Edinburgh* 1984; 29(5):281-284.

Richards TJ: Chiropractic specialists - a referral resource. *ACA Journal of Chiropractic* May 1990-26-29.

Robinson GK, Lantz CA: Videofluoroscopy in chiropractic management of cervical syndromes. *J Chiro Res Clin Invest* 1991;6(4):93-97.

Sandoz R: The choice of appropriate clinical criteria for assessing the progress of a chiropractic case. *Ann Swiss Chiro Assoc*:53-73.

Sawyer CE, Bergmann TF, Good DW: Attitudes and habits of chiropractors concerning referral to other health care providers. *J Manip Physiol Ther* 1988;11(6):480-483.

Schafer R, Faye LJ: *Motion Palpation and Chiropractic Technic,* Motion Palpation Institute, Huntington Beach, 1990.

Schafer R: *Basic Chiropractic Procedural Manual.* American Chiropractic Association, Arlington, Virginia, 1984.

Stevens RF: Treatment of adolescent scoliosis. *ACA Journal of Chiropractic,* May 1983;17:72-73.

Swezey RL, Crittenden JO, Swezey AM: Outpatient treatment of lumbar disc sciatica. *Western J Medicine* 1986;145(1):43-46.

IX. MINORITY OPINIONS

None.

Outcome Assessment

"If we are told that the serum cholesterol is 230 mg per 100 Ml, that the chest x-ray shows cardiac enlargement, and that the electrocardiogram has Q waves, we would not know whether the treated object was a dog or a person. If we were told that capacity at work was restored, that the medicine tasted good and was easy to take, and that the family was happy about the results, we would recognize a human set of responses."

(Feinstein, 1972)

Chapter Outline

I. OVERVIEW

Donabedian (1982) discussed health care quality in terms of structure (organization), process (procedures) and outcomes (benefits and harms). He defined outcomes to mean a change in a patient's current or future health status that can be attributed to antecedent health care. By using a broad operational definition of health, such things as improvement in social and psychological function can be added to the more traditional measures of physical and physiological function. Coile (1990) writes that while the history of quality care in the U.S. may have focused on the first two concepts, the current trend is swinging to assessment of outcomes as a way to hold health care practitioners accountable for their work. Ellwood (1988) agrees that outcomes are integral to definitions of quality health care.

Chiropractic clinicians and researchers have also recognized and stressed the importance of emphasizing outcome assessments (McLachlan, 1991; Hansen, 1991; Adams, 1991; Jose, 1991). This trend is consistent with chiropractic practice because the chiropractic profession has always philosophically emphasized health in its broader definitions and championed the positive potential of human beings in their environment.

The broad perspective on health outcomes leads to contemplation of a very large number of assessment or measurement procedures ranging from the social to the physical sciences. Discussion of all possible outcome assessments is beyond the scope of this chapter. The emphasis will be on outcomes related to conditions of the neuromusculoskeletal system because they represent the largest proportion of chiropractic patient complaints. General health assessment measures are very important and will also be discussed. In general, a parsimonious view of outcomes is taken, still with the idea that the needs of the patient, the practitioner and society are all important in assuring the overall quality of chiropractic care.

Outcome assessments vary considerably depending on the scope of clinical phenomena one might want to measure and the target patient population. General health outcome assessments, which have received considerable attention in recent years, attempt to measure a number of attributes deemed important to the overall concept of health. Health outcomes are important to patients, whereas physicians traditionally use more specific outcomes such as laboratory test results to assess the effects of care.

At first glance, it would seem that the results of diagnostic tests and the diagnosis itself would make ideal outcome measures. But this point of view is too narrow, emphasizing mostly physiological mechanisms more important to the practitioner's decision-making process than to the broader needs of patients and society.

There is a distinction between procedures used for diagnosis and those used for assessing the outcome of care. The purpose of a diagnosis is to label the pathological entity so that the doctor can formulate an appropriate treatment plan. Different diagnoses usually imply different treatments. In contrast, the purpose of an outcome assessment is to measure a change in patient status as a result of treatment. The same outcome assessment may be used to measure the effect of different treatments for any number of diagnoses (for example, a general health questionnaire). Also, a diagnosis may not change even though the health status of the patient may improve under care. On the other hand, if the goal of treatment is to eliminate the diagnosed disorder (i.e., "cure" the patient), then the appropriate diagnostic and outcome procedures may be one and the same.

The discussion and recommendations in the chapters on imaging, instrumentation, clinical laboratory, clinical impression, and reassessment also have a bearing on the general topic of outcome assessment. Because those chapters deal in some detail with diagnostic procedures potentially useful as outcome procedures, and with other case management considerations, some procedures may be only briefly mentioned here.

Appropriate standardized outcome assessments are useful in normal clinical practice for they can:

- Consistently evaluate the effect of care over time
- Help indicate the point of maximum therapeutic improvement
- Uncover problems related to care such as noncompliance
- Document improvement to the patient, doctor, and third parties
- Suggest modifications of the goals of treatment if necessary
- Quantify the clinical experience of the doctor
- Justify the type, dose, and duration of care
- Help provide a data-base for clinical research
- Assist in establishing standards of treatment for specific conditions.

This chapter will recommend methods of assessing outcomes of chiropractic care based upon defined criteria, scientific evidence, and expert opinion that are valid, reliable, clinically useful in chiropractic practice, and able to be interpreted by those interested in the role of chiropractic health care in society.

II. DEFINITIONS

Outcome Assessment: This term refers to a procedure or method of measuring a change in patient status over time, primarily to evaluate the effect of treatment.

Chiropractic Care: This term refers to the behaviors, methods, procedures, etc., that chiropractic practitioners employ in the case-management of patients.

Instrument: This refers to a specific tool or measuring device. It includes questionnaires filled out by patients.

General Health Assessments: These are usually questionnaires completed by patients and scored for a number of attributes deemed important to the overall concept of health.

Disease (Condition Specific) Assessments: These outcome procedures can run the gamut from physiological tests to questionnaires. They are designed to elicit information about the specific signs and symptoms and other clinical characteristics of diseases or conditions. Condition specific assessments are usually more limited in scope than general health assessments.

Meta-analysis: This refers to a type of study that statistically pools the data from many relevant single studies in order to make summary conclusions about a topic.

Spinal Manipulative Therapy (SMT): This term refers to the range of manual care delivered in chiropractic practice. It includes adjustive, manipulative and mobilization procedures.

Subluxation Syndrome: This term is defined here to mean the clinical signs and symptoms that relate to pathophysiology or dysfunction of spinal and pelvic motion segments or to peripheral joints that may be amenable to manipulative/adjustive procedures.

Definitions of Concepts for Outcome Measures

In order to make suitable recommendations with respect to outcome measurements, a number of concepts must be considered (Deyo, 1991; Bombardier, 1987).

Validity/accuracy: This concept refers to the truth. It is the answer to the question: Does this outcome procedure/instrument actually measure what it is supposed to measure? In order to evaluate validity, the outcome procedure must correlate highly with a "gold standard" of comparison. In the absence of a "gold standard," other forms of validity testing can be applied. Systematic error causes a procedure to be less than 100% valid or accurate. Scientific experimentation is very suitable for determining the validity of a procedure.

Responsiveness: This term refers to the ability of an outcome assessment to detect clinically important changes over time. Sometimes this is referred to as the sensitivity of an outcome assessment to treatment. Responsiveness is a particularly important attribute of an outcome assessment because subtle beneficial clinical effects of care should be able to be detected. Scientific experimentation, especially randomized controlled clinical trials, provide the best evidence for the responsiveness of an outcome assessment.

Reliability/precision: While distinctions of definitions between these words do exist, the general meaning here reflects the ability of an outcome procedure to consistently give the same value upon repeated measurements of the same phenomenon (e.g., patient). Random error causes a procedure to be less than 100% reliable or precise. Scientific experimentation is very suitable for determining the reliability of a procedure. Related terms are intra-observer (-examiner-rater) reliability and inter-observer (-examiner-rater) reliability. These refer respectively to the degree that one observer agrees with his own repeated measurements; and the degree that two or more observers agree with each others' measurements of the same phenomenon. Reliability must be established in order to ensure that variation in an outcome assessment over time reflects a true change rather than measurement error.

Applicability/clinical relevance: This term refers to the relevance of an outcome procedure, in other words, how it may impact upon case-management decisions. It answers the question: Is this outcome important to measure in clinical practice? Relevance also varies with health condition. Different types of patients require different types of outcome assessments. Scientific experimentation is important in determining this characteristic.

Practicality: This refers to the feasibility issues related to an outcome procedure in clinical practice. Such things as cost, time efficiency, training requirements, patient acceptance, etc., must play a role in this determination. Scientific experimentation plays a significant role here, as well as clinicians' resources and inclinations, which may vary.

Safety: Safety refers to the degree of health risk an outcome procedure may present; especially to patients, but also to doctors and their staff.

Ratings: Two separate rating scales will be employed depending upon the nature of the recommendation.

III. LIST OF SUBTOPICS

A. Functional Outcome Assessments

B. Patient Perception Outcome Assessments
- Pain
- Satisfaction

C. General Health Outcome Assessments

D. Physiological Outcomes
- Range of Motion (regional)
- Thermography
- Muscle Function
- Postural Evaluations

E. Subluxation Syndrome
- Vertebral Position Assessed Radiographically
- Abnormal Segmental Motion/Lack of Joint End-play
- Abnormal Segmental Motion Assessed Radiography
- Soft Tissue Compliance and Tenderness
- Asymmetric or Hypertonic Muscle Contraction

F. Principles of Application

IV. LITERATURE REVIEW

The outcomes of health care may be characterized as falling into one of the following categories: death, disease, disability, discomfort, dissatisfaction, and destitution (Lohr, 1988). A more positive taxonomy would simply use the opposites of these words, e.g., survival rates, lack of disease, ability, comfort, satisfaction, and thrift. While easily understood in general, operational definitions and assessment procedures for outcomes of care that match the attributes mentioned above are more difficult to obtain.

For this review, a citation search was derived from original research, review papers and books from the chiropractic, medical and scientific literature. The topic and its research base is large. A great deal of material was referenced from Interstudy, an organization devoted to the scientific development of outcome assessments. Personal experience and opinions of those conducting clinical trials in the chiropractic community were also considered.

The literature on outcome assessments can be divided into studies that have concentrated on the development of procedures, those that have tested procedures for validity and reliability, and those that have used the procedures in assessing the effects of treatment in randomized clinical trials. The latter studies provide the best information on responsiveness.

The literature review will be divided into five major subtopics, reflecting the nature of the outcome assessment procedures under discussion; 1) functional outcome assessments; 2) patient perception outcome assessments; 3) general health outcome assessments; 4) physiological outcome assessments; and 5) the subluxation syndrome as an outcome assessment.

Disease-specific physiological measurements related to treatment outcomes number in the hundreds if not thousands, so only a small number of most relevant procedures deemed important to chiropractic practice are described here. Others are described in other chapters. The subluxation syndrome as an outcome assessment has elements of function, perception and physiology, but requires special consideration because of its importance to chiropractic clinical theory and practice.

It is difficult to conceptually separate some of the physiological outcomes from those related more specifically to the subluxation syndrome. Some readers may therefore disagree with the committee's categorization and feel that some procedures under physiological outcomes should be relegated to the subluxation syndrome category. The argument exists because there are different opinions about just how comprehensive the definition of the subluxation syndrome should be in terms of encompassing different types of spinal and locomotor pathophysiology or dysfunction.

Economic outcomes (assessing the costs and cost-effectiveness of care) are becoming increasingly important. Indeed, some have argued that cost accountability is more important to third-party payers than health outcomes. Practitioners certainly are not immune to such forces and they must pay attention to the economic effects of their care. The discussion of cost outcomes will not, however, be covered in this chapter. A good discussion of economic outcome issues related to chiropractic can be found in Nyiendo (1990).

Functional Outcome Assessments

Assessing a patient's function is a logical way to assess the behavioral effects of a disease and the outcome of care. Usually, patient functioning is verbally discussed between the patient and practitioner, but new questionnaire techniques may make such information more objective. For this chapter, functional outcome assessments refer to questionnaires designed to measure a patient's limitations in performing the usual human tasks of living. Functional questionnaires seek to quantify symptoms, function and behavior directly, rather than to infer them from less relevant physiological tests.

There are a large number of functional scales described in the scientific literature. Most of them have been developed to assess the behavioral effects of diseases of the neuromusculoskeletal system and to assess the effects of treatment for those diseases. Deyo (1990) presented an excellent review and summary of many functional assessments used in back pain research. Of particular note are the *Pain Disability Index* (Tait, 1987), the *Million Disability Questionnaire* (Million, 1982), the *Oswestry Disability Questionnaire* (Fairbank, 1980), *The Roland Morris Disability Questionnaire* (Roland, 1983), the *Waddell Disability Index* (Waddell, 1982), and the *Dallas Pain Questionnaire* (Lawlis, 1989). A modification of the *Oswestry Questionnaire* to make it useful for neck function was recently published by Vernon (1991).

A very detailed discussion of the validity, reliability, responsiveness, relevance, feasibility, and safety of the many functional scales is beyond the scope of this chapter. For further information the book *Measuring Health: A Guide to Rating Scales and Questionnaires* (McDowell and Newell, 1987) is very useful. In general, while there may be some gaps in the research base for many individual functional questionnaires, the usefulness of these types of instruments is apparent.

In terms of responsiveness, which is the ability of an instrument to document changes in health status, it is instructive to examine the clinical trials with respect to manipulative/adjustive treatment methods. This is not to suggest, however, that chiropractic care is synonymous with spinal manipulative therapy. Chiropractic care encompasses a wide range of conservative therapeutics.

There are at least 28 randomized clinical trials of spinal manipulative therapy (SMT) for painful complaints in the scientific literature (Shekelle, 1991; Haldeman, 1991; Ottenbacher, 1985; Anderson, 1992). In one meta-analysis (Anderson, 1992), the authors categorized the outcome assessments in 23 randomized trials into eight categories: patient report of pain, overall clinical improvement assessed by the patient, overall clinical improvement assessed by the practitioner, range of trunk flexion, range of trunk extension, straight leg raising, work activities, and activities of daily living.

In general, the outcomes showing the greatest improvement with treatment by spinal manipulation were the functional measures (activities of daily living) and patients' report of pain. Outcome assessments in the form of ranges of trunk motion did not indicate as much improvement on the average, although improvement was certainly demonstrated in a proportion of studies. Clinical trials using the straight leg raising test as an indicator of improvement demonstrated mixed results, which is not surprising given the very mixed nature of the patients' complaints.

Most clinical trial investigators created their own functional scales and so did not use standardized outcome assessments of known validity and reliability. Berquist-Ullman (1977) used patients' reports of pain and dysfunction. Rasmussen (1979) used a measure of pain, spinal mobility, function and "fitness for work." Coxhead et al. (1981) reported measures of patient report of pain and return to work. Ongley et al. (1987) reported disability scores, and visual analog scales. MacDonald et al. (1990) used a disability scale and a linear analog pain scale. Nevertheless, most trials demonstrated a responsiveness to treatment.

Hadler et al. (1987) used the standard Roland Morris Disability scale while Meade et al. (1990) used the *Oswestry Disability Questionnaire*. Hsieh (1991) concluded that the *Roland Morris Questionnaire* and the *Oswestry Questionnaire* gave consistent but slightly different results in a chiropractic clinical trial.

Clinicians contemplating the use of functional instruments should be aware of differences between them and be able to choose the most appropriate assessment for their specific situation.

Patient Perceptions Outcome Assessments

Patient perceptions of pain and satisfaction have not traditionally been considered very important as outcomes in any quantitative fashion. This is probably because it was felt that patient perceptions were too subjective and variable to be of much use. This is despite the fact that clinical impressions of the value of treatments are most likely based on favorable comments by patients to their practitioners. Currently, however, health services researchers have discovered that patient perceptions, measured with appropriate procedures, may be an excellent way to measure many aspects of the quality of care (Donabedian, 1980; Cherkin, 1990).

Pain: Pain is a perception and most chiropractic patients have pain of the neuromusculoskeletal system. Low-back and neck pain probably represent about two thirds of all chiropractic patient concerns (Nyiendo, 1989).

In the acute stage, pain is a symptom indicating that tissue damage has occurred. In the chronic state, pain may persist in the absence of detectable tissue trauma and become a disease in its own right. It makes sense for practitioners to attempt to measure pain as a way of evaluating the success of their care (Sandoz, 1985).

There is a great deal of research in the scientific literature on pain measurement (McDowell, 1987; Melzack, 1983; Vernon, 1990). Indeed, many orthopedic and neurologic examination procedures rely upon patients' report of pain provocation. To discuss the entire range of potential assessment methods is again beyond the scope of this chapter, but details may be found in the references noted above and in other chapters.

Pain has a number of dimensions including severity (intensity), duration, and frequency. The dimension that is most commonly assessed is severity (Jensen, 1986). Methods run the gamut from single questions to complex surveys. In most cases, the patients report their own perception of pain.

Visual Analog Scales (VAS) consist of a 10 cm line anchored by two pain descriptors at either end of the line. Patients are asked to mark on the line a point that represents their perceived pain intensity. The properties of VAS have been extensively studied (Huskisson, 1982).

Numerical Rating Scales ask the patient to choose a number between 0-100 that represents their pain intensity. Another pain scale uses 11 ranked levels numbered 0-11 graphically depicted in boxes.

The so-called "Behavioral Rating Scale" has six levels, each with a description such as for the third level, "pain present, cannot be ignored, but does not interfere with everyday activities." Verbal rating scales use single word descriptors in three, four, five or more ranks.

One commonly used scale from the *McGill/Melzack Pain Questionnaire* called the Present Pain Intensity scale uses the words, "none, mild, discomforting, horrible, and excruciating."

An interesting comparison among the scales mentioned above indicated there were few differences between them, except that the "Visual Analog Scale" and the "Numerical Rating Scale" were more practical (Jensen, 1986).

Pain diaries can be useful to measure other dimensions of pain. Patients are instructed to daily indicate on a form the intensity, duration and frequency of their pain complaints. Parker (1978) used a patient report headache diary of severity, duration and frequency, and a disability score calculated from it. Pain diaries may also be very useful for single-case time-series research designs (Keating, 1985).

A famous pain measurement instrument is the *McGill/Melzack Pain Questionnaire* (Melzack, 1975). It has been used in back pain treatment research and to describe chiropractic patients (Nyiendo, 1990). The *McGill Questionnaire* consists of twenty categories of words that describe qualities of pain. Patients indicate which words apply in their case. At least six different pain variables can be calculated from the instrument. While relatively well-studied in terms of validity and reliability (McDowell, 1987), it may present some practical difficulties in clinical practice because it should be administered by an interviewer.

Most, if not all, clinical trials of SMT have utilized some way of measuring pain. For example, Coyer and Curwen (1955) used an outcome of "well" defined by lack of signs and symptoms of low-back pain presumably judged by the practitioner in consultation with the patient. Edwards (1969) assessed treatment on a five point scale of signs and symptoms judged by the doctor. Glover et al. (1974) used a scale of pain relief from 0 - 100%. Doran and Newell (1975) used a patient-reported six level pain relief scale. Koes et al. (1991) reported a randomized clinical trial for back and neck pain using severity of complaints and "global perceived effect," a subjective assessment of overall improvement. Lopes et al. (1991) in another clinical trial for cervical pain assessed pain and range of motion comparing a single manipulation to a mobilization. Both favorably affected range of motion, but pain measures favored manipulation.

Patient Satisfaction: Patient satisfaction is an important perception having not only to do with the actual effectiveness of treatment, but also the setting and the process of receiving care (Donabedian, 1980). Patient satisfaction may be an important marker of quality of care (Cleary, 1988), and it is increasingly evident that patient satisfaction is a consumer marketing target for managed care organizations.

Patient satisfaction outcomes have been studied by Ware and others (Ware, 1978; Lochman, 1983). Clearly, there are a number of dimensions that can be measured. They include: interpersonal manner, technical quality, efficacy/outcomes, accessibility/convenience, finances, continuity, physical environment, and availability. The *Patient Satisfaction Questionnaire* measures all eight dimensions (Ware, 1983). Ware also developed four questions that measure general satisfaction with care. According to Cherkin (1990), the *Visit-Specific Satisfaction Questionnaire* (Ware, 1988) is probably very appropriate for chiropractic outcomes.

Deyo (1986) developed a patient satisfaction scale specifically for patients with low-back pain. Recently, Cherkin (in press) developed and validated a back pain patient questionnaire that addressed three key dimensions of satisfaction: caring, information, and effectiveness.

One of the valuable aspects of assessing patient satisfaction is its global nature. For the great majority of ambulatory patients, certain dimensions of satisfaction may be assessed regardless of the nature of the health complaint or the diagnosis. Works by Sawyer (1991), Cherkin (1989), and Kane (1974) have suggested high levels of satisfaction with chiropractic care.

General Health Outcome Assessments

Assessment of general health status is philosophically congruent with the chiropractic viewpoint; that is, an emphasis on health as opposed to disease. General health has been notoriously difficult to define in operational terms, but progress in recent years has led to the development of a number of useful instruments that are increasingly being used as assessments of the outcome of health care (Nelson, 1989; Bronfort, 1991). A full detailed discussion of health status measurement is beyond the present scope, but an excellent review of the difficult conceptual issues and examples of various scales may be found in the book edited by Spilker entitled, *Quality of Life Assessments in Clinical Trials* (1990), and in other references (Kirschner, 1987).

The *Sickness Impact Profile* (SIP) (Bergner, 1981) is an extensively studied patient survey of a number of behavioral and psychosocial dimensions thought to reflect general health status: sleep and rest, eating, work, home management, recreation and pastimes, ambulation, mobility, body care and movement, social interaction, alertness behavior, emotional behavior, and communication. It has been used in back pain research (Deyo, 1986) as well as in other areas.

Another measure of general health was developed during the *Medical Outcomes Study* (Stewart, 1988) and has now been modified by *Interstudy* (1990). The SF36 questionnaire measures three major health attributes (functional status, well-being, and overall evaluation of health) and eight health concepts which yield eight indices: physical functioning, social functioning, role limitations due to physical problems, role limitations due to emotional problems, mental health, energy/fatigue, pain, and general health perception (*Interstudy*, 1990). The SF36 appears to be a useful way to standardize assessments across many types of clinical settings and for a variety of types of patients. The SF36 has been and is being used in several chiropractic outcome studies (Nyiendo, 1991; Kassak, 1991; Jose, 1991).

Another useful general health measure is the set of COOP Charts (Nelson, 1987). These utilize simple representative pictures as choices to answers that yield nine indices of general health. Three focus on specific dimensions of function, two are related to symptoms or feelings, three are concerned with perceptions, and one is a health covariate. They appear to be very practical, easy to administer and score and correlate well with other less practical measures.

Physiological Outcome Assessments

Range of Motion (regional): A standard examination of spinal and other joint physiology includes the measurement of the range of motion (ROM) that can be obtained by the patient. ROM is used to assess disability and impairment because of the assumed relationship to spinal function (AMA, 1988). Lack of motion is also considered a treatable dysfunction that can be addressed by a variety of manual and rehabilitative procedures. Commonly, these are SMT and exercise therapy.

In this section, regional trunk and neck mobility along with peripheral joint mobility will be considered. Segmental spinal joint mobility is addressed in the section on subluxation syndrome.

Devices and methods of measuring ROM range from the simple to the sublime. Standard joint goniometers are common, but now there are more sophisticated tools, many with electronic data recording capabilities. Mobility can be assessed with the patient actively involved, or as the passive object being mobilized. One or all planes of motion may be assessed.

The reliability of a number of common methods of measuring trunk mobility of the lumbar spine was reviewed by Liebenson (1989). He concluded that the modified Schober technique, inclinometers, flexible rulers, and spondylometers had received the most scientific support. The fingertip-to-floor method was not considered valid because of errors introduced by hip motion, hamstring flexibility and arm length. Zachman (1989) compared a simple goniometer and the "rangiometer" and assessed examiner reliability for cervical ROMs. The "rangiometer" was considered moderately reliable. Nansel (1989) concluded that taking the mean of five repeated measures of cervical lateral flexion with an inclinometer was also a reliable method.

The responsiveness of kinematic measurements of the range of regional spine motion (neck or trunk mobility) has been repeatedly demonstrated in clinical trials of manipulative therapy (Anderson, in press; Ottenbacher, 1985), and under laboratory conditions. Nansel et al. (1989) measured cervical lateral bending asymmetries with a simple goniometer and found they could be reduced by lower cervical adjustments. In additional study, rotational asymmetries in the transverse plane were reduced by upper cervical adjustments (Nansel, 1991).

Evans (1978) reported outcomes of spinal flexion, while Sims-Williams (1978,1979) used spinal mobility (goniometer), and straight leg raising. Zylbergold (1981) made use of assessments of spinal mobility, and Nwuga (1982) used measures of spinal mobility and straight leg raising. Farrell (1982) used a functional rating questionnaire and lumbar motions as outcomes. Godfrey et al. (1984) utilized spinal mobility, while Gibson (1985) measured spinal flexion.

Arkuszewski (1986) used six signs and symptoms on a three point scale: posture, gait, pain, active spinal mobility, manual examination of spine, and a neurological evaluation. Waagen (1986) used a global index of spinal mobility created by summing the results of all planes of motion. Mathews (1987) also measured spinal mobility. Hoehler (1981) used measures of spinal mobility, straight leg raising, activities of daily living, and patient report of effectiveness.

While most studies of SMT have concentrated on lumbar spinal mobility, a number of trials assessed motion in the cervical spine. Brodin (1982) measured neck pain and cervical mobility as outcomes. Nordemar (1981) and Mealy (1986) used neck pain and cervical mobility. Howe (1983) assessed measures of cervical mobility and improvement in pain and stiffness. Lopes (1991) also assessed range of motion and pain immediately after manipulation.

Training and practice are required to conduct a valid and reliable assessment of ROM. Clinicians should be aware of the range of errors inherent in a chosen method. Also, such issues as patient positioning, patient motivation and proper interpretation of the instrument must be addressed. The cost of measuring devices can range from $15.00 to many thousands of dollars depending on the sophistication. Done skillfully, measuring ROM is generally safe.

Thermography: Thermography is the recording of heat from the body. There are many devices including sophisticated computer-assisted infrared imaging procedures, liquid crystal sheets, and a variety of hand-held instruments (many traditional to chiropractic practice). Infrared and liquid crystal technologies capture entire body regions, such as the trunk and lower extremities, yielding images similar to other imaging modalities. Thermography is not an anatomical test; however, it is thought to be primarily a physiological test of the vascularization of the skin. Hand-held instruments only measure very small areas of skin at a time. It has been established that, within limits, skin temperature is symmetrical. Asymmetry of heat emission determined by comparing one side of the body to the other is considered to be abnormal (Meeker, 1986).

Thermography is a controversial topic with some organizations endorsing it (Vlasuk, 1992), and others with substantially more conservative conclusions (American Academy of Neurology, 1990). As a diagnostic procedure, thermography may have use in certain disorders of the neuromusculoskeletal system (Plaugher, 1991; Meeker, 1986). It appears to be diagnostically sensitive to some disorders, but the major criticism is that diagnostic specificity is lacking to the extent that it cannot replace other types of examination procedures. The research database on thermography has been severely criticized in one meta-analysis of the procedure for lumbar spine disorders (Hoffman, 1991), and its overall utility in clinical practice has also been questioned (Awerbuch, 1991).

There are a few limited studies of the reliability of some thermographic devices in chiropractic settings (Meeker, 1986; Plaugher, 1991; DeBoer, 1985; Keating, 1990). Nonexistent to moderate agreement above chance was generally demonstrated (depending on the instrument and the anatomy tested), but the authors were uniformly cautious about stating the technique was reliable enough for clinical purposes.

There are no randomized clinical trials using thermography as an outcome assessment, so responsiveness to treatment has not been determined. There are some published reports of thermographic changes while under conservative care (Sucher, 1990; Kelso, 1982; Diebert, 1972; Brand, 1982) but these have been uncontrolled, non-blinded, small sample observational efforts at best. Clearly, additional research is needed in this area.

Thermographic equipment can be inexpensive for the hand-held devices to many thousands of dollars for complete infrared systems. Standardized examination protocols are being established (e.g., Vlasuk, 1992) for infrared and liquid crystal procedures. Generally these are detailed and require technical expertise. Certification programs have been established to train doctors to interpret thermograms. A legally acceptable examination done by protocol may take up to an hour. Fees charged to patients and third parties may be substantial.

There is very little published standardization for the less expensive hand-held devices, which may be included in patient examinations with little inconvenience of time or cost.

Muscle Function: The evaluation of muscle function encompasses a number of parameters: strength, work and power, and endurance (Sapega, 1990). Several modes of muscle contraction can be tested separately. These are termed isotonic, isokinetic, and isometric. The distinctions center upon the nature of the applied load or by the velocity and direction of change in the length of the muscle. Concentric contractions indicate a shortening of the muscle whereas ecccentric contractions occur as the muscle is lengthening. Various sophisticated machines can now measure various combinations of these muscle function parameters in the extremities and the spine.

Quite a number of factors can affect the validity and reliability of muscle function testing. These include but are not limited to: stabilization and positioning of the body, velocity of test movements, gravitational influences, familiarity with testing procedures, inertial forces, calibration, time of day, and patient motivation (Sapega, 1990).

Most manual muscle testing procedures which are commonly used in the chiropractic profession combine elements of isometric testing with eccentric dynamic variable resistance. Manual methods are qualitative. It has been shown that examiners interpret muscular strength or weakness more on the basis of total effort they exert while overcoming a patient's resistance than on either the peak or average force (Sapega, 1990). This lessens the validity of manual tests as true tests of muscular strength (Nicholas, 1978). In one study, patients with as much as a 50% decrease in strength were rated as normal by manual methods (Watkins, 1984). Trained examiners found it difficult to detect differences of less than 25% between paired limbs (Beasley, 1956).

The reliability of manual muscle testing was assessed with a dynamometer in a chiropractic setting (Hsieh, 1990). The authors concluded that the "patient initiated" method yielded satisfactory scores for tests of the iliopsoas, the clavicular portion of the pectoral is major, and the external rotators of the hip. Dynamometers have also shown fair to good reliability in other studies (Sapega, 1990). There are no clinical reliability studies of manual muscle testing as used in some chiropractic techniques where a dichotomous decision ("strong" vs. "weak") is required. There are no clinical trials of a retrospective or prospective nature demonstrating the responsiveness of manual muscle testing to chiropractic care.

Instrumented measures of muscle function are further described in the chapter on instrumentation. Each method has advantages and disadvantages, but most have demonstrated adequate reliability when strict protocols are followed, and the ability to demonstrate changes in patients undergoing exercise or musculoskeletal rehabilitation.

Manual muscle tests are practical and generally safe. The instrumented methods can be inexpensive in the case of hand-held dynamometers to many thousands of dollars for the more sophisticated computerized measurement systems. If risks are minimized by following proper testing protocols the instrumented methods are also safe.

Posture: Postural measures are defined here to include measurements of humans of generally topographical nature. Anatomical relations include apparent limb length inequality, the shape of the spine (degree of lordosis, scoliosis, kyphosis), etc.

Apparent leg length inequality (specifically, lower limb length inequality) is often used as an indication for chiropractic care. There are many assessment methods; some are discussed in the chapter on instrumentation. The topic has been extensively reviewed by Mannello (1991). A range of clinical reliability has been established for some methods. The relationship of lower limb length to the chiropractic subluxation syndrome, however, has not been experimentally determined. There are no clinical trials using lower limb length measurements as outcome assessments, so responsiveness to care has not been established.

Two studies indicate that manipulations/adjustments may increase cervical lordosis (measured radiographically) (Leach, 1983; Owens, 1990). The clinical relevance of such changes, however, remains controversial.

Subluxation Syndrome

Historical chiropractic theory holds that manipulable lesions (subluxation syndrome) may be a cause or concomitant of some disease processes, especially dysfunctions of the locomotor system. Therefore, chiropractic care (primarily spinal adjustments and other manual procedures directed at joints) has had as one of its primary goals the reduction of clinical findings thought to be associated with such lesions.

The chiropractic subluxation syndrome (as opposed to simple joint misalignment) is described by most authorities (Haldeman, 1991; Schafer, 1989) as consisting of clinical signs and symptoms at a specific dysfunctional joint, which when manipulated or adjusted tend to diminish. Chiropractic practitioners use the concept of subluxation syndrome as a point of departure for clinical decision-making, most often to locate the site and decide on the nature of a manipulative/adjustive treatment procedure. Many practitioners have been taught that the subluxation syndrome is an adequate way to assess treatment, but this view is under increasing critical scientific scrutiny (Triano, 1990). One way to discuss the potential of using the subluxation syndrome as an outcome assessment of care is to describe some of its components.

Vertebral Position: Traditional chiropractic theory suggested that misalignment of vertebrae is a primary sign of a subluxation syndrome. The model for this deduction was probably based on notions of normal spinal geometry and symmetry, and images obtained from plane radiographs (Mootz, 1989). Palpation of bony processes could also lead to clinical conclusions of misalignment.

On plain radiographs, misalignments may be measured in many different ways; for example, by observing facet joint or vertebral body interfaces. Images can be obtained in a spinal neutral position while standing, sitting, or lying down. Radiographs have also been obtained with patients bent to the end-range in a plane of motion, for example as in lumbar lateral bending "stress" films. Many methods of "listing" or describing vertebral misalignments are common in chiropractic practice. Some methods are mostly qualitative (e.g., Gonstead) while some are quantitative (e.g., Grostic).

According to Haldeman (1991), most practitioners use the measurements of positional relationships of the spine to make a decision about the direction and nature of a manipulative/ adjustive thrust, rather than to diagnose the site of the manipulable lesion.

To be a valid outcome measure, misalignments should theoretically reduce with therapy. A number of retrospective studies (Aldis and Hill [1982], Grostic and DeBoer [1982], Anderson [1980]) suggest that changes in apparent misalignments in the upper cervical spine do occur in patients under manipulative/adjustive care. In the lumbar spine, a similar observational study suggests that mild retrolisthesis may be reduced (Plaugher, 1990). (However, all other radiographic parameters in that study did not show changes.) A clinical trial (Roberts, 1978) also did not detect radiographic changes in low-back pain patients under manipulation. In one controlled experiment, Hosek (1984) found that upper cervical changes in the adjusted group were no different than those found in the non-adjusted control group.

There are very few experimentally controlled studies indicating that manipulations/adjustments are the reason for changes in misalignments seen over time. As Owens (1991) points out, errors in measurements due to patient re-positioning in front of a radiographic apparatus, radiographic distortion, examiner reliability, as well as normal biological variability may be equally responsible for changes in misalignments as treatment. Additional experimental studies are required.

Reports by Owens (1991) and others (Bronfort, 1984) suggest that margins of error in the radiographic measurement of angular relationships between vertebrae are on the order of one to two degrees depending on the method and portion of the spine under observation. But the central question still remains. That is, what is the clinical significance of misalignments, and do they really reduce as a consequence of manipulative/adjustive care? What is the correlation between the reduction of a misalignment and improved health for the patient? These questions beg for additional research.

One study (Keating, 1990) found no reliability of palpation for misalignment of vertebrae. There are no clinical trial outcome studies using palpation of bony landmarks as indicators of misalignment.

Abnormal Spinal Segmental Motion/Lack of Joint End-play: Abnormal vertebral motion is a logical outcome assessment since adjustive and manipulative methods by definition introduce forces into the body in an attempt to make tissues move. Abnormal motion may be most commonly assessed by radiographs or by palpation. Radiographs taken at end-ranges of motion are actually static images indirectly used to ascertain if an expected range of motion in a joint occurred. Videofluoroscopy is a relatively new imaging technique that can record spinal motion in real-time on video. (Imaging procedures are discussed extensively in another chapter).

Palpation of spinal tissues is a traditional diagnostic procedure for determining the site of a manipulable lesion and many palpatory techniques have been described (Schafer, 1989). The two most commonly defined palpatory parameters for abnormal vertebral motion are range-of-motion, or more precisely the inability of a joint to demonstrate an expected amount of motion in a specific plane; and the presence (or absence) of passive joint "play." Joint "play" or "end-feel" has been defined as the manual perception of a certain elasticity or compliance when the joint has been passively stretched to its limit. Lack of joint "play" is considered an indication for adjustment or manipulation. Logically, the return of normal range and quality of movement in a joint could be a good outcome measure of manipulation. Most practitioners are convinced of the clinical value of palpation.

Several qualitative reviews have summarized the scientific literature on spinal palpation in chiropractic (Panzer, 1991; Haas, 1991). Acceptable clinical reliability has been difficult to demonstrate although rates of agreement are greater than chance. Most studies have suffered from methodological flaws, however. Validity studies have been problematic due to the lack of acceptable "gold standards," but at least one small and restricted study (Jull, 1988) indicated 100% correlation between a palpating therapist's determination of the side and level of cervical joint pathology and a determination made independently by diagnostic joint and nerve block procedures.

Jull (1987) also published motion palpation norms for 200 healthy subjects of various ages on a five point rating scale. Age was correlated with segmental hypomobility. Intra-examiner and inter-examiner reliability was assessed and indicated Pearson's correlation coefficients ranging from 0.81 to 0.98.

Haas and Nyiendo (1990, 1991) have questioned the validity and reliability of lateral lumbar bending radiographs for patients with low-back pain. There does not seem to be a greater prevalence of "abnormal" findings in persons with a history of back pain compared to those without back pain. There are only a few studies using specific vertebral motion or joint "play" as an outcome measure. One study of SI joint palpation over time as patients received adjustments suggested that as patients recovered, abnormal palpatory signs diminished (Herzog, 1990). Arkuszewski (1986) in a cohort study indicated that spinal palpatory signs also diminished to a greater extent in patients receiving manipulation compared to other treatments.

Soft-Tissue Compliance and Tenderness: Compliance refers to the attribute of flexibility or "hardness" when the soft tissues are pressed with a palpating finger or with a pressure scale. Usually in chiropractic practice, tissue compliance is assessed manually and is therefore qualitative. Compliance can also be assessed quantitatively with a pressure gauge instrument designed to measure the distance a plunger sinks into the skin at a given weight (Fisher, 1987, 1990). It is assumed that muscle tone is the primary physiology being measured, but other events, such as edema, may also play a role in compliance.

Waldorf (1991) concluded that prone segmental bilateral paraspinal tissue compliance measures (averaged together for a single segmental score) had a test/retest variation of less than 10% after two weeks in normal healthy pain-free subjects. Lawson's (1991) results also suggested good clinical reliability. Another study (Nansel, in press) using compliance as an outcome measure of cervical adjustments, demonstrated statistically significant changes in the lumbar paraspinal area. Fischer (1987) documented increases in tissue compliance in a small sample of patients undergoing physical therapy.

Tenderness refers to the sensation of pain expressed by a subject when pressure is applied to the body. Tenderness actually refers to a supposed hypersensitivity to pressure, although what this means quantitatively is rarely defined. A more precise definition is pressure pain tolerance. Tolerance can be further subdivided into threshold (the point where an initial sensation of discomfort is felt) or maximum (the point at which the patient cannot stand additional pressure stimulation). Tenderness threshold is one of the major palpatory signs used by practitioners for diagnostic and treatment assessment purposes. Most of the time clinical assessments are qualitative, but quantitative measurements of tenderness can be made with an algometer. An algometer (pressure pain meter) measures the degree of pressure a patient can endure before a pain sensation is elicited. The amount of pressure is then recorded.

Some tenderness norms have been published (Simms, 1988; Fischer, 1987), but these were with small relatively unrepresentative population samples. Clinical reliability of tenderness measures has been supported with studies by Reeves (1986) and Ohrbach (1989), who used algometers, and Keating (1990), who tested digital palpation.

Vernon (1990) measured pressure pain tolerance with an algometer in cervical paraspinal soft tissues before and after cervical adjustments in a small group of patients. Compared to a control group receiving mobilization, the adjusted group demonstrated a dramatic increase in pressure tolerance. This suggests that quantitative measurements of tenderness are responsive to manual treatments. Fischer (1988) documented

decreases in tenderness with physical therapy. In addition, Jaeger (1986) indicated decreases in sensitivity in myofascial trigger points with passive stretch therapy.

Tissue compliance and pressure pain tolerance assessments, whether measured by palpation or with suitable instruments, can be incorporated into physical examination procedures with relative ease. The assessments are safe and inexpensive and appear to be responsive to conditions and treatments commonly seen in chiropractic practice. The quantitative methods are more suitable for documenting outcomes of care.

Asymmetric or Hypertonic Muscle Contraction: Although visual observations of postural antalgia and palpation of noncompliant soft tissue suggest muscle hypertonicity, these are merely explanations for what is actually seen or felt. Actual measurements of muscle activity can be obtained with electromyographic (EMG) methods. Needle methods are invasive and generally are beyond the scope of primary care chiropractic (although there are exceptions). Surface methods, which use electrodes on the skin, are within the scope and have become somewhat popular in chiropractic practice.

There is no question that surface EMG does measure some aspects of muscle activity, but it is not very muscle specific. Surface EMG tends to pick up signals from all muscular activity below the electrode. There is also a great deal of controversy about the clinical relevance, reliability, and responsiveness of various surface EMG examination methods (Nouwen, 1984; Triano, 1991).

A number of studies have discussed the relationship between trunk EMG and back pain (Dolce, 1985). Investigators have come to conflicting conclusions; some suggest that EMG can discriminate between subjects with and without back pain, others have not been able to demonstrate discriminatory ability (Cram, 1986; Nouwen, 1984). The data are confusing because many different parameters of EMG have been studied in poorly described clinical and control populations with noncomparable research designs and with flaws in experimental design and statistical analyses.

There are no high quality controlled studies that have indicated that spinal segmentally specific measures of surface EMG activity are related to segmental pathophysiology of the spine (subluxation syndrome). In addition, at least two studies in chiropractic settings did not support the hypothesis that findings of asymmetric paraspinal EMG can differentiate between subjects with and without a history of back pain (Meeker, 1991; Leach, 1991). Certain other measurements, such as the lack of "flexion relaxation response" and thoracolumbar ratios may have clinical value (Triano, 1987; Leach, 1991).

The few reliability studies that exist have demonstrated adequate within-session results but poor between-session (over time) consistency (Ahern, 1986; Matheson, 1988). One study claiming clinical reliability with hand-held "scanning" sensors had a median Pearson's R of only 0.64 for assessments one hour apart (Cram, 1990). Biederman (1984) has been very critical of the reliability of EMG assessments and has identi-fied a number of important sources of error.

Responsiveness has been assessed in studies with biofeed-back therapy (Nouwen, 1984) and spinal manipulation (Shambaugh, 1987; Ellestad, 1988). These studies have been criticized and none have concluded that spinal segmentally specific changes have occurred as a result of treatment. Over-all EMG activity did apparently decline.

Equipment varies from relatively simple hand-held devices to computer driven recording systems that yield a multitude of data. Training is necessary to conduct a valid examination, which can be time-consuming to do properly. There is very little standardization of examination procedures at this time. Surface EMG measurements are generally safe.

Reflex Testing: A number of chiropractic approaches use putative reflexes to test for the existence of a subluxation syn-drome. Some of the more well-known are termed "isolation" tests (Activator Methods, 1985), the "arm fossa" test (De Jarnette, 1984), vertebral "challenge" (Walther, 1988), and "therapy localization" (Walther, 1988). Generally, these tests rely upon digital stimulation of spinal or paraspinal tissues to cause a change in apparent leg position or muscle function to indicate a positive finding.

Youngquist (1989) reported Kappa co-efficients over 0.50 for interexaminer agreement on the presence of a cervical subluxation complex with the "isolation test" taught by Acti-vator Methods. The study design has been criticized, however, and there are no clinical trials using the "isolation test" as an outcome assessment.

LeBouef (1990) reported that the positive results of the arm-fossa test were statistically different between lumbar symptomatic and non-lumbar symptomatic patients. Still, the percentage of false-negative test results was 40%. In addi-tional study LeBouef (1992) concluded that 18 assessment procedures including the arm-fossa test were unlikely to be reproducible enough to constitute useful clinical procedures. There are no studies of the use of the arm-fossa test as an out-come assessment of chiropractic care.

There are no peer-reviewed studies of validity, reliability, or responsiveness to care of the "challenge" or the "therapy localization" procedure.

These tests, while appearing empirically useful to some practitioners also lack a theoretical base that could explain their modes of action. Their use is hotly debated by chiropractic clinicians.

V. ASSESSMENT CRITERIA

Procedure Ratings (System I)

Established: Accepted as appropriate by the practicing chiropractic community for the given indication in the speci-fied patient population.

Promising: Given current knowledge, this technology ap-pears to be appropriate for the given indication in the specified patient population. As more evidence and experience accumu-late, this interim rating will change. This connotes provisional acceptance, but permits a greater role for the current level of clinical use.

Equivocal: Current knowledge exists to support a given in-dication in a specified patient population, though value can neither be confirmed nor denied. As more evidence and expe-rience accumulate, this interim rating will change. Expert opinion recognizes a need for caution in general application.

Investigational: Evidence is insufficient to determine ap-propriateness. Further study is warranted. Use for a given indi-cation in a specified patient population should be confined to research protocols. As more evidence and experience accumu-late this rating will change.

Doubtful: Given current knowledge, this appears to be in-appropriate for the given indication in the specified patient population. As more evidence and experience accumulate, this interim rating will change.

Inappropriate: Regarded by the practicing chiropractic community as unacceptable for the given indication in the specified patient population.

Quality of Evidence:

The following categories of evidence are used to support the ratings.

Class I:

Evidence provided by one or more well-designed controlled clinical trials; or well-designed experimental studies that ad-dress reliability, validity, positive predictive value, discriminability, sensitivity, and specificity.

Class II:

Evidence provided by one or more well-designed uncon-trolled, observational clinical studies, such as case-control, cohort studies, etc. or clinically relevant basic science studies that address reliability, validity, positive predictive value, discriminability, sensitivity, and specificity; and published in refereed journals.

Class III:

Evidence provided by expert opinion, descriptive studies or case-reports.

Procedure Ratings (System II)

Necessary: Strong positive recommendation based on Class I evidence, or overwhelming Class II evidence when cir-cumstances reflect compromise of patient safety.

Recommended: Positive recommendation based on consensus of Class II and/or strong Class III evidence.

Discretionary: Positive recommendation based on strong consensus of Class III evidence.

Unnecessary: Negative recommendation based on inconclusive or conflicting Class II, III evidence.

Quality of Evidence

The following categories of evidence are used to support the ratings.

Class I:

A. Evidence of clinical utility from controlled studies published in refereed journals.

B. Binding or strongly persuasive legal authority such as legislation or case law.

Class II:

A. Evidence of clinical utility from the significant results of uncontrolled studies in refereed journals.

B. Evidence provided by recommendations from published expert legal opinion or persuasive case law.

Class III:

A. Evidence of clinical utility provided by opinions of experts, anecdote and/or by convention.

B. Expert legal opinion.

VI. RECOMMENDATIONS

NOTE: The recommendations on the following procedures or methods refer specifically to their use as outcome assessments and not necessarily to their use for other clinical purposes such as for diagnosis, prognosis, or for designing treatment plans.

A. Functional Outcome Assessments (By Questionnaire)

As a category, functional outcome assessments of everyday tasks are very suitable for evaluating treatment of dysfunctions of the neuromusculoskeletal system. Many questionnaires could be used; choice should depend upon the validity, reliability, responsiveness, and practicality demonstrated in the scientific literature.

10.1   **Rating:** Established for assessing patients with neuromusculoskeletal disorders.
Evidence: Class I, II, III
Consensus Level: 1

B. Patient Perception Outcome Assessments

Pain: Pain measurement is generally a relevant, valid, reliable, responsive, and safe outcome assessment. Practicality may vary depending on the specific procedure used.

10.2.1   **Rating:** Established
Evidence: Class I, II, III
Consensus Level: 1

Patient Satisfaction Measures: Patient satisfaction measures are an important marker of quality and are useful in clinical practice. Satisfaction is best assessed using standard questionnaires measuring a number of dimensions. Scales may be found in the scientific literature. Although additional research as satisfaction relates to chiropractic practice is required, validity, reliability, responsiveness, relevance, safety and practicality are scientifically supported.

10.2.2   **Rating:** Established
Evidence: Class I, II, III
Consensus Level: 1

C. General Health Outcome Assessments

As a category of outcomes, general health is possible and desirable to assess. Depending on the particular scale chosen, validity, reliability, and responsiveness have been demonstrated. The measures are safe; some are more practical than others. General health assessments should be used along with condition specific assessments.

10.3.1   **Rating:** Established
Evidence: Class I, II, III
Consensus Level: 1

D. Physiological Outcomes

Range of Motion: Depending upon the method applied, assessment of range of motion is a valid, reliable, responsive, safe outcome assessment. Depending on the level of automation, practical considerations may vary.

10.4.1   **Rating:** Established
Evidence: Class I, II, III
Consensus Level: 1

Thermography: Thermographic exams of the trunk and extremities with infrared or liquid crystal may be valid for certain diagnoses of the neuromusculoskeletal system. The validity of the numerous single and dual probe type hand-held instruments is less clear. The few reliability studies that exist are not particularly encouraging. There is very little scientific data to support the responsiveness of thermographic measurements to changes in health status. The procedures are generally safe, but the practicality of thermography depends upon the equipment and the examination procedures used. Thermograms should be interpreted by those trained in the procedure.

10.4.2 **Rating:** Investigational to equivocal as an outcome assessment for patients with neuromusculoskeletal conditions.
Evidence: Class II, III (For minority opinion, see Section IX, 10.7.1)
Consensus Level: 3

Muscle Function: There are many methods of assessing the parameters of muscle function. Manual methods have not been explored adequately enough to assure validity, reliability, relevance and responsiveness to care. Manual methods, however, are practical and generally safe and tend to be popular. Studies with automated methods (e.g., Cybex, etc.) have suggested a greater level of confidence, but require expert training, and are time-consuming.

10.4.3 **Rating:** Established for instrumented methods to measure muscle function.
Evidence: Class I, II, III
Consensus Level: 1

10.4.4 **Rating:** Equivocal for manual methods to measure muscle function.
Evidence: Class II, III
Consensus Level: 1

Postural Evaluations: Certain postural parameters may be responsive to treatment, but validity, reliability and relevance issues still need to be addressed scientifically. Depending on the method, postural observations are probably practical and safe.

10.4.5 **Rating:** Promising
Evidence: Class II, III
Consensus Level: 1

E. Subluxation Syndrome

The subluxation syndrome provides decision-making information for application of chiropractic treatment methods, primarily adjustments and manipulations. Regarding outcome assessments, the various components must be considered separately. These are discussed below.

Vertebral Position Assessed Radiographically: The clinical relevance of small changes in vertebral position is scientifically controversial. Responsiveness of vertebral position to manipulative/adjustive treatment care has been established in some cases. Observational studies have not ruled it out. Many practitioners accept measurement of vertebral position as routine and customary. The risk/benefit ratio of using radiographs for measuring vertebral position as an outcome assessment should be carefully considered.

10.5.1 **Rating:** Equivocal
Evidence: Class II, III
Consensus Level: 1

Abnormal Segmental Motion/Lack of Joint End-play Assessed by Palpation: There are a few validity studies of joint palpation although the existing literature on reliability is disappointing. There are studies suggesting that palpatory signs diminish with treatment, but the degree of responsiveness has been difficult to quantify. In skilled hands, palpation is safe.

10.5.2 **Rating:** Equivocal to Promising (as an outcome assessment for patients with neuromusculoskeletal conditions)
Evidence: Class II, III
Consensus Level: 1

Abnormal Segmental Motion Assessed Radiographically: There are few validity studies, reliability has been questioned, and the relevance is controversial. While responsiveness of segmental motion to treatment has not been confirmed experimentally, observational studies have not ruled it out. The risk/benefit ratio of radiographs to assess this outcome must be seriously considered.

10.5.3 **Rating:** Investigational (as an outcome assessment for patients with neuromusculoskeletal conditions).
Evidence: Class II, III
Consensus Level: 1

Soft-Tissue Compliance and Tenderness: Clinical studies indicate a relationship between tenderness and painful neuromusculoskeletal conditions. Clinical reliability has been established. Compliance and tenderness appear to be responsive to treatment. Algometers, tissue compliance meters, and palpatory methods appear to be practical and safe.

10.5.4 **Rating:** Promising (as an outcome measure for patients with neuromusculoskeletal conditions).
Evidence: Class I, II, III
Consensus Level: 1

Asymmetric or Hypertonic Muscle Contraction: There is no question that surface EMG procedures measure some aspects of muscle activity. However, clinical relevance and reliability have been more difficult to demonstrate scientifically. The responsiveness of EMG measurements to treatment has not been confirmed experimentally to any great degree. Surface methods are safe.

10.5.5 **Rating:** Equivocal for fixed electrodes as an outcome assessment for patients with neuromusculoskeletal conditions.
Evidence: Class I, II, III
Consensus Level: 1

10.5.6 **Rating:** Investigational to Equivocal for scanning EMG as an outcome assessment for neuromusculoskeletal conditions
Evidence: Class II, III (For minority opinion see Section IX, 10.7.2)
Consensus Level: 3

F. Principles of Application

The subluxation syndrome should be used as an outcome assessment only when the actual parameters being measured have been explicitly identified.

10.6.1 **Rating:** Recommended
Evidence: Class II, III
Consensus Level: 1

Outcome assessments should only be performed and interpreted by appropriately trained and qualified individuals.

10.6.2 **Rating:** Necessary
Evidence: Class II, III
Consensus Level: 1

When outcome assessments are used, consideration must be made for their established test properties, for patient compliance, and for the nature of the condition(s) being assessed.

10.6.3 **Rating:** Necessary
Evidence: Class II, III
Consensus Level: 1

Patient outcomes should be assessed at appropriate intervals during case management depending upon the nature of the condition and the patient's progress.

10.6.4 **Rating:** Necessary
Evidence: Class II, III
Consensus Level: 1

Generic functional and health status outcome measurements are essential for comparing outcomes across different patient populations and treatment interventions, while disease or condition-specific measures assess the special concerns of patients with certain diagnoses. Outcome information is very valuable to doctors of chiropractic, and to the chiropractic profession. Therefore, whenever feasible, a general health outcome of chiropractic care should be assessed by a standardized, commonly accepted method; and whenever feasible, a condition specific outcome of chiropractic care should be assessed by a standardized, commonly accepted method.

10.6.5 **Rating:** Recommended
Evidence: Class II, III
Consensus Level: 1

VII. COMMENTS, SUMMARY OR CONCLUSION

None.

VIII. REFERENCES

Activator Methods Chiropractic Technique Seminar Workbook. Willmar, MN, 1985.

Adams A: Methodological considerations in the selection of outcome measures for chiropractic practice. *Proceedings of the 1991 International Conference on Spinal Manipulation.* April 12, 1991, Arlington, Virginia. Foundation for Chiropractic Education and Research.

Ahern D, Follick M, Council J, Laser-Wolston N: Reliability of lumber paravertebral EMG assessment in chronic low-back pain. *Arch Phys Med Rehabil* 1986, 67:762.

Aldis G, Hill JM: Analysis of a chiropractor's data. Journal and Proceedings, Royal Soc, New South Wales. 1979, 112:93. (Reprinted in *J Manip Physiol Ther* 1980, 3(3):177.)

American Academy of Neurology, Therapeutics and Technology Assessment Subcommittee: Assessment: Thermography in neurologic practice. *Neurology* 1990, 40:523.

Anderson R, Meeker W, Wirick B, Mootz R, Kirk D, Adams A: A Meta-Analysis of Clinical Trials of Spinal Manipulation. *J Manip Physiol Ther* 1992, 15(3)00.

Anderson R: Anatomic rotation at the atlanto-occipital joint. Eleventh Annual Biomechanics Conference on the Spine. Boulder, CO, Dec.6, 1980. pp.113.

Arkuszewski A: The efficacy of manual treatment in low-back pain: a clinical trial. *Manual Medicine* 1986, 2:68-71.

Assendelft W, Koes B, Van den Heijden G, Bouter L: *The Efficacy of Spinal Manipulative Therapy for Treatment of Low-back and Neck Pain: A Criteria Based Meta-Analysis.* (In Press). Presented at the World Chiropractic Congress, Toronto, Canada, 1991.

Awerbuch M: Thermography-Its current diagnostic status in musculoskeletal medicine. *Med J Aust* 1991, 154(7):441.

Beasley W: Influence of method on estimates of normal knee extensor force among normal and postpolio children. *Phy Ther Rev* 1956, 36:21-41.

Bergmann TF (ed): Proceedings of the March 1990 Consensus Conference on Validation of Chiropractic Methods. *Chiropractic Technique* 1990, 2(3):71-161.

Bergner M, Bobbitt R, Carter W, Gilson B: The sickness impact profile: Development and final revision of a health status measure. *Medical Care* 1981, 19(8):787.

Bergquist-Ullman M, Larrson U: Acute low-back pain in industry. *Acta Orthop Scan*d (Suppl) 1977, 170:1-110.

Biederman H: Comments on the reliability of muscle activity comparisons in EMG biofeedback research with back pain patients. *Biofeed Self-Regul* 1984, 9(4):451.

Bombardier C, Tugwell P: Methodological Considerations in Functional Assessment. *J Rheum* (Suppl 15) 1987, 14:6.

Brand N, Gizoni C: Moire contourography and infrared thermography: Changes resulting from chiropractic adjustments. *J Manip Physiol Ther* 1982, 5:113.

Brodin H: Cervical pain and mobilization. *Int J Rehab Research* 1984, 7:190-191.

Bronfort G, Jochumsen O: The functional radiographic examination of patients with low-back pain: A study of different forms of variation. *J Manip Physiol Ther* 1984, 7(2):89.

Bronfort G: An overview of short multi-dimensional health status outcomes instruments. *Proceedings of the 1991 International Conference on Spinal Manipulation.* April 12, 1991, Arlington, Virginia. Foundation for Chiropractic Education and Research.

Cherkin D, Deyo R, Berg A: Evaluation of a physician education intervention to improve primary care for low-back pain. II. Impact on patients. *Spine* (in press).

Cherkin D, MacCornack F: Patient evaluations of low-back pain care from family physicians and chiropractors. *West J Med* 1989, 150:351.

Cherkin D: Patient satisfaction as an outcome measure. *Chiro Tech* 1990, 2(3):138.

Cleary P, McNeil B: Patient satisfaction as an indicator of quality care. *Inquiry* 1988, 25:25.

Coile RC: *The New Medicine: Reshaping Medical Practice and Health Care Management.* Rockville, MD, Aspen Publishers, 1990.

Coxhead CE, Inskip H, Meade TW, North WRS, Troup JDG: Multicentre trial of physiotherapy in the management of sciatic symptoms. *Lancet* 1981, 1:1065-1068, May 16.

Coyer AB, Curwen IHM: Low-back pain treated by manipulation. *Br Med J* 1955, 1:705-707.

Cram J, Engstrom D: Patterns of neuromuscular activity in pain and nonpain patients. *Clinical Biofeedback and Health* 1986, 9(2):106.

Cram J, Lloyd J, Cahn T: The reliability of EMG muscle scanning. *International Journal of Psychosomatics* 1990, 37:68.

DeBoer K, Harmon R, Chambers R, Swank L: Inter- and intra-examiner reliability study of paraspinal infrared temperature measurements in normal students. *Research Forum,* Autumn: 4, 1985.

DeJarnette M: *Sacro-occipital technic.* Nebraska City, Nebraska: Privately Published, 1984.

Deyo R, Diehl A: Patient satisfaction with medical care for low back pain. *Spine* 1986, 11:28.

Deyo R, Diehr P, Patrick D: Reproducibility and responsiveness of health status measures. *Controlled Clinical Trials* 1991, 12: 142S.

Deyo R: Comparative validity of the sickness impact profile and shorter scales for functional assessment in low-back pain. *Spine* 1986, 11(9):951.

Deyo R: Measuring the functional status of patients with low-back pain. *Arch Phys Med Rehab* 1988, 69:1044.

Deibert P, England R: Crystalligraphic study: thermal changes and the osteopathic lesion. *J Am Osteo Assoc* 1972, 72:223.

Dolce J, Raczynski J: Neuromuscular activity and electromyography in painful backs: Psychological and biomechanical models in assessment and treatment. *Psychological Bulletin* 1985, 97(3):502.

Donabedian A: The Quality of Medical Care. In: Graham NO (ed): *Quality Assurance in Hospitals.* Rockville, MD, Aspen Publishers, 1982.

Doran DML, Newell DJ: Manipulation in the treatment of low-back pain: a multicentre study. *Br Med J* 1975, 2:161-164.

Edwards BC: Low-back pain resulting from lumbar spine conditions: a comparison of treatment results. *Aust J Physiother* 1969, 15:104-110.

Ellestad S, Nagle R, Boesler D, Kilmore M: Electromyographic and skin resistance responses to osteopathic manipulative treatment for low-back pain. *J Amer Osteo Ass* 1988, 88(8):991.

Ellwood P: Outcomes management: a technology of patient experience. *N Eng J Med* 1988, 318:23.

Evans, DP, Burke MS, Lloyd KN, Roberts EE, Roberts GM: Lumbar spinal manipulation on trial: Part 1-clinical assessment. *Rheumatology and Rehabilitation* 1978, 17:46-53.

Fairbanks J, Davies J, Couper J, O'Brien J: The Oswestry low-back pain disability questionnaire. *Physiotherapy* 1980, 66:271.

Farrell JP, Twomey LT: Acute low-back pain: comparison of two conservative treatment approaches. *Med J Aust* 1982, 1:160-164.

Feinstein AR: The need for humanized science in evaluating medication. *Lancet* 1972, 2:241-243.

Fischer A: Tissue compliance meter for objective, quantitative documentation of soft tissue consistency and pathology. *Arch Phys Med Rehabil* 1987, 68:122-125.

Fischer A: Clinical use of tissue compliance meter for documentation of soft tissue pathology. 1987, *Clin J Pain* 3:23-30.

Fischer A: Pressure algometry over normal muscles. Standard values, validity and reproducibility of presssure threshold. *Pain* 1987, 30:115-126.

Fischer A: Application of pressure algometry in manual medicine. *Manual Medicine* 1990, 5:145-150.

Fischer A: Pain and spasm alleviation by physiotherapy. *Arch Phys Med Rehabil* 1988, 69:735.

Gibson T, Grahame R, Harkness J, Woo P, Blagrave P, Hills R: Controlled comparison of shortwave diathermy treatment with osteopathic treatment in non-specific low-back pain. *Lancet:* 1985, 1258-1261.

Giles L, Taylor J: Low-back pain associated with leg length inequality. *Spine* 1981, 6(5):510.

Glover JL, Morris JG, Khosla T: Back pain: a randomized clinical trial of rotational manipulation of the trunk. *Br J Ind Med* 1974, 31:59-64.

Godfrey CM, Morgan PP, Schatzker J: A randomized trial of manipulation for low-back pain in a medical setting. *Spine* 1984, 9:301-304.

Grostic J, DeBoer: Roentgenographic measurement of atlas laterality and rotation: A retrospective pre- and post-manipulation study. *J Manip Physiol Ther* 1982, 5(2):63.

Guides to the evaluation of permanent impairment. 3rd edition. Chicago, American Medical Association, 1988.

Haas M, Nyiendo J, Peterson C, Thiel H, Sellers T, Cassidy D, Yong-Hing K: Interrater reliability of roentgenoloical evaluation of the lumber spine in lateral bending. *J Manip Physiol Ther* 1990, 13(4): 179.

Haas M, Nyiendo J: Lumbar motion trends and correlation with low-back pain. A roentgenological evaluation of quantitative segmental motion in lateral bending. *Proceedings of the 1991 World Chiropractic Congress,* April 29, 1991, Toronto. World Federation of Chiropractic.

Haas M: The reliability of reliability. *J Manip Physiol Ther* 1991, 14:199.

Hadler NM, Curtis P, Gillings B, Stinnett S: A benefit of spinal manipulation as adjunctive therapy for acute low-back pain: a stratified controlled trial. *Spine* 1987, 12:703-706.

Haldeman S, Phillips R: Spinal manipulative therapy in the management of low-back pain. In: Frymoyer J (ed.)*: The adult spine: Principles and practice.* New York: Raven Press, 1991.

Hansen D: Outcomes assessments in clinical decision making. *Proceedings of the 1991 International Conference on Spinal Manipulation.* April 12, 1991, Arlington, Virginia. Foundation for Chiropractic Education and Research.

Herzog W, Conway P, Wilcox B: Effects of different treatment modalities on gait symmetry and clinical measures for sacroiliac joint patients. *J Manip Physiol Ther* 1991, 14(2):104.

Hoehler FK, Tobis JS, Buerger AA: Spinal manipulation for low-back pain. JAMA 1981, 2245: 1835-1838.

Hoffman R, Kent D, Deyo R: Diagnostic accuracy and clinical utility of thermography for lumbar radiculopathy: A meta-analysis. *Spine* 1991, 16(6):675.

Hosek R et al.: A triple-blind study of the effects of specific upper cervical adjusting. Presented at the Conservative Health Science Conference, Pasadena, TX, November 17-18, 1984.

Howe DH, Newcombe RG, Wade MT: Manipulation of the cervical spine -a pilot study. *Journal of the Royal College of General Practitioners* 1983, 33:574-579.

Hsieh J, Phillips R: Reliability of manual muscle testing with a computerized dynamometer. *J Manip Physiol Ther* 1990, 13(2):72.

Hsieh J: Functional outcomes of low-back pain: A comparison of four treatment groups in a controlled randomized trial. *Proceedings of the World Federation of Chiropractic,* April 29, 1991, Toronto. World Federation of Chiropractic.

Huskisson S: Measurement of pain. *J Rheumatol* 1982, 9:768.

Interstudy: An introduction to Interstudy's Outcomes Management System Development Plans. October, 1990. Interstudy, Excelsior, MN.

Interstudy: User's Manual SF-36 Health Status Questionnaire. April 10, 1989. Interstudy, Excelsior, MN.

Jaeger B, Reeves JL: Quantification of changes in myofascial trigger point sensitivity with the pressure algometer following passive stretch. *Pain* 1986, 27:203-210.

Jansen R, Nansel D, Slosbert M: Normal paraspinal tissue compliance: The reliability of a new clinical and experimental instrument. *J Manip Physiol Ther* 1990, 13(5):243.

Jensen M, Karoly P, Braver S: The measurement of clinical pain intensity: A comparison of six methods. *Pain* 1986, 27:117.

Jose W, Adams A, Meeker W: The three-site outcomes assessment project: Status report. *Proceedings of the 1991 International Conference on Spinal Manipulation.* April 12, 1991, Arlington, Virginia. Foundation for Chiropractic Education and Research.

Jose W: What is outcomes assessment and why should we do it? *Proceedings of the 1991 International Conference on Spinal Manipulation.* April 12, 1991, Arlington, Virginia. Foundation for Chiropractic Education and Research.

Jull G, Bogduk N, Marsland A: The accuracy of manual diagnosis for cervical zygapophysial joint pain syndromes. *Med J Aust* 1988, 148:233.

Jull G, Bullock M: A motion profile of the lumbar spine in an ageing population assessed by manual examination. *Physiotherapy Practice* 1987, 3:70-81.

Kane R, Olsen D, Leymaster C, et al.: Manipulating the patient: A comparison of the effectiveness of physician and chiropractor care. *Lancet* 1974, 1 (June):1333.

Kassak K: Outcomes measurement assessment: The experience of NWCC. *Proceedings of the 1991 International Conference on Spinal Manipulation.* April 12, 1991, Arlington, Virginia. Foundation for Chiropractic Education and Research.

Keating J, Bergmann T, Jacobs G, Finer B, Larson K: Interexaminer reliability of eight evaluative dimensions of lumbar segmental abnormality. *J Manip Physiol Ther* 1990, 13(8):463.

Keating J, Giljum K, Menke M, Lonczak R, Meeker W: Toward an experimental chiropractic: Time-series designs. *J Manip Physiol Ther* 1985, 8(4):229.

Kelso A, Johnston W: Use of thermograms to support assessment of somatic dysfunction or effects of osteopathic manipulative treatment: A preliminary report. *J Am Osteo Assoc* 1982, 82:182.

Kirschner B, Guyatt G: A Methodologic Framework for Assessing Health Indices. *J Chron Dis* 1987, 38:27.

Koes B, Bouter L, Mameren, Essers A, Hofhuizen D, Houben J, Verstegen G, Knipschild: A randomized clinical trial of physiotherapy and manual therapy for chronic back and neck complaints: Results of the physical outcome measures. *Proceedings of the 1991 World Chiropractic Congress.* April 29, 1991, Toronto. World Federation of Chiropractic.

Lawlis G, Cuencas R, Selby D, McCoy C: The development of the Dallas Pain Questionnaire. An assessment of the impact of spinal pain on behavior. *Spine* 1989, 14(5):511.

Lawson D, Sanders G: Stability of paraspinal tissue compliance measurements. *Proceedings of the 1991 International Conference on Spinal Manipulation.* April 12, 1991, Arlington, Virginia. Foundation for Chiropractic Education and Research.

Leach R: An evaluation of the effect of chiropractic manipulative therapy on hypolordosis of the cervical spine. *J Manip Physiol Ther* 1983, 6:17.

Leach R: Thoraco-lumbar asymmetry detected in low-back pain patients with hand-held post-style electrodes. *Proceedings of the 1991 International Conference on Spinal Manipulation,* April 12, Arlington, VA. Foundation for Chiropractic Education and Research.

LeBoeuf C: The sensitivity of seven lumbo-pelvic orthopedic tests and the arm-fossa test. *J Manip Physiol Ther* 1990, 13(3):138.

LeBoeuf C: The reliability of specific sacro-occipital technique diagnostic tests. *J Manip Physiol Ther* 1991, 14(9):512.

Liebenson C, Phillips R: The reliability of range of motion measurements for human spine flexion: A review. *Chiro Tech* 1989, 1(3):69.

Lochman J: Factors related to patients' satisfaction with their medical care. *J Commun Health* 1983, 9(2):91.

Lohr K: Outcomes measurement: Concepts and questions. *Inquiry* 1988, 25(1):37.

Lopes A, Cassidy D, Yong-Hing K: The immediate effect of manipulation versus mobilization on pain and range of motion in the cervical spine: A randomized controlled trial. *Proceedings of the 1991 World Chiropractic Congress.* April 29, 1991, Toronto. World Federation of Chiropractic.

MacDonald RS, Bell CM: An open controlled assessment of osteopathic manipulation in nonspecific low-back pain. *Spine* 1990, 15(5):364.

Mannello D: Leg Length Inequality: A Review. *Proceedings of the Sixth Annual Conference on Research and Education.* June 21-23, Monterey, CA. Consortium for Chiropractic Research.

Matheson D, Jordan P, Murray M: Reliability of scanning EMG of the paraspinal muscles within and between sessions. *Psychophysiology* 1988, 25:467.

Mathews JA, Mills B, Jenkins VM, Grimes AM, Morkel MJ, Mathews W, Scott CM, Sittampalam Y: Back pain and sciatica: controlled trials of manipulation, traction and sclerosant and epidural injections. *Br J Rheumatol* 1987, 26:416-423.

McDowell I, Newell C: *Measuring Health: A guide to rating scales and questionnaires.* New York, Oxford Press, 1987.

McLachlan C: Enhanced patient decision-making: A role for outcomes management systems. *Proceedings of the 1991 International Conference on Spinal Manipulation.* April 12, 1991, Arlington, Virginia. Foundation for Chiropractic Education and Research.

Meade TW, Dyer S, Browne W, Townsend J, Frank AO: Low-back pain of mechanical origin: Randomised comparison of chiropractic and hospital outpatient treatment. *Brit Med J* 1990, 300(6737):1431-37.

Mealy K, Brennan H, Fenelon GCC: Early mobilization of acute whiplash injuries. *Br Med J* 1986, 292:656-657.

Meeker W, Gahlinger P: Neuromusculoskeletal thermography: A valuable diagnostic tool? *J Manip Physiol Ther* 1986, 9:257.

Meeker W: Inter and intra-examiner reliability of thermography. *Proceedings of the Fifth Annual Conservative Health Science Research Conference.* Davenport, Iowa, October 17, 1986. Palmer College of Chiropractic and the Foundation for Chiropractic Education and Research.

Meeker W, Matheson D, Wong: Lack of evidence for a relationship between low-back pain and asymmetrical muscle activity using scanning electromyography. *Proceedings of the Scientific Symposium of the 1991 World Chiropractic Congress,* April 29, 1991 Toronto, Canada. World Federation of Chiropractic.

Melzack P (ed): *Pain measurement and assessment.* New York, Raven Press, 1983.

Melzack R: The McGill Pain Questionnaire: Major properties and scoring methods. *Pain* 1975, 1:277.

Million R, Hall W, Nilsen K, Baker R, Jayson M: Assessment of progress of back pain patients. *Spine* 1982, 7:204.

Mootz R, Meeker W: Minimizing radiation exposure to patients in chiropractic practice. *ACA Journal of Chiropractic* April, 1989.

Nansel D, Cremata E, Carlson, Szlazak M: Effect of unilateral spinal adjustments on goniometrically-assessed cervical lateral end-range asymmetries in otherwise asymptomatic subjects. *J Manip Physiol Ther* 1989, 12(6):419.

Nansel D: Side-specific and level-specific effects of spinal adjustments on cervical lateral-flexion and rotational passive end-range asymmetries. *Proceedings of the 1991 World Chiropractic Congress.* April 29, 1991, Toronto. World Federation of Chiropractic.

Nansel D, Waldorf T, Cooperstein R: Effect of cervical spinal adjustments on lumbar paraspinal muscle tone-Evidence for facilitation of intersegmental tonic neck reflexes. *J Manip Physiol Ther* (in press).

Nelson E, Berwick D: The measurement of health status in clinical practice. *Medical Care* 1989, 27(3):S77.

Nelson E, Wasson J, Kirk J: Assessment of function in routine clinical practice: Description of the COOP Chart method and preliminary findings. *J Chronic Dis* 1987, 40 (S1):55S.

Nicholas J, Sapega A, Kraus H, Webb J: Factors influencing manual muscle tests in physical therapy. The magnitude and duration of force applied. *J Bone Joint Surg* 1978, 60A:186-190.

Nordemar R, Thorner C: Treatment of acute cervical pain: a comparative group study. *Pain* 1981, 10:93-101.

Nouwen A, Bush C: The relationship between paraspinal EMG and chronic low-back pain. *Pain* 1984, 20:109.

Nwuga VBC: Relative therapeutic efficacy of vertebral manipulation and conventional treatment in back pain management. *Am J Phys Med* 1982, 61:273-278.

Nyiendo J: A comparison of low-back pain profiles of chiropractic teaching clinic patients with patients attending private clinicians. *J Manip Physiol Ther* 1990, 13(8):437.

Nyiendo J, Haas M, Jones R: Using the Low-back Pain Type Specification Protocol in a Pilot Study of Outcome Assessment for Low-back (Chiropractic) Patients. *Proceedings of the 1991 International Conference on Spinal Manipulation.* April 12, 1991, Arlington, Virginia. Foundation for Chiropractic Education and Research.

Nyiendo J, Haas M, Jones R: Using the SF36D (General health status questionnaire) in a pilot study of outcome assessment for low-back pain (chiropractic) patients. *Proceedings of the 1991 International Conference on Spinal Manipulation.* April 12, 1991, Arlington, Virginia. Foundation for Chiropractic Education and Research.

Nyiendo J, Phillips R, Meeker W, Konsler G, Jansen R, Menon M: A Comparison of patients and patient complaints at six chiropractic teaching clinics. *J Manip Physiol Ther* 1989, 12(2):79.

Nyiendo J: Economic measures used in determining effectiveness and efficiency of chiropractic methods. *Chiro Tech* 1990, 2(3):143.

Ohrbach R, Gale E: Pressure pain threshold in normal muscles: reliability, measurement effects, and topographic differences. *Pain* 1989, 37:257-263.

Ongley MJ, Klein RG, Dorman TA, Eek B, Hubert LJ: A new approach to the treatment of chronic low-back pain. *Lancet* 1987, 2:143-146.

Ottenbacher K, DiFabio R: Efficacy of spinal manipulation/mobilization therapy: A meta-analysis. *Spine* 1985, 10(9):833.

Owens E, Leach R: Changes in cervical curvature determined radiographically following chiropractic adjustment. *Proceedings of the 1991 International Conference on Spinal Manipulation.* April 12, 1991, Arlington, Virginia. Foundation for Chiropractic Education and Research.

Owens E: Line drawing analyses of static cervical x-ray used in chiropractic. *Proceedings of the Sixth Annual Conference on Research and Education.* June 21-23, 1991, Monterey, CA. Consortium for Chiropractic Research.

Panzer D: Lumbar motion palpation: A literature review. *Proceedings of the Sixth Annual Conference on Research and Education.* June 21-23, 1991, Monterey, CA. Consortium for Chiropractic Research.

Parker G, Tupling H, Pryor D: A controlled trial of cervical manipulation for migraine. *Aust NZ J Med* 1978, 8:589.

Phillips R, Howe J, Bustin G, Mick T, Rosenfeld I, Mills T: Stress x-rays and the low-back patient. *J Manip Physiol Ther* 1990, 13(3):127.

Plaugher G: Skin temperature assessment for neuromusculoskeletal abnormalities of the spinal column: A Review. *Proceedings of the Sixth Annual Conference on Research and Education.* June 21-23, 1991, Monterey, CA. Consortium for Chiropractic Research.

Plaugher G, Lopes M, Melch P, Cremata E: The inter and intra-examiner reliability of a paraspinal skin temperature differential instrument. *J Manip Physiol Ther* 1991, 14(6):361.

Plaugher G, Cremata E, Phillips R: A retrospective consecutive case analysis of pretreatment and comparative static radiological parameters following chiropractic adjustments. *J Manip Physiol Ther* 1990, 13(9):498.

Rasmussen TG: Manipulation in treatment of low-back pain (a randomized clinical trial). *Manuelle Med* 1978, 1:8-10.

Reeves J, Jaeger B, Graff-Radford S: Reliability of the pressure algometer as a measure of myofascial trigger point sensitivity. *Pain* 1986, 24:313-321.

Roberts F, Roberts E, Lloyd K, Burke M, Evans D: Lumbar spinal manipulation on trial. Part ll. Radiological assessment. *Rheumatol Rehabil* 1978, 17:54.

Roland M, Morris R: Study of natural history of back pain. Part 1: Development of reliable and sensitive measure of disability in low back pain. *Spine* 1983, 8:141.

Sandoz R: The choice of appropriate clinical criteria for assessing the progress of a chiropractic case. *Annals of the Swiss Chiropractic Association* 1985, 8:53.

Sapega A: Muscle performance evaluation in orthopedic practice. *J Bone Joint Surg* 1990, 72A(10):1562-1574.

Sawyer C: Patient Satisfaction as a Chiropractic Research Outcome. *Proceedings of the 1991 International Conference on Spinal Manipulation.* April 12, 1991, Arlington, Virginia. Foundation for Chiropractic Education and Research.

Schafer R, Faye L: *Motion palpation and chiropractic technic: Principles of dynamic chiropractic.* Huntington Beach, CA: The Motion Palpation Institute, 1989.

Shambaugh P: Changes in electrical activity in muscle resulting from chiropractic adjustment: A pilot study. *J Manip Physiol Ther* 1987, 19(6):300.

Shekelle P, Adams A, Chassin M, Hurwitz, Phillips R, Brook R: *The appropriateness of spinal manipulation for low-back pain.* Publication R-4025/1-CCR/FCER. Rand Corporation, 1991.

Simms R, Goldenberg K, Felson D, Mason J: Tenderness in 75 anatomic sites. *Arthritis Rheum* 1988, 31:182-187.

Sims-Williams H, Jayson MIV, Young SMS, Baddeley H, Collins E: Controlled trial of mobilization and manipulation for patients with low-back pain in general practice. *Br Med J* 1978, 2:1338-1340.

Sims-Williams H, Jayson MIV, Young SMS, Baddeley H, Collins E: Controlled trial of mobilization and manipulation for low-back pain: hospital patients. *Br Med J* 1979, 2:1318-1320.

Spilker B (ed): *Quality of life assessments in clinical trials.* New York, Raven Press, 1990.

Stewart A, Hays R, Ware J: The M.O.S. short form general health survey: Reliability and validity in a patient population. *Medical Care* 1988, 26(7):724.

Sucher B: Thoracic outlet syndrome-A myofascial variant: Part 1. Pathology and diagnosis. *JAOA* 1990, 90(8):686.

Tait R, Pollard C, Margolis R, Duckro P, Krause S: Pain disability index: Psychometric and validity data. *Arch Phys Med Rehabil* 1987, 68:438.

Terret T, Vernon H: Manipulation and pain tolerance: A controlled study of the effect of spinal manipulation on paraspinal pain tolerance levels. *Am J Phys Med* 1984, 63(5):217.

Triano J, Schultz A: Correlation of objective measures of trunk motion and muscle function with low-back disability ratings. *Spine* 1987, 12(6):561.

Triano J: The subluxation syndrome: Outcome measure of chiropractic diagnosis and treatment. *Chiro Tech* 1990, 2(3):114.

Vernon H: Applying research-based assessments of pain and loss of function to the issue of developing standards of care in chiropractic. *Chiro Tech* 1990, 2(3):121.

Vernon H, Aker P, Burns, Viljakaanen, Short: Pressure pain threshold evaluation of the effect of spinal manipulation in the treatment of the effect of chronic neck pain: A pilot study. *J Manip Physiol Ther* 1990, 13(1):13.

Vernon H, Mior S: The neck disability index: A study of reliability and validity. *J Manip Physiol Ther* 1991, 14(7):409.

Vlasuk S: Standards for thermography in chiropractic practice. In: Vear H (ed): *Chiropractic Standards of Practice and Quality of Care.* Gaithersburg, Maryland: Aspen Publishers, 1991.

Waagen GN, Haldeman S, Cook G, Lopez D, DeBoer KF: Short term of chiropractic adjustments for the relief of chronic low-back pain. *Manual Medicine* 1986, 2:63-67.

Waddell G, Main C: Assessment of severity in low-back disorders. *Spine* 1984, 9:204.

Waldorf T, Devlin L, Nansel D: The comparative assessment of paraspinal tissue compliance in asymptomatic female and male subjects in both prone and standing positions *J Manip Physiol Ther* 1991, 14(9):457-461.

Walther D: *Applied Kinesiology Synopsis*. Pueblo, CO, Systems DC, 1988.

Ware J, Davies-Avery A, Stewart A: The measurement and meaning of patient satisfaction. *Health and Medical Care Services Review* 1978, 1:1.

Ware J, Hays R: Methods for measuring patient satisfaction with specific medical encounters. *Medical Care* 1988, 26:393.

Ware J, Snyder M, Wright W, et al.: Defining and measuring patient satisfaction with medical care. Evaluation and Program Planning 1983, 6:247.

Watkins M, Harris B, Kozlowski B: Isokinetic testing in patients with hemiparesis. A pilot study. Phys Ther 1984, 64:184-189.

Youngquist M, Fuhr A, Osterbauer P: Interexaminer reliability of an isolation test for the identification of upper cervical subluxation. *J Manip Physiol Ther* 1989, 12(2), 93.

Zachman Z, Traina A, Keating J, Bolles S, Braun-Porter L: Interexaminer reliability and concurrent validity of two instruments for the measurement of cervical ranges of motion. *J Manip Physiol Ther* 1989, 12(3):205.

Zylbergold RS, Piper MC: Lumbar disc disease: Comparative analysis of physical therapy treatment. *Arch Phys Med Rehabil* 1981, 62:176-179.

IX. MINORITY OPINIONS

Thermography: Thermographic exams of the trunk and extremities with infrared or liquid crystal may be valid for certain diagnoses of the neuromusculoskeletal system. The validity of the numerous single and dual probe type hand-held instruments is less clear. The few reliability studies that exist are not particularly encouraging. There is very little scientific data to support the responsiveness of thermographic measurements to changes in health status. The procedures are generally safe, but the practicality of thermography depends upon the equipment and the examination procedures used. Thermograms should be interpreted by those trained in the procedure. (For majority recommendation see 10.4.2.)

10.7.1 **Rating:** Equivocal as an outcome assessment for patients with neuromusculoskeletal conditions

Asymmetric or Hypertonic Muscle Contraction: There is no question that surface EMG procedures measure some aspects of muscle activity. The responsiveness of EMG measurements to treatment has not been confirmed experimentally to any great degree. Surface methods are safe. (For majority recommendation see 10.5.6.)

10.7.2 **Rating:** Equivocal
Evidence: Class I, II, III

Collaborative Care

Chapter Outline

I. OVERVIEW

All patients of all primary health care providers have the right to expect health care services at the highest level of quality. The preservation of patient trust and confidence depends on this. When the needs of the patient demand the inclusion of other providers[1] or institutions in the program of care, extra caution and extra effort are required to ensure that no gaps in service or conflicts will be allowed to jeopardize the quality of care. The chiropractic practitioner should be aware of programs of cooperation and/or collaboration which can assist the patient.

Relationships between health care professionals can only become more complex, and possibly more contentious as we presently enter an era of great change and instability in health care. Concepts such as "managed care," "preferred provider" and "gatekeeper physician" are becoming the new currency of health care policy. As efforts to control health care costs center more and more on the managed care theory of cost and utilization containment, a credible protocol for interaction becomes an urgent necessity.

To ensure that all requirements for patient care can truly be addressed, this new model must consider cooperative relationships in all settings, including institutional settings such as the hospital, nursing home, and hospice, and among all health care professionals. The model to be devised must be comprehensive, clear to all parties involved, and flexible and dynamic enough to adapt to the daily realities of practice.

Finally, as competition for the health care dollar intensifies, it is particularly important that the chiropractic profession take steps to ensure that relationships with other providers are not tainted by economic self-interest or professional rivalry. Likewise, we must carefully safeguard the rights of chiropractic patients and ensure that other providers are conscious of the need to conduct patient care in a totally objective and professional manner. When professions interact in the delivery of health care services, economic and social factors as well as professional territorialism should never be allowed to override the fundamental obligation to the patient. There is no place for such distractions in the delivery of quality health care.

II. DEFINITIONS

Case Management: the process of evaluating patient needs or indicated care so as to provide service at the optimum level. All providers make case management decisions for each patient using a variety of variables and indicators. This concept takes on additional meaning in managed health care plans, where a professional "gatekeeper" or "key physician" is designated by the patient or by the plan, and has responsibility to determine what care should be provided for a given episode. In such managed health care plans it is the role of the managing "gatekeeper" to provide or authorize only such care as is truly needed. This care is from the most appropriate provider having regard to considerations of quality control and cost-containment.

Clinically Necessary: services or supplies which are determined to be:

(1) appropriate and necessary for the symptoms, diagnosis/clinical impression or care/treatment of the patient condition, and,

(2) provided for the diagnosis/clinical impression or direct care and treatment of the health care condition, and,

(3) according to standards of good primary health care practice within the organized professional community, and,

(4) not primarily for the convenience of the patient, or one or more of the patient's providers, and,

(5) the most appropriate supply or level of service. For hospital stays, this means that acute care as an inpatient is necessary due to the kind of services the patient is receiving or the severity of the patient's condition, and that safe and adequate care cannot be received as an outpatient or in a less intensified clinical setting.

Collaborative Care: the reciprocal interprofessional interaction of two or more health care providers in the management of the patient's current health status.

Emergency: onset of a medical/health condition manifesting itself by acute symptoms of sufficient severity that the absence of immediate attention could reasonably result in:

1. permanently placing the patient's health in jeopardy;
2. causing other serious health consequences;
3. causing serious impairment to bodily functions; or
4. causing serious and permanent dysfunction of any bodily organ or part.

Gatekeeper: Health care professional designated to exercise responsibility for, and control of, the utilization of health care services. (The concept of "gatekeeper physician" is the cornerstone of HMO/prepaid plan efforts to deliver care at the optimum level, thus avoiding both underutilization and overutilization.)

MHCO (Managed Health Care Organization): An organized system for providing health care in a geographic area, accepting the responsibility to provide or otherwise assure the delivery of an agreed upon set of services to a voluntarily enrolled group of persons (e.g., HMO, PPO, etc.).

Overutilization: The provision of more than an appropriate or adequate amount of care in a given case. (See "underutilization".)

Patient Satisfaction: Degree of confidence and gratification accompanying the delivery of health care services. Patient satisfaction relates strongly to perceptions on the part of the patient that his/her wishes are being carried out, that quality care is being delivered, and that patient sensitivities are being respected. These perceptions are based on subjective patient feelings, and may or may not deal with issues of technical appropriateness of care or outcomes.

Doctor Visit: a visit to the doctor of medicine, chiropractic, osteopathy or other physician for the purpose of examination, diagnosis, treatment/care, or advice.

Primary Care Doctor:

(1) any health care provider capable of providing first level contact and intake into the health delivery system (portal-of-entry provider).

(2) any health care provider licensed to receive patient contact in the absence of physician referral.

Quality of Care: the degree to which care is provided in an appropriate manner, within an appropriate time frame.

Referral: the direction of a patient to another health care professional or institution for evaluation, consultation or care. Referrals may be made or received for purposes of consultation, concurrent care, post-chiropractic care, the administration of diagnostic procedures, the evaluation of diagnostic findings, emergency care or because a clear determination has been made on the part of the practitioner that a patient condition is outside his/her scope of professional experience.

Underutilization: the provision of less than an appropriate or adequate amount of care in a given case.

Utility: significant benefit to both the patient and clinician resulting from a reduction in uncertainty pertaining to the case.

III. LIST OF SUBTOPICS

Reasonable Patient Expectations in the Cooperative and Collaborative Care Setting

A. **The Patient and the Primary Care Provider**
B. **Freedom of Choice and Informed Consent**
C. **Professional Knowledge and Understanding**
D. **Referrals**
E. **Exchange of Information and Records between Providers**
F. **Professional Interaction in the Hospital or Other Institutional Setting.**
G. **Economic Considerations**

IV. LITERATURE REVIEW

Collaboration can be defined as the reciprocal interprofessional interaction of two or more health care providers. Collaborative care involves this interaction in the management of the patient's current health status. Collaborative care,

therefore, includes care in a private practitioner's office, where interaction exists on a daily basis between the practitioner and his/her assistants, as well as care within a complex institutional setting such as a medical specialty ward in a hospital[2] and care within a managed care setting. Various specialty fields exist within chiropractic and are available as a resource.[3]

Hospitals and other institutional inpatient settings represent to some degree a new frontier for chiropractic. Chiropractic has an enormous contribution to make in this context. As well, hospitals are of great social, political and economic importance in North America. It is here that the largest publicly-supported concentration of leading-edge diagnostic equipment is to be found. Hospitals are also the scene of the vast majority of clinical information gathering and research.[4,5]

Collaborative care is neither new nor unique to this generation of providers,[1, 6, 7] though cooperative relationships between the medical and chiropractic professions have been less frequent in the past. The federal court judgment in 1987 in Wilk et al. vs. AMA et al.,[8] which effectively eliminated formal barriers previously established to the collaboration of the chiropractic and medical professions, has been a key factor in increasing cooperation. However, as greater emphasis is now being placed on the concept of nominating one primary care doctor as a "gate-keeper"[9] whose function is to ensure appropriate care yet contain specialist and other costs,[10] new effort is required to understand the appropriate role of different health disciplines. This is a difficult task for a number of reasons.

Firstly, from an organizational viewpoint, much of modern medicine is based on a "problem-oriented model" rather than one based either on the management of chronic, incurable illness or disease prevention. The problem-oriented model is less conducive to an interdisciplinary team approach than a "goal-oriented model" where the patient's achievement of highest possible level of health is the goal of all concerned. [11]

Secondly, as a number of authors have observed, coordination of health services has become a major characteristic of primary care. [12] As a result, an information system which fosters effective communication between health care professionals is essential.[13, 14] This is a particularly pertinent issue for chiropractic practice, where terms unique to the profession have been perpetuated in an effort to maintain an identity and philosophy. [15] As noted by Anderson, however, terms that are precise and accurate should be used because in interprofessional relationships, communication may well be frustrated by simple language barriers alone. If the principal goal is to aid the patient in the most appropriate and cost-effective manner, language preferences must be secondary to effective communication in the collaborative care setting.

Thirdly, overlap in knowledge and skills between the providers in any given case can result in confusion of roles. Which professional is to assume responsibility for which facets of individual care?[16] Role disagreement has been cited as an important factor in several arenas, from nurse practitioner/doctor in the Western world[17] to physicians/lay providers in the health care team in third world countries.[18] It has been shown that there are significant differences both in time under care and the choice of diagnostic and therapeutic techniques provided to a patient depending upon the professional specialty of the provider.[19]

Clarity of roles is vital. This clarity is dependent to some extent on the probability of a successful treatment outcome and to some extent upon the provider chosen. This should be understood when clinical policies and guidelines are made on decision-making in patient management.[20] Dixon[21] has noted that while policies can be helpful in simplifying complex clinical dilemmas, they have at times been adopted without evidence of benefit and that research studies using appropriate clinical methodology should be encouraged in order to prevent useless or even dangerous algorithms of treatment.

The development of wise patient care guidelines, incorporating the many approaches available in health care today, should provide for the most effective balance of resources for the patient's needs. Determining the role of each profession in the various algorithms for patient management should reflect the varying and unique needs of each individual patient. Developing such algorithms, which are currently not in place nationwide, may reasonably be expected to have a significant impact on health outcomes in general, as well as on the difficult interprofessional issue of cost-containment. To that end, for example, Wennenberg[22] has stated that patients' understanding of their treatment options is anticipated to be a major contributing factor in their treatment selection. He noted that health care allocation by patient preference is likely to be cost-effective because patients prefer and select less invasive, less expensive treatments. It is in the best interest, therefore, of all concerned that the health care system have all its professional resources, and ready information on them, available to all patients.

Initially, as the chiropractic profession explores the arena of collaborative care more fully, documents generated by practitioners engaging in this work and setting out interprofessional referral protocols can serve as guidelines. [23,24,25] As part of the health care system at large, however, the chiropractic profession must now begin to focus more of its resources in researching and developing clinical standards relevant to collaborative care. As noted earlier, such efforts are needed to meet the many and varied needs of all patients. [26]

V. ASSESSMENT CRITERIA

Procedure Ratings (System II):

Necessary: Strong positive recommendation, based on Class I evidence, or overwhelming Class II evidence, when circumstances reflect compromise of patient safety.

Recommended: Positive recommendation, based on consensus of Class II and/or strong Class III evidence, expert opinion.

Discretionary: Positive recommendation, based on consensus of Class III evidence.

Unnecessary: Negative recommendation, based on inconclusive or conflicting Class II, Class III evidence.

Quality of Evidence

The following categories of evidence are used to support the ratings.

Class I:

A. Evidence of clinical utility from controlled studies published in refereed journals.

B. Binding or strongly persuasive legal authority such as legislative or case law.

Class II:

A. Evidence of clinical utility from the significant results of uncontrolled studies published in refereed journals.

B. Evidence provided by recommendations from published expert legal opinion or persuasive case law.

Class III:

A. Evidence of clinical utility provided by opinions of experts, anecdote and/or by convention.

B. Expert legal opinion.

VI. RECOMMENDATIONS

A. The Patient and the Primary Care Provider

1. Patients are entitled to a clear explanation of why the participation of other health professionals has been determined to be necessary.

> 11.1.1 **Rating:** Necessary
> Evidence: Class II, III
> **Consensus Level:** 1

B. Freedom of Choice and Informed Consent

1. All health care professionals should recognize and respect the right of the patient to select his/her own method of health care and the setting in which that care is delivered, as well as the right of the patient to change providers at will.

> 11.2.1 **Rating:** Necessary
> Evidence: Class III
> **Consensus Level:** 1

2. Primary health care providers should supply sufficient information to enable the patient to make an informed decision regarding choices in treatment/care and of providers.

11.2.2 **Rating:** Necessary
Evidence: Class III
Consensus Level: 1

C. Professional Knowledge and Understanding

1. Chiropractic practitioners should be familiar with medical procedures and terminology as needed, so as to effectively understand and relate medical care delivered to or recommended to a patient.

11.3.1 **Rating:** Recommended
Evidence: Class II, III
Consensus Level: 1

2. Chiropractic practitioners should make every reasonable effort to be familiar with alternative health care providers whose care may have implications for the care of their patients, and should strive to communicate such information, as appropriate, to the patient.

11.3.2 **Rating:** Recommended
Evidence: Class III
Consensus Level: 1

D. Referrals

1. Primary health care providers should consult or refer if the needs of the patient so indicate.

11.4.1 **Rating:** Necessary
Evidence: Class I, II, III
Consensus Level: 1

2. Chiropractic practitioners should accept referrals from other health care providers.

11.4.2 **Rating:** Recommended
Evidence: Class III
Consensus Level: 1

E. Exchange of Information and Records between Providers

1. Chiropractic practitioners referring a patient to a peer or another professional should take all necessary steps to provide information from the case history and diagnostic findings to the practitioner receiving the referral in an effort to minimize unnecessary testing or repetition of diagnostic procedures.

11.5.1 **Rating:** Recommended
Evidence: Class III
Consensus Level: 1

2. Postreferral communication between referring and receiving practitioners should be complete and adequately detailed. Appropriate records of clinical findings or recommendations should be exchanged.

11.5.2 **Rating:** Recommended
Evidence: Class III
Consensus Level: 1

3. Questions about care decisions made or recommended by another provider should be addressed directly to that provider in a constructive manner. Relying on the patient to be an effective messenger of critical information is inappropriate.

11.5.3 **Rating:** Recommended
Evidence: Class III
Consensus Level: 1

4. Response to requests for records should occur in a timely fashion. Likewise, records requested by the practitioner that are another practitioner's property should be returned in a timely fashion.

11.5.4 **Rating:** Recommended
Evidence: Class III
Consensus Level: 1

F. Professional Interaction in the Hospital or Other Institutional Setting

1. In a collaborative or cooperative care setting, every effort should be made to develop and present to the patient a consensus among all participating practitioners on the recommended course of care.

11.6.1 **Rating:** Recommended
Evidence: Class III
Consensus Level: 1

2. Practitioners should seek access to other health care facilities and institutions as necessary to meet the needs of their patients. This may include authority to admit or co-admit the patient into the appropriate clinical setting or hospital.

11.6.2 **Rating:** Recommended
Evidence: Class III
Consensus Level: 1

3. In the process of concurrent care, each professional party should be aware of the care decisions made by other participants, and fully coordinate activities and information for the patient's benefit.

11.6.3 **Rating:** Recommended
Evidence: Class III
Consensus Level: 1

4. The resolution of disputes between members of different professions on the course of care for a given patient should be based on: a) the best professional judgment of the practitioners involved; b) the objective evaluation of appropriate clinical

options and intervention alternatives; and c) responsible family involvement where appropriate.

Informed consent on the part of the patient continues to be necessary.

11.6.4 **Rating:** Recommended
Evidence: Class III
Consensus Level: 1

5. To facilitate patient access to the widest possible range of health care resources and options, practitioners are encouraged to seek participation in managed health care organizations (e.g., HMOs, PPOs, etc.).

11.6.5 **Rating:** Recommended
Evidence: Class III
Consensus Level: 1

G. Economic Considerations

1. No referral should be sought or made on the basis of economic considerations and no financial relationship should exist between parties in a referral process. No fee, rebate or commission should be paid to any referring provider for the referral.

11.7.1 **Rating:** Necessary
Evidence: Class III
Consensus Level: 1

2. Primary providers should cooperate to secure proper insurance payment for all clinically-indicated health care services.

11.7.2 **Rating:** Recommended
Evidence: Class III
Consensus Level: 1

VII. COMMENTS, SUMMARY, OR CONCLUSION

Professional behavior should be governed by the principles of the art and science of chiropractic, and a strict set of ethical canons which go beyond the legal obligations of licensure. Ethical requirements are as compelling and imperative to the delivery of quality care as any clinical indications.

Interaction between professions in a hospital or other institutional setting will be governed by the laws and regulations of the jurisdiction within which the facility operates and the rules and bylaws of the hospital or facility. Recognition of the degree to which professional roles are specified by such regulations should eliminate much of the confusion and concern surrounding the participation of chiropractic practitioners in the hospital setting.

In situations where patients need or request diagnostic outpatient services or inpatient care, the practitioner should provide a full and accurate explanation of his/her professional ac-

cess to such facilities. It is important that degrees of institutional access be understood by all parties in a collaborative care situation. Under no circumstances should any chiropractic practitioner overlook or minimize the need to employ outside services because he/she does not have access, referral or staff privileges at a specific facility. It is incumbent upon the practitioner to find a means to meet patient needs on a timely basis, all such considerations notwithstanding.

VIII. REFERENCES

1. Sawyer C, Bergmann T, Good, D: Attitudes and habits of chiropractors concerning referral to other health care providers. *J Manip Physiol Ther* 1988; 11:480-483.

2. Cassidy J, Mierau D, Nykoliation J, Arthur, B: Medical chiropractic correspondence. *J Can Chiro Assoc.*, 1985; 29:29-31.

3. Richards T: Chiropractic specialists: A referral resource, *ACA J Chirop*, 1990; 27:26-29.

4. Krantz KC: *Chiropractic and Hospital Privileges Protocol,* International Chiropractors' Association, Arlington, Virginia, 1987.

5. Krantz KC, Hendrickson RM: *Chiropractic and the HMO-PPO Challenge,* International Chiropractors' Association, Arlington, Virginia, 1988.

6. Banks R, Leboeuf C, Webb M: Recently graduated chiropractors in Australia: Part 3. Interprofessional referrals. *J Australian Chiro Assoc.,* 1988; 18:14-16.

7. Denton D: Wave of the future: equality and cooperation. *ACA J Chirop*, 1988; 25:23-25.

8. Wilk et al., vs. AMA et al.: US Federal Court for the Northern District of Illinois, Eastern Division, No 76C3777, Judgement dated August 27, 1987.

9. Eisenberg JM: The Internist as Gatekeeper: Preparing the General Internist for a New Role. *Annals of Internal Medicine*, 1985; 102:537-543.

10. Somers AR: And who shall be the gatekeeper? The role of the primary physician in the health care delivery system. *Inquiry*, 1983; 20:301-313.

11. Mold JW, Blake GH, Becker LA: Goal-Oriented Medical Care. *Family Medicine,* 1991; 23:46-51.

12. Starfield BH, Simborg DW, Horn SD, Yourtee SA: Continuity and coordination in primary care: their achievement and utility. *Medical Care,* 1976; 14:625-636.

13. Jamison J: Chiropractic's functional integration into conventional health care: some implications. *J Manip Physiol Ther* 1987; 10:5-10.

14. Neff S: Taxonomy of neurodiagnostic modalities. *J Manip Physiol Ther* 1989; 12:120-130.

15. Anderson R: Standards for Interprofessional Relations: *Chiropractic Standards of Practice and Quality of Care*, Vear HJ, ed., Aspen, Gaithersburg 1991; pp 163-178.

16. Demetrious J: What is the primary objective in sub-specialty care? *ACA J Chirop*, 1989; 26:20-21.

17. Davidson RA, Fletcher RH, Earp JA: Role disagreement in primary care practice. *J Community Health*, 1981; 7:93-102.

18. Chen PC: Providing Primary Health Care with Non-Physicians. *Annals of Internal Medicine*, Singapore, 1984; 13:264-271.

19. Greenwald HP, Peterson ML, Garrison LP, Hart LG, Moscovice IS, Hall TL, Perrin EB: Interspecialty variation in office-based care. *Medical Care*, 1984; 22:14-29.

20. Haney P, Mootz R: A case report on non-resolving conservative care of low-back pain and sciatic radicular syndrome. *J Manipulative Physiol Ther* 1985; 8:109-114.

21. Dixon AS: The Evolution of Clinical Policies. *Medical Care* 1990; 28:201-220.

22. Wennenberg JE: Outcomes Research, Cost-Containment, and the Fear of Health Care Rationing. *New Eng J Med.* 1991; 323:1202.

23. Mootz RD: *Interprofessional Referral Protocol.*

24. American Chiropractic Association: *Code of Ethics,* 1990-1991, Arlington, Virginia.

25. International Chiropractors' Association. *Policy Handbook and Code of Ethics*, Arlington, Virginia, ed 2, 1991.

26. Harrison JD: *Chiropractic Practice and Liability: A Practical Guide to Successful Risk Management*, International Chiropractors' Association, Arlington, Virginia, 1990.

IX. MINORITY OPINIONS

None.

Contraindications and Complications

Chapter Outline

I. OVERVIEW

Most forms of treatment carry some risk of harm to the patient. While chiropractic procedures are considered comparatively safe, special caution is warranted with certain conditions. These include, for example, vertebral artery syndrome, herniated disc, and bone weakening processes.

Prevention of complications from treatment is facilitated when good professional judgment is exercised and quality care is provided. Elements common to all primary care practitioners include sufficient history taking and record keeping, thorough examination, timely re-evaluation procedures throughout the course of case management, good communication with the patient and appropriate response in the event that an unexpected incident does occur. With serious manipulative accidents, it is of critical importance that the intervention or procedure associated with the onset of the complication not be repeated.

Some of the complications reported in the literature could have been prevented. The development of acceptable preventative strategies to minimize future risk should be directed by methods of consensus, illuminated by continuous evaluation of research, protocol experience, and risk management and peer review programs. The expected goal of establishing guidelines for standards of practice is to assist practitioners to set and abide by standards which improve all aspects of patient care.

The scope of manipulative incidents and reactions may range from short-term pain and stiffness to cerebrovascular accidents arising from a dissecting aneurysm. This review of complications of and contraindications to high-velocity thrust procedures outlines various clinical conditions requiring treatment modification. Other manual procedures (e.g., soft tissue and low force technique procedures) are not addressed in this chapter. Guidelines for sound clinical management and prevention are recommended.

II. DEFINITIONS

Complication: The unexpected aggravation of an existing disorder or the onset of an unexpected new disorder as a result of treatment.

Classification of Complications.
a) **Adverse Effect:** Any detrimental result of an action or treatment.
b) **Reaction:** A slight or benign adverse effect of short duration usually lasting no more than a few days.
c) **Accident or Incident:** An unexpected event occurring by chance, unknown causes, carelessness, negligence, or a combination thereof, resulting in serious or permanent impairment, injury, or fatality. The onset of signs and symptoms may be immediate or a day or two following the treatment.

d) **Indirect Complication:** Delay of diagnosis and appropriate treatment as a consequence of using a procedure or treatment that, in retrospect, has proven to be of no benefit for the condition.

Contraindication—Absolute: Any circumstance which renders a form of treatment or clinical intervention inappropriate because it places the patient at undue risk.

Contraindication—Relative: Any circumstance which may place the patient at undue risk unless treatment approach is modified.

Effectiveness: Effectiveness refers to the potential any given procedure or group of procedures has to produce a desired effect under actual conditions of use.

Iatrogenesis: Disorders or complications caused by health care providers.

Instability: An unstable joint condition resulting in damage or symptoms under the influence of physiologic loading.

Joint Dysfunction (Manipulable lesion, subluxation, functional spinal lesion): Decreased or aberrant joint mobility for which manipulation is indicated. In this context the term excludes states of hypermobility or instability.

Management: A plan of action for treatment of the patient in accordance with diagnosis, progress, and expectations of outcome.

Manual Therapy: Broadly described as a skilled manual method of movement of the soft tissues and articulations. May include all manual procedures, such as massage, muscle energy and strain-counterstrain techniques, trigger point therapy, joint mobilization, manipulation, and articular adjustment.
a) **Stretching:** Techniques that attempt selectively to apply tensile forces along the length of specific ligaments or muscles. Loads used are quasistatic and are thought to bring about increased flexibility of the appropriate joint through passive means. Relaxation of muscle spasm and creep deformity of the elastic elements in connective tissues are commonly assumed mechanisms of action.
b) **Mobilization:** Passive movement within the physiologic joint space, administered by a clinician for the purpose of increasing overall range of joint motion.
c) **Soft Tissue Procedures:** A variety of manual techniques for soft tissue. As muscles and noncontractile structures lose function and elasticity, they have an effect on joint function. Most soft tissues are richly innervated with a variety of proprioceptive mechanisms, and often chiropractic application of soft tissue procedures will follow a traditional chiropractic rationale of attempting to improve a clinically identifiable aberrant neurologic reflex or pain pattern. Such work may be used in conjunction with other adjustive or manipulative approaches. Some practitioners use a

variety of soft tissue procedures for nonarticular purposes as well (e.g., abdominal pressure points may be stimulated in a constipated patient).

    d) **High-Velocity Thrusting:** Techniques involving movement of the selected joint to its end range of voluntary motion, followed by the application of an impulse loading. These methods are among the most common in chiropractic practice and are often referred to as "manipulation" or "adjustment" to differentiate them from less dynamic procedures.

Motion Segment: The smallest functional unit, made up of two adjacent articulating surfaces and contiguous and intervening soft tissues.

Negligence: Breach of the legal duty of care placed on all practitioners to exercise reasonable care and skill in the circumstances.

Risk Management: A systematic preventative strategy to minimize patient harm and practitioner liability through education and the development of guidelines for practice.

Safety: Safety refers to a judgment of the acceptability of any risk in a specified situation during the application of a specific procedure or group of procedures provided by an individual with specified and appropriate training.

Specialist: A health care provider who has obtained a professionally accepted or recognized level of additional training and competence with respect to specific procedures or disorders.

III. LIST OF SUBTOPICS

Conditions selected have come from a review of the scientific and medicolegal literature as well as insurance claim information.

A. Articular Derangements

1. Arthritides
    i) Acute arthropathies
    ii) Subacute and chronic ankylosing spondylitis
    iii) Degenerative joint disease
    iv) Spondylolysis and spondylolisthesis
2. Dislocation, fractures, instability
3. Os odontoideum
4. Articular hypermobility
5. Postsurgical joint
6. Acute joint injury
7. Scoliosis

B. Bone Weakening and Destructive Disorders

1. Juvenile osteochrondroses
2. Osteoporosis, osteomalacia
3. Bone tumors
4. Malignancy
5. Infection of bone and joint

C. Circulatory and Cardiovascular Disorders

1. Vertebrobasilar, etc.
2. Aneurysm
3. Bleeding disorders

D. Neurological Disorders

1. Myelopathy, cauda equina syndrome

IV. LITERATURE REVIEW

Over the past two decades there has been a rapid growth of literature on manipulation-induced accidents or injuries. (Dvorak 1991; Patjin, 1991; Schmitt, 1991; Terrett, 1990, 1987; Grieve, 1986; Gotlib and Thiel, 1985; Schmidely and Koch, 1984; Gutmann, 1983; Dvorak and Orelli, 1982; Ladermann, 1981; Gatterman, 1981; Jaskoviak, 1980; Kleynhans, 1980; Livingston, 1971). There can be little doubt that the elevated level of reporting arises from a general increase in awareness of complications by all professionals interested in spinal manipulative therapy. Because some alleged "consequences" are consistent with the natural history of a condition, anecdotal or polemic reports must be distinguished from those that provide objective evidence of true manipulation-induced injuries. Some case reports of injury have proven to be unfounded upon further unbiased inquiry.

Complications that do occur in a chiropractic office setting may be attributed to the following (Shekelle et al. 1991):

- misdiagnosis
- presence of coagulation dyscrasias
- cervical manipulation
- presence of a herniated nucleus pulposus
- improper technique application

The relative harm caused by therapeutic procedures used by chiropractic practitioners may be appreciated by reviewing claims of malpractice. The National Chiropractic Mutual Insurance Company listed the six most common claims in 1990 as:

- disc problems - 29%
- failure to diagnose - 13%
- fracture - 9%
- soft tissue - 7%
- cerebrovascular accidents - 6%
- aggravation of prior condition - 4%

A review of claims made in Canada from 1978 to 1985 revealed that cervical injuries represented 34% of the frequency and 50% of the total cost of claims. The second most reported claim was lumbar injury accounting for a frequency of 19% and cost of 26% of all claims made. Common reasons for malpractice claims against practitioners were inappropriate treatment and poor patient communication. Aside from the treatment of functional disorders of the spine and extremities, other co-existing and unrecognized conditions are a significant factor in some accident claims. (Canadian Chiropractic Protective Association — CCPA Claims Review, to 1985).

A more recent CCPA Claim Review, for the period January 1986 to December 1990, revealed the following:

Lumbar spine injury	36 (23% of claims)
Rib Fracture	29 (19%)
Neck Injury	24 (16%)
Soft tissue/non-spinal injury	26 (13%)
CVA	12 (8%)
Other *	24 (16%)

(* fee dispute, patient perception of general injury, failure to diagnose, improper treatment, practitioner concern over lawsuit)

With respect to the frequency of complications, Ladermann (1980) identified 135 case reports of serious complications over a 30 year period from 1950-1980, a time period during which tens of millions of manipulations were administered by a variety of practitioners. Kleynhans (1980), analyzing some of these case studies, outlined a number of likely practitioner-related causes of adverse reactions and suggested three main factors: lack of knowledge or diagnostic error; lack of technique skill; and lack of rational clinical attitude in case management. These causes could well account for a number of iatrogenic injuries reported in the literature, e.g., pathological fractures (Austin, 1985; Holta, 1942), ruptured abdominal aneurysms (Kornberge, 1988), electrotherapy burns and injuries, etc.

Jaskoviak (1981) and Terrett (1987) specifically dealt with case reviews on the adverse effect of cervical manipulation where vertebrobasilar insufficiency was evident. Gutmann (1984), Terrett (1987), Theil (1991) and Schmitt (1991) have recently described or studied the biomechanical effects of head and neck movement and cervical manipulation in association with vertebral artery injury. Manipulation has been identified as only one of many activities or health care procedures that may result in damage to the vertebral artery. However, it has been the one most extensively reviewed and discussed. (Pratt-Thomas and Berger, 1947; Gutmann 1957, 1962, 1971, 1984; Smith and Estridge, 1962; Maigne, 1969; Houle, 1972; Lewit, 1972; Giles, 1977; Henderson, 1979, 1991; George et al., 1981; Terrett, 1982, 1983, 1987; Hulse, 1983; Fast et al., 1987; Henderson and Cassidy, 1988; Martienssen and Nilsson, 1989; Raskind and North, 1990).

It is thought that cervical rotation combined with extension and traction may have some obstructive effect on perfusion of the vertebral artery on the contralateral side of rotation. If the ipsilateral artery is diseased or hypoplastic, symptoms of hind brain ischemia may occur because the dominant healthy artery is under partial physiological compression, resulting in a loss of sufficient or compensatory blood flow. If trauma to the arterial wall does occur, thrombus formation may be the result. Further, this may lead to stroke or stroke-like complications in susceptible patients. While incidence figures vary, it is generally agreed that the risk of serious neurological complications is extremely low, and is approximately one or two per million cervical manipulations. Structural abnormalities, particularly where mechanical instability, pathological bone disorders, dislocations and fractures of the cervical spine are present may also lead to mechanical strain of the vertebral arteries (Terrett, 1987; Kleynhans, 1980; Jaskoviak, 1981; Ladermann, 1981).

Other cervical manipulative complications, which are rare but have either been reported or described in the literature, include Horner's syndrome, diaphragmatic paralysis, cervical myelopathy secondary to meningeal hemorrhage, pathological fracture of a cervical vertebra and cervical disc protrusions (Dabert et al., 1970; Rinsky et al., 1976; Krewalramani, 1982; Hefner, 1985; Grayson, 1987; Gatterman, 1991). Dislocation in the upper cervical spine due to inflammatory or traumatic rupture of the transverse atlantal or alar ligaments warrants particular caution (Yochum and Rowe, 1980, 1987; Jeffreys, 1980; Sandman, 1981; Redlund-Johnell, 1984).

Though rarely reported in the literature, empirically the most common complaint of manipulation of the thoracic region occurs when forceful or poorly applied manipulations cause costovertebral strains, rib fractures and costochondral separations (Grieve, 1986). Excessive thoracolumbar torque in the side posture position as well as inappropriately applied posterior to anterior techniques may cause thoracic cage injuries particularly in the elderly.

Lower back injury alleged to have occurred following spinal manipulative therapy has been reported in patients with pre-existing disc herniation or prolapse (CCPA Claim Review, 1990; Bromley, 1989; Gallinaro and Cartesegna, 1983). While it is suggested that the forces required to cause a disruption of the annular fibers of the healthy intervertebral disc well exceed that of a rotational manipulative thrust (Adams and Hutton, 1981, 1983; Farfan, 1983; Gilmore, 1986; Triano, 1991), some disc herniation/protusion may certainly be aggravated by an inappropriately applied manipulative maneuver, as it may be by other simple activities of daily living such as bending, sneezing, lifting. The most frequently described severe complication is compression of the cauda equina by massive midline nuclear herniation at the level of third, fourth or fifth intervertebral disc (Lehmann et al., 1991; Malmivivaara and Pohjola, 1982; Kleynhans, 1980; Hooper, 1973).

Of the thirty cauda equina complications associated with manipulation reported in the French, German and English literature over an 80 year period, only eight were allegedly related to chiropractic treatment (Ladermann, 1980). Had these patients not been manipulated, the outcome may have been the same with menial effort or impulsive strain replacing the rupturing effect alleged to arise from the manipulation. However, this clinical outcome does stress the need for particular care in this susceptible subgroup of patients.

Psychological factors including pain intolerance, hysteria conversion reactions, hypochondriasis, malingering, etc., require special consideration, since the presence of neuromusculoskeletal symptoms may be of secondary importance. Aside from the risk of creating a dependency for care that may or may not be indicated, treatment itself may aggravate or contribute to real or imagined harm.

V. ASSESSMENT CRITERIA

Complications may occur spontaneously or arise as a result of chiropractic treatment. The risk of these complications may vary within subgroups of patients based on their clinical presentation. The main focus for the prevention of complications is the recognition of well known and established indicators or "red flag" signs and symptoms, which may require careful assessment and reassessment, changes in treatment plan, or other appropriate action such as emergency care or referral to another health care specialist. Ignoring these "red flag" indicators increases the likelihood of patient harm.

The literature and clinical experience show that the most common therapeutic procedure in chiropractic practice, and the one most likely to result in complications, is the adjustment or high-velocity manipulative thrust. The following assessment criteria and recommendations relate to this procedure applied to, or adjacent to, the anatomical site of pathology.

Assessment criteria developed and used in this chapter relate to:

a) Rating of conditions
b) Severity of complication
c) Quality of evidence
d) Level of contraindication: based on the above factors and the probability of complication

A. Rating of Conditions:

Type I:

A condition for which high-velocity thrust procedures have been shown to be comparatively safe and effective so long as an adequate diagnosis has been made and a therapeutic trial is rationally applied (e.g., upper cervical dysfunction/subluxation associated with tension headaches).

Type II:

A type I condition is present but may be coincident with another related or unrelated condition requiring modification of procedures and/or further diagnostic assessment (e.g., upper cervical joint dysfunction/subluxation accompanied by

widening of the atlantodental interval or inflammatory causes affecting the area). Careful clinical judgment is required as high-velocity thrust procedures may be relatively or absolutely contraindicated.

Type III:

Type I or II conditions are present but considered negligible compared with clinical evidence of another pathological problem requiring further diagnostic assessment and referral to another health care professional (e.g., cervical joint dysfunction/subluxation and local metastatic bone tumor). As the risk of serious harm far outweighs benefit, the therapeutic procedure may be absolutely contraindicated.

B. Severity of Complication:

Minimal Level:

Any complications of high-velocity thrust procedures may be considered minimal, with slight objective evidence of worsened signs usually lasting a maximum of several days. (Reactions such as short term pain and stiffness or, infrequently, a mild chronic pain disorder alleged to arise from aggravation of a pre-existing problem). These reactions are rarely reported in the literature/claim reviews, given the brief duration of mild symptoms experienced by patients and the superimposed natural history of the presenting complaint. High-velocity thrust procedures are not generally contraindicated. Treatment modifications may have to be anticipated in exceptional cases.

Moderate Level:

Level of harm is generally moderate, characterized by more-or-less serious but usually reversible harm lasting weeks to months. Effects are temporary and/or residual in nature (e.g., broken rib, uncomplicated disc herniation, radiculopathy, foot drop). Depending on all factors (e.g., frequency of complications, benefits) high-velocity thrust procedures may be relatively or absolutely contraindicated.

High Level:

Evidence suggests risk of a high level of harm. The complication or accident may be serious and/or permanent, particularly in susceptible patients. (e.g., stroke, cauda equina syndrome). High-velocity thrust procedures may be relatively contraindicated with careful treatment modification, or absolutely contraindicated given patient history, diagnostic tests and/or other information obtained during a trial of therapy.

C. Quality of Evidence:

Evidence on the risk of complication arising from chiropractic treatment and particularly high-velocity thrust procedures comes from case reports, surveys, literature reviews, and insurance and legal claims records. There needs to be further systematic study of the incidence, severity and management of complications. Present classification of quality of evidence is:

Class I:

Evidence provided by surveys, systematic studies, literature reviews, and detailed clinical case reports published in refereed journals.

Class II:

Evidence provided by other case studies or reviews, or consensus expert opinion from legitimate consensus-building efforts.

Class III:

Evidence provided by expert opinion and one or more case reports.

D. Level of Contraindication:

Having regard to all of the individual assessment criteria already discussed, the following overall ratings are used:

No Contraindication

Relative Contraindication: high-velocity thrust procedures may be used with appropriate care and/or modification.

Relative to Absolute Contraindication: careful clinical judgment dictates whether contraindication is relative or absolute with each specific patient.

Absolute Contraindication

Example: As an example of the complete rating system:

Noncomplicated Low-Back Pain:
No contraindication to high-velocity thrust procedures.

Risk-of-Complication Rating:
Severity (if harm did occur): Minimal
Rating of Condition: Type I
Quality of Evidence: Class I

This rating system assumes no negligence or error on the part of the practitioner. Tolerance to treatment may sometimes, but not always, be estimated by provocative or premanipulative testing.

In the examples below it is assumed that traditionally and commonly used high-velocity, low-amplitude thrusts (adjustment/manipulation) are administered to, or immediately adjacent to, the segmental level where both the manipulable subluxation/dysfunction and/or the condition has primarily manifested itself.

VI. RECOMMENDATIONS

Note: General health problems which have been described in the literature as either contraindications to or complications of high-velocity thrust procedures include the following con-

ditions. It should be understood that the listed conditions are not necessarily those for which high-velocity thrust procedures are intended. Rather they may be coincidentally present in a patient undergoing treatment. The fundamental object of treatment is a manipulable joint lesion (subluxation, dysfunction, blockage).

A. Articular Derangements:

1. Acute rheumatoid, rheumatoidlike and nonspecific arthropathies including acute ankylosing spondylitis characterized by episodes of acute inflammation, demineralization, ligamentous laxity with anatomic subluxation or dislocation, represent an **absolute contraindication** to high-velocity thrust procedures in anatomical regions of involvement.

> **12.1.1** **Risk-of-Complication Rating:**
> Severity: Moderate to High Condition Rating:
> Type III
> Quality of Evidence: Class II, III
> **Consensus Level: 1**

2. Sub-acute and/or chronic ankylosing spondylitis and other chronic arthropathies in which there are no signs of ligamentous laxity, anatomic subluxation or ankylosis are **not contraindications** to high-velocity thrust procedures applied to the area of pathology.

> **12.1.2** **Risk-of-Complication Rating:**
> Severity: Minimal
> Condition Rating: Type I, II
> Quality of Evidence: Class II, III
> **Consensus Level: 1**

3. Degenerative joint disease, osteoarthritis, degenerative discopathy and spondyloarthrosis are **not contraindications** to high-velocity thrust procedures to the area of pathology but treatment modification may be warranted during active inflammatory phases.

> **12.1.3** **Risk-of-Complication Rating:**
> Severity: Minimal
> Condition Rating: Type I, II
> Quality of Evidence: Class II
> **Consensus Level: 1**

4. In patients with spondylolysis and spondylolisthesis caution is warranted when high-velocity thrust procedures are used. These conditions are **not contraindications**, but with progressive slippage they may represent a **relative contraindication**.

> **12.1.4** **Risk-of-Complication Rating:**
> Severity: Minimal to Moderate
> Condition Rating: Type I, II
> Quality of Evidence: Class II
> **Consensus Level: 1**

5. Acute fractures and dislocations, or healed fractures and dislocations with signs of ligamentous rupture or instability, represent an **absolute contraindication** to high-velocity thrust procedures applied to the anatomical site or region.

12.1.5   **Risk-of-Complication Rating:**
Severity: High
Condition Rating: Type III
Quality of Evidence: Class III
Consensus Level: 1

6. Unstable os odontoideum represents an **absolute contraindication** to high-velocity thrust procedures to the area of pathology.

12.1.6   **Risk-of-Complication Rating:**
Severity: High
Condition Rating: Type III
Quality of Evidence: Class III
Consensus Level: 1

7. Articular hypermobility, and circumstances where the stability of a joint is uncertain, represent a **relative contraindication** to high-velocity thrust procedures to the area of pathology.

12.1.7   **Risk-of-Complication Rating:**
Severity: Minimal
Condition Rating: Type I, II
Quality of Evidence: Class II, III
Consensus Level: 1

8. Postsurgical joints or segments with no evidence of instability are **not a contraindication** to high-velocity thrust procedures but may represent a **relative contraindication** depending on clinical signs (e.g., response, pretest tolerance or degree of healing).

12.1.8   **Risk-of-Complication Rating:**
Severity: Minimal
Condition Rating: Type II
Quality of Evidence: Class III
Consensus Level: 1

9. Acute injuries of osseous and soft tissues may require modification of treatment. In most cases, high-velocity thrust procedures to the area of pathology are **not contraindicated.**

12.1.9   **Risk-of-Complication Rating:**
Severity: Minimal to moderate
Condition Rating: Type I, II
Quality of Evidence: Class I, II
Consensus Level: 1

10. The presence of scoliosis is **not a contraindication** to high-velocity thrust procedure.

12.1.10   **Risk-of-Complication Rating:**
Severity: Minimal
Condition Rating: Type I, II

Quality of Evidence: Class II, III
Consensus Level: 1

B. Bone Weakening and Destructive Disorders

1. Active juvenile avascular necrosis, specifically of the weight bearing joints (e.g., Perthes' disease) represents an **absolute contraindication** to high-velocity thrust procedures to the area of pathology.

12.2.1   **Risk-of-Complication Rating:**
Severity: High
Condition Rating: Type III
Quality of Evidence: Class III
Consensus Level: 1

2. Demineralization of bone warrants caution with the use of high-velocity thrust procedures. This represents a **relative contraindication** to high-velocity thrust procedures to the area of pathology.

12.2.2   **Risk-of-Complication Rating:**
Severity: Minimal to Moderate
Condition Rating: Type II
Quality of Evidence: Class II, III
Consensus Level: 1

3. Benign bone tumors may result in pathological fractures and therefore represent a **relative to absolute contraindication** to high-velocity thrust procedures to the area of pathology.

12.2.3   **Risk-of-Complication Rating:**
Severity: Low to Moderate
Condition Rating: Type II, III
Quality of Evidence: Class III
Consensus Level: 1

4. Malignancies represent conditions for which high-velocity thrust procedures to the area of pathology are **absolutely contraindicated** .

12.2.4   **Risk-of-Complication Rating:**
Severity: Moderate to High
Condition Rating: Type III
Quality of Evidence: Class II, III
Consensus Level: 1

5. Infection of bone and joint represents an **absolute contraindication** to high-velocity thrust procedures to the area of pathology.

12.2.5   **Risk-of-Complication Rating:**
Severity: Minimal to High
Condition Rating: Type III
Quality of Evidence: Class II
Consensus Level: 1

C. Circulatory and Cardiovascular Disorders

1. Clinical manifestations of vertebrobasilar insufficiency syndrome warrant particular caution and represent a **relative to absolute contraindication** to cervical high-velocity thrust procedures to the region of pathology.

    12.3.1   **Risk-of-Complication Rating:**
           Severity: Minimal to High
           Condition Rating: Type II, III
           Quality of Evidence: Class I, II, III
           Consensus Level: 1

2. When a diagnosis of a significant aneurysm involving a major blood vessel has been made, a **relative to absolute contraindication** may exist for high-velocity thrust procedures within the area of pathology.

    12.3.2   **Risk-of-Complication Rating:**
           Severity: High
           Condition Rating: Type III
           Quality of Evidence: Class III
           Consensus Level: 1

3. Bleeding is a potential complication of anticoagulant therapy or certain blood dyscrasias. Patients with these disorders represent a **relative contraindication** to high-velocity thrust procedures.

    12.3.3   **Risk-of-Complication Rating:**
           Severity: Minimal to High
           Condition Rating: Type II
           Quality of Evidence: Class III
           Consensus Level: 1

D. Neurological Disorders

1. Signs and symptoms of acute myelopathy or acute cauda equina syndrome represent an **absolute contraindication** to high-velocity thrust procedures applied to the anatomic site of involvement.

    12.4.1   **Risk-of-Complication Rating:**
           Severity: High
           Condition Rating: Type II, III
           Quality of Evidence: Class I, II
           Consensus Level: 1

* Most dysfunctions or disease processes have variations or phases. Levels of severity and probability have been assigned on the basis that the condition displays usual and classical signs and symptoms. The difficulty in precisely detailing the degree or severity and probability of an individual patient's overall physical and psychological response both to the condition and therapeutic procedure (subtleties of force, amplitude, direction, patient positioning, etc.) is acknowledged. Nevertheless, ratings have been assigned based on the literature and the current consensus process. These provide a starting point which will require ongoing review and refinement.

Some conditions, such as scoliosis, are not level-specific and high-velocity thrust procedures used apply more to a region than a level.

VII. COMMENTS, SUMMARY OR CONCLUSION

This chapter provides an analytical framework and specific interim guideline recommendations with respect to complications of and contraindications to manipulative thrust procedures. At present, detailed systematic studies on this subject are lacking and the recommendations made are based on information from clinical reviews and case reports, as well as from expert opinion and consensus methods. One objective of this chapter is to encourage productive debate leading to firmer commitment on risk management protocols.

The recommendations made must be continuously re-evaluated in light of ongoing research and clinical experience. Cooperative intradisciplinary and interdisciplinary research will be necessary to determine the true extent of the nature and occurrence of iatrogenic complications in chiropractic practice. The development of a central registry system capable of generating comprehensive research data would be valuable, and would facilitate the establishment of more detailed and refined guideline recommendations in the future.

VIII. REFERENCES

Adams MA, Hutton WC: The mechanical function of the lumbar apophyseal joints. *Spine* 1983; 8(3):327-30.

Adams MA, Hutton WC: The relevance of torsion to the mechanical derangement of the lumbar spine. *Spine* 1981; 6:241-8.

Austin RT: Pathological vertebral fractures after spinal manipulation. *Br Med J* 1985; 291:1114-1115.

Bromley W: The National Chiropractic Mutual Insurance Company: stronger than ever. *ACA J Chirop* 1989; 26:52.

Dabert O, Freeman, DG, Weis AJ: Spinal meningeal hematoma, warfarin therapy and chiropractic adjustment. *JAMA* 1970; 214(11):2058.

Campbell LK, Ladenheim CJ, Sherman RP, Sportelli L: Risk management in chiropractic. Fincastle, Virginia. Health Services Publication, 1990.

Canadian Chiropractic Protective Association: Data from claim reviews, Canadian Chiropractic Association. 1978-85; 1986-90.

Dvorak J, Orelli F: How dangerous is manipulation of the cervical spine? *J Manual Medicine.* 1982; 20:44-8.

Dvorak J: Inappropriate indications and contraindications for manual therapy. *J Manual Medicine.* 1991; 6(3):85-88.

Dvorak J, Baumgertner H, Burn L, Dalgaard JB, et al.: Consensus and recommendations as to the side effects and complications of manual therapy of the cervical spine. *J Manual Medicine,* 1991; 6(3):117-8.

Farfan HF: Biomechanics of the lumbar spine. In: Kirdaldy-Willis WH (ed.) *Managing low back pain.* New York, Churchill-Livingstone, 198:109-127.

Fast A, Zincola DF, Marin EL: Vertebral artery damage complicating cervical manipulation. *Spine* 1987; 12:840-1.

Jeffreys E: *Disorders of the cervical spine.* London, Butterworths, 1980:106-118.

Gallinaro P, Cartesegna M: Three cases of lumbar disc rupture and one of cauda equina associated with spinal manipulation (chiropraxis). *Lancet* 1983; Feb 19:411.

Gatterman MI: Contraindications and complications of spinal manipulative therapy. *ACA J Chiro* 1981; 15:75-86.

Gatterman MI: Contraindications and complications of spinal manipulative therapy. In: Gatterman MI, (ed.): *Chiropractic Management of Spine Related Disorders.* Baltimore, Williams and Wilkins, 1990, pp 231-232.

George PE, Silverstein HT, Wallace H, Marshall M: Identification of the high risk prestroke patient. *ACA J Chiro* 1981; 15:26-8.

Giles LGF: Vertobrobasilar artery insufficiency. *J Can Chiro Assoc.*, 1977; 21:112-7.

Gilmore KL: Biomechanics of the lumbar motion segment. In: Grieve GP, (ed.): *Modern manual therapy of the vertebral column.* New York, Churchill-Livingstone, 1986; 103-11.

Gotlib A, Thiel H: A selected annotated bibliography of the core biomechanical literature pertaining to stroke, cervical spine, manipulation and head/neck movement. *J Can Chiro Assoc.*, 1985; 29:80-9.

Grayson MF: Horner's syndrome after manipulation of the neck. *Br Med J.*, 1987; 295:1382.

Grieve GP: Incidents and accidents of manipulation. In: Grieve GP (ed.): *Modern Manual Therapy.* Churchill Livingstone, New York 1986; pp 873-889.

Gutmann G, Tiwisina T: *Zum problem der irritation der arteria vertebralis.* Stuttgart, Hippokrates-Verlag GmgH 1957; 15.

Gutmann G: Halswirlebsaule und durchbu-lutungsstorrungen in der vertebralis-basilaris-strombahn. In:...*Die wirbelsaule in forschung und praxis.* Stuttgart, Hippokrates 1962; 25:138-55.

Gutmann G: Durchbluntungsstorungen der arteria vertebrails im zusammenhang mit Halswirbel-sauleenverletzungan. *Manuelle Medlizlin* 1971; 5:112-6.

Gutmann G, ed: *Arteria vertebralis - traumatologie und funtionelle pathologie.* Berlin/Heidelberg: Springer-Verlag, 1984.

Gutmann G: Injuries to the vertebral artery caused by manual therapy. *Manuelle Medizin* 1983; 21:2-14.

Hefner JE: Diaphragmatic paralysis following chiropractic manipulation of the cervical spine. *Arch Intern Med.*, 1985; 145:562-563.

Henderson DJ: Significance of vertebral dyskinesia in relation to the cervical syndrome. *J Manip Physiol Ther.*, 1979; 2:3-15.

Henderson DJ, Cassidy JD: Vertebrobasilar vascular accidents associated with cervical manipulation. In:...Vernon H, (ed.): *Upper cervical syndrome - chiropractic diagnosis and treatment.* Baltimore, Williams & Wilkins, 1988; 194-206.

Henderson DJ: Vertebral artery syndrome. In: Vear HJ, (ed.): *Chiropractic standards of practice and quality of care.* Gaithersburg, Maryland, Aspen Publishers, Inc. 1992: 115-143.

Holta O: Hemangioma of the cervical vertebra with fracture and compression myelomalacia. *Acta Radiol.*, 1942; 23:423.

Hooper J: Low-back pain and manipulation: paraparesis after treatment of low-back pain by physical methods. *Med J Australia* 1973; Mar 17:549-551.

Houle JOE: Assessing hemodynamics of the vertebrobasilar complex through angiothlipsis. *J Can Chiro Assoc.*, 1972; 41:35-6, 41.

Hulse M: *Die zervikalen gleichgewichtsstorungen.* Berlin, Sprinder-Verlag. 1983:4-9.

Jaskoviak PA: Complications arising from manipulation of the cervical spine. *J Manip Physiol Ther* 1980; 3:213-9.

Kewalramani LS, Kewalramani DL, Krebs M, Saleem A: Myelopathy following cervical spine manipulation. *Am J Physical Med.*, 1982; 61:165-175.

Kleynhans AM: The prevention of complications from spinal manipulative therapy. In: Idezak RM, (ed.): *Aspects of manipulative therapy.* Melbourne, Lincoln Institute of Health Sciences -Conference Proceedings. 1980; 133-141.

Kleynhans AM: Complication and contraindications to spinal manipulative therapy. In: Haldeman S, (ed.): *Modern developments in the principles and practice of chiropractic.* New York, Appleton-Century-Crofts, 1980: 133-41.

Kornberge E: Lumbar artery aneurysms with acute aortic occlusion resulting from chiropractic manipulation: a case report. *Surgery* 1988; 103(1) : 122-124.

Ladermann JP: Accidents of spinal manipulation. *Ann Swiss Chiro Assoc.*, 1981; 7:162-208.

Lehmann OJ, Mendoza ND, Bradford R: Beware the prolapsed disc. *Br J Hosp Med.*, 1991; 46-52.

Lewit K: Komplikationen nach chiropraktischen manipulationen. *Dtsch Med Wschr* 1972; 97:784.

Livinston CP: Spinal manipulation causing injury. A three-year study. *Clin Ortho Rel Res.* 1971; 81:82-86.

Maigne R: Manipulations vertebralis et les thromboses vertebro basilares. *Angeiologie* 1969; 21:287.

Malmivivaara A, Pohjola R: Cauda equina syndrome caused by chiropraxis on a patient previously free of lumbar spine symptoms. *Lancet.* 1982; Oct 30:986-987.

Martienssen J, Nillson N: Cerebrovascular accidents following upper cervical manipulation: the importance of age, gender and technique. *Amer J Chiro Med.*, 1989; 2(1):10-3.

National Chiropractic Mutual Insurance Company: Claim information, 1990.

Patjin J: Complications in manual medicine: a review of the literature. *J Manual Medicine.* 1991;6(3);89-92.

Pratt-Thomas HR, Berger KE: Cerebellar and spinal injuries after chiropractic manipulation. *JAMA* 1947; 133:600-3.

Quon JA, Cassidy JD, O'Conner SM: Kirkaldy-Willis. Lumbar intervertebral disk herniation; treatment by rotational manipulation. *J Manip Physiol Ther.*, 1989; 12:220-227.

Raskind R, North CM: Vertebral artery injuries following chiropractic manipulation. *Angiology* 1990; 41(6):445-52.

Redlund-Johnell I: Atlanto-occipital dislocation in rheumatoid arthritis. *Acta Radiol Diagn.*, 1984; 25:165-168.

Rinsky LA, Reynolds GG, Jameson RM, Hamilton RD: A cervical spinal cord injury following chiropractic manipulation. *Paraplegia* 1976; 13:223-227.

Sandman TD, Sandman KB: Rheumatoid arthritis of the cervical spine; examination prior to chiropractic manipulative therapy. *J Manip Physiol Ther.*, 1981; 4(1)19-20.

Sandoz R: The nature of a spinal degenerative lesion. *Ann Swiss Chiro Assoc.* 1989; 9:149-192.

Schmidley JW, Koch T: The non-cerebrovascular complications of chiropractic manipulation. *Neurology* 1984;34:684-685.

Schmitt HP: Anatomical structure of the cervical spine with reference to the pathology of manipulation complications. *J Manual Medicine* 1991;6(3):93-101.

Smith RA, Estridge MN: Neurological complications of head and neck manipulations. *JAMA* 1962; 182:528.

Terrett AGJ, Webb M: Vertebrobasilar accidents following cervical spine adjustment manipulation. *J Aust Chiro Assoc.*, 1982; 12:24-7.

Terrett AGJ: Importance and interpretation of tests designed to predict susceptibility to neurocirculatory accidents from manipulation. *J Aust Chiro Assoc.*, 1983; 13:29-34.

Terrett AGJ: Vascular accidents from cervical spine manipulation: report of 107 cases. *J Aust Chiro Assoc.*, 1987; 17:15.

Terrett AGJ: Vascular accidents from cervical spine manipulation. *J Aust Chiro Assoc.*, 1987; 17:131-44.

Terrett AGJ: It is more important to know when not to adjust. *Chiro Tech.*, 1990; 2:1-9.

Thiel HW: Gross morphology and pathoanatomy of the vertebral arteries. *J*

Manip Physiol Ther., 1991; 14(2):133-141.

Triano JJ, Hyde T: Nonsurgical treatment of sports-related spine injuries-manipulation. In: Hochschuler SH (ed). *Spine-Spinal Injuries in Sport.* Hanley & Belfus, Inc., Philadelphia, 1990; 4(2):446-453.

Triano JJ: *Proceedings of the American Society of Biomechanics,* Phoenix, AZ., 1991.

Yochum TR, Rowe LJ: *Essentials of skeletal radiology.* Baltimore, Williams & Wilkins, 1987.

Yochum TR, Rowe LJ: Arthritides of the upper cervical complex. In: Idozak RM, (ed.): *Aspects of manipulative therapy.* Victoria, Lincoln Institute of Health Sciences, 1980:22-32.

IX. MINORITY OPINION

None.

13

Preventive/Maintenance Care and Public Health

Chapter Outline

I. OVERVIEW

The practice of chiropractic deals with acute therapeutic intervention and long-term care plans. This chapter focuses on the latter, which includes wellness or preventative care (designed to reduce the future incidence of illness or impairment) and health promotion (based upon optimal function).

Some confusion arises from the use of various terms to describe such care - including supportive care, maintenance care, and preventive care. In this chapter, it is called "preventive/maintenance care."

Long-term ongoing health management has been a significant component of the holistic chiropractic model of health. Surrounding this is a wellness paradigm that recognizes related influences on health, emphasizes drugless, non-surgical management, and takes a positive dynamic view of health. In addition to periodic passive care, the model looks to the whole individual and requires active patient participation.

Active care efforts emphasize patient responsibility and may include exercise programs, weight loss, dietary counseling, life style modifications, education on body postures and mechanics, coordination training, safety habits, modification of life stressors, etc.

This type of management program, which combines health promotion, preventive/maintenance care, and patient participation, is gaining much more widespread understanding and acceptance in today's more health conscious society.

II. DEFINITIONS

These definitions are intended to clarify inconsistency in professional, legal and contractual terminology. It is expected that they will become standard.

Active Care: Modes of treatment requiring "active" involvement, participation, and responsibility on the part of the patient.

Passive Care: Application of treatment procedures by the care giver to the patient who "passively" submits to and receives care.

Supportive Care: Treatment for patients who have reached maximum therapeutic benefit, but who fail to sustain this benefit and progressively deteriorate when there are periodic trials of withdrawal of treatment. Supportive care follows appropriate application of active and passive care including rehabilitation and life style modifications. It is appropriate when alternative care options, including home-based self-care, have been considered and attempted. Supportive care may be inappropriate when it interferes with other appropriate primary care, or when the risk of supportive care outweighs its benefits, i.e., physician dependence, somatization, illness behavior, or secondary gain.

Preventative/Maintenance Care: Any management plan that seeks to prevent disease, prolong life, promote health and enhance the quality of life. A specific regimen is designed to provide for the patient's well-being or for maintaining the optimum state of health.

Risk Factors: Health characteristics increasing the probability that an individual, or group of individuals will develop a given disease or disorder.

III. LIST OF SUBTOPICS

A. Preventive /Maintenance Care
1. Disclosure
2. Chiropractic adjustments used in preventive/maintenance regimen
3. Health Screening
4. Health Promotion
5. Wellness Care

B. Public Health Considerations
6. Community Based Screening
7. Public Health Education

IV. LITERATURE REVIEW

From the very beginning, the chiropractic model of health has had as its foundation the maxim that a human being is an ecologically and biologically unified organism. The relationship between a patient's internal and external environment must be understood. A major premise is that the inherent recuperative power of the body aids restoration and maintenance of health. These assumptions comprise a wellness paradigm embraced by the great majority of the chiropractic profession. The spinal lesion, along with other factors such as poor nutrition, stress, trauma, heredity, congenital weaknesses, fatigue, environmental stressors and sedentary lifestyles, are viewed as lowering resistance and creating physical disharmony. The chiropractic model requires active patient participation.[1,2,3]

Patients presenting with a musculoskeletal problem often obtain a swift and favorable result. Then they may look to the practitioner for other health care needs.[4]

Some patients require ongoing long-term care, others choose it. Insurance constraints, however, mandate that the practitioner indicate when maximum therapeutic benefit has been achieved. The effectiveness of chiropractic preventive/maintenance care has not been subjected to study by randomized trial, a process that presents major methodological and financial challenges, but is supported by evidence from case studies.[5,6] However, its long-term benefits have not been clearly demonstrated.

Third party payers have typically resisted reimbursements for long-term preventive/maintenance care. Nonetheless, there is growing consumer demand for this and chiropractic care generally, despite increases in out-of-pocket expenses.[7,8,9]

Preventive/maintenance care is for patients without substantive manifestations. Therapeutic necessity is absent by definition. Clinically there is a need to distinguish for each patient when therapeutic and supportive care stops, and when preventive/maintenance care begins. The latter is considered safe and effective when used discriminately, so as not to foster physician dependence and chronicity.

The overall efficacy of preventive health care is subject to considerable debate.[10] In addition, the chiropractic profession has a specific role in the prevention of complaints of spinal origin. This includes identifying principles of spinal hygiene, and therapeutic strategies to avoid the need for more radical interventions, such as surgery.

But enhanced public awareness of environmental, psycho-social, and physiological issues through education and community action has forced preventive care into the public health agenda as the number one priority. Smoking cessation, weight control, nutritional considerations, stress reductions, and advice about exposure to environmental pollutants are examples of initiatives affecting the chiropractic patient population. [11]

Coile [3] offers this historical input: "Thirty years ago, Rene Dubos, a research microbiologist, suggested in *Mirage of Health* that the advancements he and others had made in the development of antibiotics and therapeutics had less to do with the real health of populations than a variety of economic, social, nutritional, and behavioral factors. Five years later, the U.S. Surgeon-General's landmark report clearly revealed the links between smoking and diseases such as emphysema, chronic bronchitis, hypertension and lung cancer.

"A new awareness of the contribution of lifestyle, environment, and genetics infused medicine in the decade following. Sometimes called the 'wellness movement,' this new orientation broadened the paradigm of traditional biomedicine. Since Dubos' essay on health, a body of research findings has accumulated that demonstrates the validity of a more comprehensive approach to health, one which recognizes the many antecedents and co-factors in the disease and healing process.

"Although not fully accepted by all physicians, the holistic concept of health is gaining stature. Dozens of studies by employers have begun to quantify the beneficial impact of health promotion programs in terms of reduced health care utilization and lower health care costs."

Long-term care concepts and considerations in chiropractic have been discussed by a number of authors (Coulter, [1] Jamison,[2] Coile [3]). Jamison [2] offers a comprehensive overview of the current trends in chiropractic, and worksheets for health care assessment. McDowell and Newell [12] describe general health care indicators and instruments. Jamison [13] reviews the improvement of basic health status by alteration of behavior, especially through health education.

Some recent surveys focus upon musculoskeletal chiropractic practice (Phillips,[14] Wardwell,[8] Shekelle and Brook [4]), but other current literature takes a firm stance on the importance of maintaining a focus on prevention and health promotion (Coulter,[1] Sportelli,[9] Caplan [7]).

Areas with new significance for chiropractic long-term care include the management of osteoporosis (Stacey [5]), and hypertension and stress management (Yates, et al.[6]).

No study yet addresses what specific impact preventive/maintenance care has on overall health or health care costs, or if preventive care enhances longevity or quality of life. Now, however, research into such complex issues as these is becoming more feasible (Nyiendo,[15] Kassak,[16] Jose [17]).

Notwithstanding the challenges of research in the field of prophylactic care there must be publication of valid clinical studies before chiropractic long-term preventive/maintenance care gains widespread public acknowledgement as an important component of health maintenance and wellness.

V. ASSESSMENT CRITERIA

Procedure Ratings (System I)

Established: Accepted as appropriate by the practicing chiropractic community for the given indication in the specified patient population.

Promising: Given current knowledge, this appears to be appropriate for the given indication in the specified patient population. As more evidence and experience accumulates, this interim rating will change. This connotes provisional acceptance, but permits a greater role for the level of current clinical use.

Equivocal: Current knowledge exists to support a given indication in a specified patient population, though value can neither be confirmed or denied. As more evidence and experience accumulates this interim rating will change. Expert opinion recognizes a need for caution in general application.

Investigational: Evidence is insufficient to determine appropriateness. Further study is warranted. Use for a given indication in a specified patient population should be confined largely to research protocols. As more evidence and experience accumulates this interim rating will change.

Doubtful: Given current knowledge, this appears to be inappropriate for the given indication in the specified patient population. As more evidence and experience accumulates this interim rating will change.

Inappropriate: Regarded by the practicing chiropractic community as unacceptable for the given indication in the specified patient population.

Quality of Evidence

The following categories of evidence are used to support the ratings.

Class I:

Evidence provided by one or more well-designed controlled clinical trials; or well-designed experimental studies that address reliability, validity, positive predictive value, discriminability, sensitivity, and specificity.

Class II:

Evidence provided by one or more well-designed uncontrolled, observational clinical studies, studies such as case control, cohort studies, etc.; or clinically relevant basic science studies that address reliability, validity, positive predictive value, discriminability, sensitivity, and specificity; and published in refereed journals.

Class III:

Evidence provided by expert opinion, descriptive studies or case reports.

Suggested Strength of Recommendation Ratings

Type A. Strong positive recommendation. Based on Class I evidence or overwhelming Class II evidence when circumstances preclude randomized clinical trials.

Type B. Positive recommendation based on Class II evidence.

Type C. Positive recommendation based on strong consensus of Class III evidence.

Type D. Negative recommendation based on inconclusive or conflicting Class II evidence.

Type E. Negative recommendation based on evidence of ineffectiveness or lack of efficacy based on Class I or Class II evidence.

Safety and Effectiveness

Safety: A judgment of the acceptability of risk in a specified situation, e.g., for a given health problem, by a provider with specified training (at a specific stage of the disorder, etc.).

Effectiveness: Producing a desired effect under conditions of actual use.

VI. RECOMMENDATIONS:

A. Preventive/Maintenance Care

1. Disclosure:
Preventive/maintenance care is discretionary and elective on the part of the patient. When recommended, it is necessary for the practitioner to clearly identify the type and nature of this care and to give proper patient disclosure.

13.1.1   **Rating:** Established
Evidence: Class III
Consensus Level: 1

2. Use of Chiropractic Adjustments:
The clinical experience of the profession developed over a period of nearly 100 years suggests that the use of chiropractic adjustments in a regimen of preventive/maintenance care has merit.

13.1.2   **Rating:** Equivocal
Evidence: Class III
Consensus Level: 1

3. Health Screening:
The importance of health preventive strategies is widely recognized. These services may have value in identifying early or potential manifestations of a health problem.

13.1.3   **Rating:** Promising to Established
Evidence: Class II, III
Consensus Level: 1

4. Health Promotion:
Preventive orientation to health through health promotion is well established. Health promotion provides the opportunity for chiropractic practitioners to promote health through assessment, education, and counseling on topics such as nutrition, exercise, stress reduction, life style patterns, weight reduction, smoking cessation, and ergonomics, among others.

13.1.4   **Rating:** Established
Evidence: I, II, III
Consensus Level: 1

5. Wellness Care:
Chiropractic is the largest of the holistic-oriented professions. Wellness and health management lifestyle strategies have gained popularity and acceptance. Chiropractic practitioners may choose to expand their practices to include those interventions that may influence a person's attainment of optimum performance and behavior, and in so doing, improve health status. This kind of care is performance specific (i.e., quality of life) rather than condition (e.g., symptom) specific.

13.1.5   **Rating:** Equivocal
Evidence: Class III
Consensus Level: 1

B. Public Health Considerations

6. Community Screening:
Community-based screening programs are commonly used by all disciplines to promote public health. Spinal screening and blood pressure checks offer excellent examples of such programs.

13.2.1   **Rating:** Promising
Evidence: Class II, III
Consensus Level: 1

7. Public Health Considerations:
The chiropractic profession has recognized the need to engage in the local, state, national and international agendas of public health. Such programs provide opportunities for educa-

tion and understanding programs regarding spinal health, nutrition, exercise and life styles, drugs, alcohol, tobacco, and infectious disease, as well as environmental and other social issues.

13.2.2 **Rating:** Promising
Evidence: II, III
Consensus Level: 1

VII. COMMENTS, SUMMARY, OR CONCLUSION

In this chapter a distinction has been drawn between two kinds of long-term chiropractic care: supportive care which has therapeutic necessity; and preventive/maintenance care which is elective and focuses upon patient participation and wellness.

At present there has been insufficient research into the effectiveness and cost-effectiveness of most forms of preventive care. Better study methods and greatly increased public awareness of the importance of healthy lifestyle and health promotion have produced the climate in which the needed research can be started.

The chiropractic profession, which has always had a wellness paradigm and has stood at the forefront of the health promotion movement, must participate in this research and better evaluate the basis of preventive/maintenance care.

VIII. REFERENCES

1. Coulter Ian D: The patient, the practitioner, and wellness: paradigm lost, paradigm gained. *J Manip Physiol Ther* 1990; 13(2): 107-111.

2. Jamison Jennifer R: *The Chiropractor as Health Information Resource, Health Promotion for Chiropractic Practice.* Gaithersburg, Maryland, Aspen Publishers, Inc., 1991: 35-36.

3. Coile Jr, Russell C: *Promoting Health, The New Medicine: Reshaping Medical Practice and Health Care Management.* Rockville, Maryland, Aspen Publishers, Inc., 1990: 151-166.

4. Shekelle PG, Brook RH: A community-based study of the use of chiropractic services. *Am J Pub Health* 1991; 81(4):439-442.

5. Stacey TA: Osteoporosis: exercise therapy, pre- and post-diagnosis. *J Manip Physiol Ther* 1989; 12(3):211-219.

6. Yates RG, Lamping DL, Abram NL, Wright C: Effects of chiropractic treatment on blood pressure and anxiety: A randomized, controlled trial. *J Manip Physiol Ther* 1988; 11(6):484-488.

7. Caplan RL: Health care reform and chiropractic in the 1990s. *J Manip Physiol Ther* 1991; 14(6):341-354.

8. Wardwell WI: The Connecticut survey of public attitudes toward chiropractic. *J Manip Physiol Ther* 1989; 12(3):167-173.

9. Sportelli L (Commentary): The future of health and health care: Contradictions and dilemmas. *J Manip Physiol Ther* 1985; 8(4):271-182.

10. Kaplan RM: Behavior as the central outcome in health care. *American Psychologist* 1990; 45:1211-1220.

11. Karl SV: The Detection and Modification of Psychosocial and Behavioral Risk Factors. *Applications of Social Science to Clinical Medicine and Health Policy, Chapter 17.* Rutgers University Press, New Brunswick, NJ., 1986.

12. McDowell I, Newell C: *Measuring Health: A Guide to Rating Scales and Questionnaires.* Oxford University Press, New York, 1987.

13. Jamison J: Preventive chiropractic and the chiropractic management of visceral conditions: Is the cost to chiropractic acceptance justified by the benefits to health care? *Chiropr J Austr.* 1991; 9(3):95-101.

14. Phillips RB, Butler R: Survey of chiropractic in Dade County, Florida. *J Manip Physiol Ther* 1982; 5(2):83-89.

15. Nyiendo J, Jaas M, Jones R: Using the SF-36D (General Health Status Questionnaire) in a Pilot Study of Outcome Assessment for Low-Back (Chiropractic) Patients. *Proceedings: International Conference on Spinal Manipulation.* Arlington, VA., 1991.

16. Kassak K: Outcomes Measurement Assessment: The Experience of NWCC. *Proceedings: American Public Health Association.* Atlanta, 1991.

17. Jose WS: Health Objectives for the Year 2000: A Challenge to the Chiropractic Profession. *Proceedings: American Public Health Association.* Atlanta, 1991.

18. Balduc H: *How Chiropractic Care Can Promote Wellness* (Northwestern College of Chiropractic).

19. Feinstein AR: Problems, pitfalls, and opportunities in long-term randomized trials. *Drug Res* 1989; 39:980-985.

IX. MINORITY OPINIONS

None

14

Professional Development

Chapter Outline

I. OVERVIEW

The chiropractic profession has evolved and continues to develop within a similar dynamic process as have other professions. Research in the areas of professional education and continuing education has delineated characteristics of professionalism. These characteristics focus upon the central themes of education, credentialing, professional organizations, ethical considerations and legal reinforcement. Each characteristic speaks to the dynamic development of a profession as it moves toward greater organization, influence, and responsibility to the public that it serves.

This chapter will relate these common characteristics of professionalism to the chiropractic profession and will present models to be used for future development.

II. DEFINITIONS

Assessment Outcomes: Assessment of the impact of a continuing education or postgraduate program on a practitioner's knowledge, attributes, practice performance and patient care.

Continuing Education: Voluntary and/or mandatory ongoing instruction for facilitation of clinical performance.

Credentialing: A formal means by which the capabilities of the individual practitioner to perform duties at an acceptable level are certified.

Graduate Education: Education beyond undergraduate degree level usually denoting a masters degree or Ph.D.

Postgraduate Education: Education beyond first professional degree usually leading to specialty or certification status.

III. LIST OF SUBTOPICS

    A. Continuing Education
    B. Postgraduate Education
    C. Graduate Education
    D. Professional Organizations
    E. Ethics/Standards of Conduct
    F. Research

IV. LITERATURE REVIEW

The literature search was conducted through primary sources, printed indexes, computerized bibliographic databases and in a library card catalog. Printed indexes searched included the *Index to Chiropractic Literature* 1980-1990, the *Chiropractic Literature Index* 1970-1979, and the *Chiropractic Research Archives Collection* (Vols 1-3). The computerized database searched was Medline, the National Library of Medicine's current medical literature database. Finally, searches for relevant materials were conducted in the card catalog of the David D. Palmer Health Sciences Library.

Both specific thesaurus terms and "keyword" terms were searched in these resources. A sampling of thesaurus, keyword terms and concepts searched included: professional development; continuing education; credentialing; continuing competency; life-long learning programs; diplomate/specialization programs; certification programs; extern programs; preceptorship; residency programs; performance measurement; licensure; licensure and reciprocity; professional associations; ethics and advertising; social responsibility; professional responsibility; peer review; information literacy.

A. Chiropractic Education

The practitioner is educated in the basic and clinical sciences as well as in related health subjects. Chiropractic science concerns itself with the relationship between structure and function as that relationship may affect the restoration and preservation of health. The purpose of chiropractic professional education is to prepare the practitioner to serve as a portal of entry to the health care delivery system. He/she must be well educated to evaluate and diagnose, to provide care, and to consult with or refer to other health care providers.

All applicants to chiropractic colleges must have successfully completed a minimum of 60 semester hours, or equivalent, of college credits from a nationally recognized accrediting body.

The Council of Chiropractic Education, a national accrediting agency for chiropractic colleges, produces a standards document specifying guidelines for chiropractic educational institutions and programs. However there is no CCE standard regarding residency specialty programs. At present, standards with regard to postgraduate education are at the discretion of the colleges, and the individual institutions hold the printed materials relevant to their postgraduate residency offerings. National organizations have established specialty councils but specific guidelines and requirements are then subject to determination by the council.

The needs of society require that chiropractic practitioners be able to carry out their duties according to the highest possible standards of character, competence and practice. Chiropractic is an art based on the application of a complex body of scientific knowledge. Competence in solving problems, capacity to use complex knowledge and a sensitive awareness of ethical problems are related to the entire lifelong learning process of the individual practitioner.

B. Credentialing

Credentialing is a formal means by which the capabilities of the individual practitioner to perform duties at an acceptable level are recognized. The major instrument for licensure within the chiropractic profession is the state government which fulfills this function with guidance from the profession in setting examination policies and testing the applicants.

In all states an applicant for license to practice must supply evidence of successful completion of an approved program of chiropractic education leading to the doctor of chiropractic degree, and proficiency by passing required examinations to demonstrate mastery of basic and practical elements of chiropractic as defined in that state.

National testing for the profession is conducted by the National Board of Chiropractic Examiners. The National Board examinations address basic and clinical sciences. The examination scores are recognized by all states in partial fulfillment of licensure requirements. A subsequent component of licensure is continuing education. The purpose of continuing professional education is to update theoretical knowledge, technique skills and clinical applications. To be effective continuing education should enhance successful clinical performance of practitioners. In addition, continuing education must be truly "continuing," not sporadic or opportunistic, and must be self-directed, with each professional being the ultimate monitor of his or her own learning. The ultimate test of a continuing education program is in the improvement of clinical outcomes and thus the quality of service.

Currently most states (42) require evidence of board-approved continuing education for license renewal. This requirement may range from 24 to 40 hours every two years with some states requiring specific areas of focus for credit hours. While it is recognized that mandatory continuing education requirement for license renewal does not equate with continuing competency, it is the consensus of licensing boards that practitioners need to remain knowledgeable and maintain skills current with standards within the profession.

Postgraduate continuing education is offered in many fields including orthopedics, neurology, sports injuries, nutrition, and occupational health. These courses are taught and monitored by chiropractic educational institutions and have specific requirements for practitioners to meet board certification status. However, postgraduate specialty programs and credentialing requires individual evaluation with respect to reliability, standardization of education, and its implication regarding quality of care.

C. Professional Organizations

Formal association with other chiropractic professionals enhances creation of a professional identity, fostering a relationship which nurtures distinct attributes for its members. Membership in a professional association could be restricted to those who have met rigorously defined requirements or perhaps open to anyone who wishes to participate.

Practitioners should participate in interprofessional organizations that bring a variety of health care providers together. In this way practitioners can educate other health providers and at the same time have an opportunity to be aware of other health care services that may impact on chiropractic practice and the interests of patients. Communication and understanding between chiropractic practitioners and other health care professionals must be facilitated and enhanced for the benefit of the health care consumer.

D. Ethical Considerations

Ethical principles in chiropractic care focus on patient rights. A code of ethics addresses the professional principles each practitioner should adopt in all interactions with patients, the public, and other practitioners.

Fundamental values and ethical principles in health care focus around three main principles: beneficence, justice and respect for persons. Respect for persons encompasses a central theme of treating patients as individuals with rights. Patients have the right to know, the right to privacy, and the right to acknowledge and make choices about treatment. Central to this concept is informed consent, confidentiality and presenting patients with information regarding conditions and remedial treatment. This concept also speaks to the practitioner's need to maintain the patient's autonomy by sharing knowledge, providing self-help measures, and avoiding physician dependency. Justice demands universal fairness. Health care resources and opportunities for treatment should be available regardless of race, creed, and/or economic status. Inherent in this concept is the practitioner's responsibility to maintain standards of quality care, including the consistency of treatment. Beneficence focuses on the doctor's duty to care. Inherent in this responsibility is the duty "to do good and avoid doing harm."

Both national chiropractic associations and all state chiropractic associations have codified ethics for their members. State licensing boards have laws and administrative rules that include ethical considerations which the practitioner must adhere to for continued licensure.

The practitioner's demeanor and behavior impact greatly on the patient. There is a moral, ethical and professional obligation to treat each patient with skill, dedication and respect. Health care professionals should remain aware of those issues if they are to establish appropriate patient-provider relationships. A therapeutic relationship is generated by an honest, caring and concerned attitude.

Advertising and marketing are common within all health care professions. Promotion of chiropractic should be in a responsible, informative, and professional manner. State law dictates that advertising should not be false, misleading or deceptive. In addition, promises of cure or statements that would create unjustified expectations of beneficial treatment should be avoided.

E. Research

Chiropractic researchers, clinicians, and administrators have emphasized the paucity of well-designed research studies in the field of chiropractic practice, and the importance of clinical research to the profession. Individual practitioners have important roles to play in research. Practice experience provides the opportunity to report on clinical phenomena and observations and propose diagnostic and treatment outcomes in the literature. Clinicians, professional organizations, and chiropractic academic personnel should continue to be involved in and supportive of research activities conjoint with other health care professionals.

V. ASSESSMENT CRITERIA

Procedure Ratings (System II)

Necessary: Strong positive recommendation based on Class I evidence, or overwhelming Class II evidence when circumstances reflect compromise of patient safety.

Recommended: Positive recommendation based on consensus of Class II and/or strong Class III evidence.

Discretionary: Positive recommendation based on strong consensus of Class III evidence.

Unnecessary: Negative recommendation based on inconclusive or conflicting Class II and Class III evidence.

Quality of Evidence

The following categories of evidence are used to support the ratings.

Class I:

  A. Evidence of clinical utility from controlled studies published in refereed journals.
  B. Binding or strongly persuasive legal authority such as legislation or case law.

Class II:

  A. Evidence of clinical utility from the significant results of uncontrolled studies in refereed journals.
  B. Evidence provided by recommendation from published expert legal opinion or persuasive case law.

Class III:

  A. Evidence of clinical utility provided by opinions of experts, anecdote and/or by convention.
  B. Expert legal opinion.

VI. RECOMMENDATIONS

A. Continuing Education

1. It is expected that every practitioner shall participate in continuing education.

  14.1.1 **Rating:** Necessary
           Evidence: Class I, II, III
           Consensus Level: 1

2. Continuing education should be ongoing and should facilitate successful clinical performance.

  14.1.2 **Rating:** Recommended
           Evidence: Class I, II, III
           Consensus Level: 1

3. Completion of mandatory continuing education requirements for license renewal does not necessarily assure continuing competency. Those requirements should include assessment of outcomes by administering institutions/organizations to evaluate the effectiveness of their programs.

  14.1.3 **Rating:** Recommended
           Evidence: Class I, II, III
           Consensus Level: 1

4. Continuing education should allow for a variety of instructional formats.

  14.1.4 **Rating:** Recommended
           Evidence: Class II, III
           Consensus Level: 1

5. Practitioners should continue to educate themselves through critical reading and review of clinical and/or scientific literature.

  14.1.5 **Rating:** Recommended
           Evidence: Class II, III
           Consensus Level: 1

B. Postgraduate Education

1. All chiropractic colleges are encouraged to provide residency programs for qualified graduates for the purpose of advanced research, education and clinical practice.

  14.2.1 **Rating:** Recommended
           Evidence: Class II, III
           Consensus Level: 1

2. Colleges should provide opportunities for postgraduate programs for professional development which may lead to certification or specialty status.

  14.2.2 **Rating:** Recommended
           Evidence: Class II, III
           Consensus Level: 1

3. Practitioners are encouraged to participate in certification or specialty postgraduate education programs (e.g., specialty programs).

  14.2.3 **Rating:** Discretionary
           Evidence: Class II, III
           Consensus Level: 1

4. Where such postgraduate programs exist the impact and outcome should be measured appropriately.

14.2.4 **Rating:** Recommended
Evidence: Class II, III
Consensus Level: 1

5. Proprietary programs should affiliate with accredited educational institutions for the purposes of development, evaluation and implementation.

14.2.5 **Rating:** Recommended
Evidence: II, III
Consensus Level: 1

C. Graduate Education

1. Practitioners are encouraged to participate in programs providing graduate education (e.g., masters or doctorate) offered by accredited educational institutions.

14.3.1 **Rating:** Discretionary
Evidence: Class II, III
Consensus Level: 1

D. Professional Organizations

1. Practitioners should be members of one or more professional associations.

14.4.1 **Rating:** Recommended
Evidence: Class II, III
Consensus Level: 1

Comment: Professional organizations and associations provide a structure of responsibility through which members develop and maintain awareness of professional developments and gain enhanced professional competence. Practitioners also develop leadership abilities by participating in sponsored conventions, conferences, workshops and other gatherings; receive publications pertinent to the profession; support and encourage legislative programs and otherwise influence public policy in the interests of the public and the profession.

E. Ethics/Standards of Conduct

1. Practitioners should conduct themselves in a manner consistent with a professional code of ethics which addresses morality, honesty and all aspects of professional conduct.

14.5.1 **Rating:** Necessary
Evidence: Class I, II, III
Consensus Level: 1

2. Practitioners who advertise should do so in a responsible, ethical and professional manner.

14.5.2 **Rating:** Necessary
Evidence: Class I, II, III
Consensus Level: 1

Comment: The responsibility for regulation of advertising lies with professional associations and licensing boards. Professional organizations can assist by enforcing guidelines established for the membership; the state licensing boards promulgate rules to aid the profession and safeguard the public. Violation of state or provincial laws can result in fines or suspension or revocation of a license.

F. Research

1. Practitioners are encouraged to participate in research and support institutions/organizations conducting research, for the purposes of professional development and improved patient care. Valid research requires appropriate research protocols as approved by recognized institutional review boards.

14.6.1 **Rating:** Recommended
Evidence: Class I, II, III
Consensus Level: 1

VII. COMMENTS, SUMMARY OR CONCLUSION

None.

VIII. REFERENCES

1. Council on Chiropractic Education. *Standards for Chiropractic Institutions.* West Des Moines, IA, Council on Chiropractic Education, 1990.

2. Davis I. Ethics: an analysis and a theory. *J Chiro* Apr 1990; 27(4):20-23.

3. Federation of Chiropractic Licensing Boards. *Official Directory of the Federation of Chiropractic Licensing Boards.* Kremmling, CO, Federation of Chiropractic Licensing Boards, 1989. Annual.

4. Haldeman S, ed. *Modern Developments in the Principles and Practice of Chiropractic:* based on a conference sponsored by the International Chiropractors Association, Anaheim, CA. Feb 1979. New York, Appleton-Century-Crofts, 1980. 390 pp.

5. Haldeman S. Philosophy and the future of chiropractic. *J Chiro* 1990 Jul; 27(7):23-28.

6. Hildebrandt R. Chiropractic continuing education: a critical review. *Am J Chiro Med* 1989 Sep; 2(3):89-92.

7. Houle CO. *Continuing Learning in the Professions.* San Francisco, Jossey-Bass, 1980. 390 pp.

8. Kelner M, Hall O, Coulter I. *Chiropractors: Do They Help? A Study of Their Education and Practice.* Toronto, Fitzhenry & Whiteside, 1980. 303 pp.

9. Kumerow RP. *Inspector General Report Regarding State Licensure and Discipline of Chiropractors,* 1989.

10. Lawrence DJ. Research and responsibility. *J Manipulative Physiol Ther* 1984 Sep; 7(3):179-181.

11. Mauer EL. *Selected Ethics and Protocols in Chiropractic.* Gaithersburg, MD, Aspen Publishers, Inc. 1991. 273 pp.

12. Rosenthal SF. *A Sociology of Chiropractic.* Lewiston, NY, Edwin Mellen Press, 1986. 15 pp.

13. Thompson IE. Fundamental ethical principles in health care. *Br Med J* (Clin Res) 1987 Aug 8; 295(6594):388-9.

14. Vear HJ, ed. *Chiropractic Standards of Practice and Quality of Care.* Gaithersburg, MD, Aspen Publishers, Inc., 1991. 303 pp.

IX. MINORITY OPINIONS

None.

Epilogue

EVOLUTION OF THE CONSENSUS PROCESS

The consensus process which resulted in the publication of these guidelines should be considered part of an ongoing process rather than a final prescription for the practice of chiropractic. The recommendations voted on at the Mercy Conference are the product of two years of literature review, consultation, debate and compromise. This resulted in the most comprehensive set of guidelines ever established for the chiropractic profession.

The guidelines outlined in this document can and will be used to assist practitioners to improve their practice parameters. They should not, however, be considered set in stone. The practice of chiropractic is dynamic. There is an increasing amount of research being done both at chiropractic colleges and within private practices, hospitals and universities. This research can be expected to impact the practice of chiropractic on a continuous basis ensuring that there is progression and growth in knowledge and understanding of the benefits and role of chiropractic in the health care delivery system. As the results of such research begin to have a practical impact, the practice of chiropractic will change and future guidelines will have to take such changes into account.

In addition, there are rapid changes in all fields of health care which are likely to affect the practice of chiropractic. Legislation and legal precedent can be expected to influence the expectations and responsibilities of the profession. The attitude of practitioners toward patients, insurance carriers and government agencies will have to adapt in response to these changes. In addition, there is increasing debate and emphasis on ethics by all health care professionals and future consensus processes within chiropractic should follow the example of this Commission and attempt to give guidance on these issues.

RESEARCH AND THE CONSENSUS PROCESS

It can be anticipated that additional consensus conferences will be held every few years to update these guidelines and bring the recommendations in line with the results of future research and the normal evolution of the role of the chiropractic profession in the delivery of health care. The primary rationale for such conferences and modification of these guidelines should be the incorporation of research knowledge into established chiropractic practice.

A number of practitioners may disagree with individual recommendations and specific guidelines which were included in these proceedings. The proper course for them to take is to accumulate research or literature which may not have been considered at the Mercy Conference. Where there is no published literature or research, then it is the responsibility of those practitioners with a specific opinion on the guidelines to initiate such research. It is only through published research that significant advances in the practice of chiropractic can occur. There are numerous techniques and diagnostic methods which have been discussed in these guidelines which could not be given a high rating due to the lack of research on the topic. Many of these techniques and methods are fairly widely practiced. The failure of these methods to gain a high recommendation rating can be expected to be of concern to those individuals who believe them to be of value. The guidelines should serve as an incentive to develop and finance the research necessary to establish the credibility of a greater number of techniques and procedures.

Many manufacturers and suppliers of diagnostic and therapeutic equipment, as well as practitioners who have developed methods of adjusting or treating patients, may feel that their particular procedure or method has value which was not recognized by the conference delegates. It is incumbent upon these individuals or companies to take the initiative to establish a research base for future consensus conferences. When such a conference is convened the justification for such procedures must be made available in the form of research papers published in peer reviewed journals. Failure to present research at future consensus conferences can lead to the dismissal of a technique or method from the chiropractic therapeutic armamentarium.

GUIDELINES FOR EVALUATION

The following are offered as guidelines for the evaluation of the appropriateness/clinical usefulness of tests and treatment procedures in chiropractic practice.

I. Guides for Determining the Clinical Usefulness of a Test:[1]

A. There have been independent, blind comparisons with an acceptable gold standard of diagnosis based on the best available methods of determination.

B. The test has been evaluated in a patient sample that included patients with an appropriate spectrum of mild and severe, treated and untreated disorders, plus individuals with different but commonly confused disorders.

C. The setting for the evaluation, as well as the criteria by which study patients were included, were adequately described.

D. The reproducibility of the test result (precision) and its interpretation (observer variation) have been determined.

E. The reference (normal) has been defined sensibly as it applies to the test being evaluated.

F. If the test is advocated as part of a cluster or sequence of tests, its individual contribution to the overall validity of the cluster or sequence has been determined.

G. The tactics for carrying out the test have been described in sufficient detail to permit their replication.

H. The utility of the test has been determined.

I. The test is documented by publication in refereed journals.

II. Guides for Determining the Clinical Usefulness or Appropriateness of a Treatment Procedure

An evaluator should consider the following points:

A. Design
1. The strength of the study design (randomized, controlled, cohort, case-control, case studies: prospective, retrospective).
2. Evaluation of the assignment of patients to intervention.
3. Biases in the intervention.
4. Biases in the outcome.

B. All clinically relevant outcomes (e.g., both morbidity and mortality) are reported.

C. Sample
1. Biases in the sample.
2. The characteristics of the sample are known for all intervention groups and their characteristics are comparable and appropriate for the interventions studied.

D. Significance
1. Clinical significance is demonstrated.
2. Statistical significance is demonstrated.
3. There is appropriate review for Type I error and Type II error.

E. Dropouts and subjects lost to follow-up are acknowledged and dealt with appropriately.

F. The procedure is documented by publication in refereed journals.

FUTURE CONSENSUS CONFERENCES

It is unlikely that any substantial revision of these guidelines will occur and be sponsored by a credible portion of the profession within the next two or three years. It takes approximately two years from the time of the initial considering of a commission to the publication of the final document. This should be ample time for any group of practitioners or manufacturers to begin developing research projects to establish whether there is value in a particular method or technique. Such research is best performed by independent investigators in the chiropractic colleges or in recognized universities or research institutions. The research should then be submitted to peer reviewed journals in order that it can be debated and considered on its scientific merit.

Future consensus processes may be comprehensive or have limited scope. Because the guidelines produced by this commission were extremely comprehensive, addressing the entire practice of chiropractic, it was not possible to address each area of practice in the degree of detail which may be desirable. It may become necessary to develop consensus processes for specific areas of practice such as treatment of the elderly or children, rehabilitation, the use of specific adjusting techniques or the management of specific conditions such as cervical injuries or headaches. Guideline parameters on these topics would be of great value to practicing chiropractors treating specific groups of patients.

When the next commission is established to revise these guidelines there must be a sufficient period of time allowed for the profession to have input to any changes that may be considered. As was the case in the development of these guidelines, the process must be widely advertised and input from a wide cross section of the profession invited. At no time, however, must political consideration be allowed to supersede basic scientific principles and health care ethics. As was repeatedly stressed by the participants in this Commission, the only justification for any guideline is the advancement of the health of the millions of patients who seek the care and advice of the chiropractic profession every year.

Anyone who would like to submit comments regarding these Guidelines please see Appendix C on page 217.

REFERENCES:

1. Sackett DL, Haynes RB, Guyatt GH, Tugwell P: *Clinical Epidemiology—A Basic Science for Clinical Medicine*. 2nd ed. Little, Brown and Company, Boston, 1991, p 20.

Appendix A

Endorsement by the Federation of Chiropractic Licensing Boards

RESOLUTION #3

Myrtle Beach, South Carolina
April 11, 1992

WHEREAS, The establishment and continuing review of chiropractic practice guidelines is important with respect to quality of care and the public interest; and

WHEREAS, National guidelines are important to the regulation of chiropractic practice and the better coordination of the work of the chiropractic licensing boards; and

WHEREAS, In order to provide national practice guidelines the Congress of Chiropractic State Associations created a Commission for the establishment of guidelines for chiropractic quality assurance and standards of practice in December of 1989; and

WHEREAS, The work of the Commission was subsequently sponsored by most major chiropractic associations in North America including the American Chiropractic Association, the Canadian Chiropractic Association, International Chiropractors Association, Association of Chiropractic Colleges and the Federation of Chiropractic Licensing Boards; and

WHEREAS, The Consensus Panel established by the Commission included chiropractors who represent the chiropractic profession as a whole in a fair and equitable manner; and

WHEREAS, It is appreciated that the Commission was the first national effort by the chiropractic profession to establish comprehensive practice guidelines and that these guidelines are imperfect, incomplete and will require revision; and

WHEREAS, Due to the nature of the consensus process itself it is recognized that diversity of opinion exists, but that most chiropractors will agree with the majority of the guidelines. Now therefore, be it

RESOLVED, That the Federation of Chiropractic Licensing Boards hereby endorses the work of the Commission in the legitimate consensus process representing as closely as practicable the views of the entire chiropractic profession, and the Federation of Chiropractic Licensing Boards endorses the Guidelines appearing in the proceedings of the Commission and encourages the chiropractic profession to continue with the ongoing process of establishing valid and useful guidelines for the practice of chiropractic.

Appendix B

Summary of Recommendations (Guidelines)

The recommendations are the most important part of these proceedings. Each of these recommendations was voted on by the entire Commission with varying degrees of consensus. The practitioner who wishes to utilize the guidelines will want to read and understand the entire document but will be looking to the recommendations to evaluate specific aspects of his or her practice. At all times, however, it must be kept in mind that the recommendations should not be perceived as free floating statements. Each recommendation must be placed in the context of the entire document. The scientific and theoretical base of a recommendation must be kept in mind, as well as its relationship to other recommendations.

For easy reference the recommendations have been summarized in table format. The tables which follow list each of the recommendations under chapter titles. The first column lists the recommendation number. The second column lists the subject of each recommendation in abbreviated form. The actual recommendation or guideline is considerably longer in most cases and must be read in detail for a full understanding of its meaning.

The next three columns provide the ratings for the recommendations—the rating (e.g., "necessary"), the quality of evidence in support, and for Chapters 3 and 8 a strength of rating. The rating systems are discussed in detail at the beginning of this text. (See "Introduction and Guide to Use" Section C.) The evidence upon which these ratings were derived appears in the chapter discussion.

The final column lists the level of consensus. (For explanation of consensus levels see "Introduction and Guide to Use" Section E.) Any minority opinion or report is noted at end of the table. In the text minority opinions appear at the end of each relevant chapter.

In order to understand these tables fully it is necessary to read the "Introduction and Guide to Use of These Guidelines" and follow the procedure given in Section G.

	CHAPTER 1 HISTORY AND PHYSICAL EXAMINATION				
Rec #	**Recommendation**	**Rating System I & II**	**Quality of Evidence**	**Strength**	**Consensus Level**
	A. HISTORY				
1.1.1	The Process	Necessary	II,III	—	1
1.1.2	The Role	Established	I,II,III	—	1
1.1.3	The Components	Necessary	I,II,III	—	1
	B. EXAMINATION				
1.2.1	All DX Procedures	Necessary	II,III	—	1
1.2.2	Regardless of CC	Recommended	III	—	1
1.2.3	Cranial Complaints	Established	II,III	—	1
1.2.4	CNS Evaluation	Established	II,III	—	1
1.2.5	Neck & Adjacent	Established	II,III	—	1
1.2.6	Thoracic/Chest	Established	II,III	—	1
1.2.7	Low Back	Established	I,II,III	—	1
1.2.8	Extremity	Established	I,II,III	—	1
1.2.9	ICE	Recommended	II	—	1

CHAPTER 2
DIAGNOSTIC IMAGING

Rec #	Recommendation	Rating System I	Quality of Evidence	Strength	Consensus Level
2.1.1	Sequence of Services	Established	III	—	1
2.2.1	Patient Selection	Established	I,II,III	—	1
2.3.1	Interpretation & Report	Established	II,III	—	1
2.4.1	Legal Issues	Established	III	—	1
2.5.1	Technology & Protection	Established	I,II,III	—	1
2.6.1	Plain Film	Established	I,II,III	—	1
2.6.2	Postural & Biomech	Promising	II,III	—	1
2.7.1	Full Spine-Scoliosis	Established	I,II,III	—	1
2.7.2	Full Spine-Biomech & Postural	Promising	II,III	—	1
2.8.1	Stress—DJD, Trauma, or Instability	Established	I,II,III	—	1
2.8.2	Stress—Other Uses	Equivocal	II,III	—	1
2.9.1	V Fluoro Kinematic & Biomechanical	Promising	II,III	—	1
2.9.2	V Fluoro Instab Wrist & Contrast	Established	I,II,III	—	1
2.10.1	Plain Film Contrast	Established	I,II,III	—	1
2.11.1	CT Scanning	Established	I,II,III	—	1
2.12.1	MRI	Established	I,II,III	—	1
2.13.1	Radionucleotide BS	Established	I,II,III	—	1
2.14.1	Diag Ultrasound	Established	I,II,III	—	1

CHAPTER 3
INSTRUMENTATION

Rec #	Recommendation	Rating System I	Quality of Evidence	Strength	Consensus Level
3.1.1	Instrumentation Questionnaires	Established	I,II	A	1
3.1.2	Screening Questionnaires	Equivocal	II,III	C	1
3.1.3	Pressure Algometry	Promising	II,III	B	1
3.2.1	Plumbline Analysis	Established	II,III	B	1
3.2.2	Scoliometry	Established	I,II	A	1
3.2.3	Photogrammetry	Established	I,II,III	A	1
3.2.4	Moire Topography	Promising	II,III	B	1
3.2.5	Bilateral Weights	Equivocal	II,III	C	1
3.2.6	Automated Posture	Promising	II,III	B	1
3.3.1	Goniometry	Established	I,II	A	1
3.3.2	Inclinometers	Established	I,II	A	1
3.3.3	Optical Systems	Established	II	B	1
3.3.4	Computer ROM	Promising	II,III	B	1
3.4.1	Manual Strength Test	Established	I,II	A	1
3.4.2	Isometric	Established	I,II	A	1
3.4.3	Isokin-Sport	Established	II,III	B	1
3.4.4	Isokin-Post Injury	Promising	II,III	C	1
3.5.1	Isoinertial Thermocouples	Doubtful	II,III	D	3
3.5.2	Infrared Thermograph	Equiv/Prom	II,III	C	3
3.6.1	Galvanic Skin Resp	Investigational	II,III	D	1
3.6.2	GSR Acupuncture	Doubtful	II,III	E	1
3.7.1	EMG Scanning	Investigational	II,III	C	2
3.7.2	EMG Flexion-Relax/Mean-Median Freq	Promising	II,III	B	1
3.7.3	Surface Electro DX	Established	I,II	A	1
3.7.4	Needle Electro DX	Established	I,II	A	1
3.7.5	ECG	Established	I,II	A	1
3.8.1	Clinical Laboratory	Established	I,II,III	A	1
3.9.1	Doppler Ultrasound	Established	II,III	B	1
3.9.2	Plethysmog Diff Dx	Established	II,III	B	1
3.9.3	Plethysmog Monitor Spine	Investigational	II,III	D	1
3.9.4	Spirometry	Established	I,II	A	1
3.10.1	Thermocouples	Equivocal	II	C	Minority Report
3.10.2	Infrared Thermograph	Promising	II,III	B	Minority Report

CHAPTER 4
CLINICAL LABORATORY

Rec #	Recommendation	Rating System I	Quality of Evidence	Strength	Consensus Level
4.1.1	Role of Laboratory	Established	III	—	1
4.1.2	Lab Selection	Established	III	—	1
4.1.3	Office Laboratories	Established	III	—	1
4.1.4	Patient Preparation	Established	III	—	1
4.1.5	Specimen Collection	Established	III	—	1
4.1.6	Need for Lab Testing	Established	I,II,III	—	1
4.1.7	Test Selection-DX	Promising	I,II,III	—	1
4.1.8	Test Selection-Screen	Established	I,II,III	—	1
4.1.9	Test Selection-Patient Mgt.	Established	II,III	—	1
4.1.10	Interpretation of Reference Values	Established	I,II,III	—	1
4.1.11	Integration of Data	Established	I,II,III	—	1
4.1.12	Communication with Patients	Established	III	—	1
4.1.13	Recording Results	Established	III	—	1
4.1.14	Consultation	Established	III	—	1
4.1.15	Organ Profiles	Established	I,II,III	—	1
4.1.16	Investigational Tests	Established	I,II,III	—	1
4.1.17	Novel Applications	Established	I,II,III	—	1
	GUIDELINES FOR ORDERING:				
4.2.1	Urinalysis	Established	I,II,III	—	1
4.2.2	CBC	Established	I,II,III	—	1
4.2.3	ESR	Established	I,II,III	—	1
4.2.4	Biochem Profiles	Established	I,II,III	—	1
4.2.5	Serum or Plasma Glu	Established	I,II,III	—	1
4.2.6	Serum Urea Nitro & Creatinine	Established	I,II,III	—	1
4.2.7	Serum Calcium	Established	II,III	—	1
4.2.8	Serum Inorg Phos	Established	II,III	—	1
4.2.9	Serum Prot & Albumin	Established	II,III	—	1
4.2.10	Serum Cholesterol	Established	I,II,III	—	1
4.2.11	Alk Phos	Established	I,II,III	—	1
4.2.12	Prostatic Acid Phos	Established	I,II,III	—	1
4.2.13	Prostate Specific Antigen	Established	I,II,III	—	1
4.2.14	AST	Established	I,II,III	—	1
4.2.15	CK	Established	I,II,III	—	1
4.2.16	Thyroid Function	Established	I,II,III	—	1
4.2.17	Uric Acid	Established	I,II,III	—	1
4.2.18	Rheumatoid Factor	Established	I,II,III	—	1
4.2.19	ANA	Established	I,II,III	—	1

		Rating System I	Quality of Evidence	Strength	Consensus Level
Rec #	**Recommendation**				
4.2.20	HLA-B27	Established	I,II,III	—	1
4.2.21	CRP	Established	I,II,III	—	1
4.2.22	Potassium	Established	I,II,III	—	1
4.2.23	Sodium	Established	I,II,III	—	1
4.2.24	Iron	Established	I,II,III	—	1
4.2.25	Fecal Occult Blood	Established	II,III	—	1
4.2.26	Ferritin	Established	I,II,III	—	1
4.3.1	Hair Analysis	Investigational	I,II,III	—	1
4.3.2	Live Cell Analysis	Investigational	III	—	1
4.3.3	Biochem Biopsy	Investigational	I,II,III	—	1
4.3.4	Optimal Values w/o accept. proced.	Investigational	I,II,III	—	1
4.4.1	Cytotoxic	Inappropriate	I,II,III	—	1
4.4.2	Reams Testing	Inappropriate	III	—	1

CHAPTER 4
CLINICAL LABORATORY - CONTINUED

CHAPTER 5
RECORD KEEPING AND PATIENT CONSENTS

Rec #	Recommendation	Rating System II	Quality of Evidence	Strength	Consensus Level
5.1.1	Pt File, Initial	Necessary	I,II,III	—	1
5.1.2	Pt File, Archive	Recommended	II,III	—	1
5.1.3	Dr/Clinic ID	Necessary	I,II,III	—	1
5.1.4	Patient IDq	Necessary	I,II,III	—	1
5.1.5	Patient Demographs Sex & Occupation	Necessary	I,II,III	—	1
5.1.6	Marital Status, Race, Dependents, Employer, Spouse Occupation	Discretionary	I,II,III	—	1
5.1.7	Health Coverage	Discretionary	III	—	1
5.1.8	Health Hist Date, CC, Description, Rev Sys, Tx, Signature	Necessary	I,II,III	—	1
5.1.9	Questionnaires, Drawings and Other Patient Information	Recommended	I,II,III	—	1
5.1.10	Exam Findings	Necessary	I,II,III	—	1
5.1.11	Special Studies	Recommended	I,II,III	—	1
5.1.12	Misc Assess Outcome Instruments	Recommended	I,II,III	—	1
5.1.13	Clinical Impression	Necessary	I,II,III	—	1
5.1.14	Treatment Plan	Recommended	I,II,III	—	1
5.1.15	Chart/Progress Notes	Necessary	I,II,III	—	1
5.1.16	Clinical Info	Necessary	I,II,II	—	1
5.1.17	Adj/Man Tech	Necessary	II,III	—	1
5.1.18	Initials, Other than Attending	Necessary	I,II,III	—	1
5.1.19	Reexam/Reassess	Necessary	I,II,III	—	1
5.1.20	Financial Records	Necessary	I,III	—	1
5.1.21	Info Storage & Retrieval	Discretionary	III	—	1
5.1.22	Internal Memoranda	Discretionary	I,III	—	1
5.2.1	Direct Correspondence	Recommended	II,III	—	1
5.2.2	Health Records	Recommended	II,III	—	1
5.2.3	Dx Imaging	Recommended	II,III	—	1
5.2.4	External Reports	Recommended	II,III	—	1
5.3.1	Gen Chart File Org	Necessary	I,II,III	—	1
5.3.2	Preprinted Forms	Discretionary	II,III	—	1
5.3.3	Legibility & Clarity	Necessary	I,II	—	1
5.3.4	Abbreviations/Symbols	Recommended	II,III	—	1
5.4.1	Confidentiality	Necessary	I,II	—	1
5.4.2	Records Retention	Necessary	I,II	—	1
5.4.3	Beyond Legal Time Limits	Discretionary	III	—	1
5.4.4	Admin. Records	Necessary	I,II,III	—	1
5.4.5	Records Transfer	Necessary	I,II,III	—	1

CHAPTER 5
RECORD KEEPING AND PATIENT CONSENTS - CONTINUED

Rec #	Recommendation	Rating System II	Quality of Evidence	Strength	Consensus Level
5.4.6	Staff Responsibility	Necessary	I,II,III	—	1
5.5.1	Consent to Tx General	Necessary	I,II,III	—	1
5.5.2	Consent to Tx Competence	Necessary	I,II,III	—	1
5.5.3	Authorization	Necessary	I,II,III	—	1
5.5.4	Financial Assignments	Discretionary	III	—	1
5.5.5	Consent Research	Necessary	I,II,III	—	1
5.5.6	Consent Records Photo/Video	Recommended	I,II,III	—	1
5.5.7	Consent Research Pub/Photo/Video	Necessary	I,II,III	—	1
5.5.8	Consent Observers	Necessary	I,II,III	—	1

	CHAPTER 6 **CLINICAL IMPRESSION**				
Rec #	**Recommendation**	**Rating System** **I & II**	**Quality of** **Evidence**	**Strength**	**Consensus** **Level**
6.1.1	Necessity	Necessary	I,II,III	—	1
6.2.1	Initial Responsibility	Necessary	I,II,III	—	1
6.3.1	Subsequent Responsibility	Necessary	I,II,III	—	1
6.4.1	Terminology	Recommended	II,III	—	1
6.5.1	Content—Unrelated Impressions	Recommended	II,III	—	1
6.5.2	Content—Intensity & Region	Recommended	II,III	—	1
6.5.3	Content—Sub/Obj Findings	Established	I,II,III	—	1
6.6.1	Timely Diagnosis	Necessary	I,II,III	—	1
6.6.2	Appropriate Consultation	Recommended	II,III	—	1
6.6.3	Impression Recorded	Necessary	I,II,III	—	1
6.7.1	Working sypothesis	Necessary	I,II,III	—	1
6.8.1	Communication	Necessary	I,II,III	—	1

	CHAPTER 7 MODES OF CARE				
Rec #	Recommendation	Rating System I	Quality of Evidence	Strength	Consensus Level
	MAN MANIP & ADJ PROCEDURES **SPECIFIC CONTACT THRUST**				
7.1.1	Hi Vel-LBP	Established	I,II,III	—	1
7.1.2	Hi Vel Other NMS	Established	II,III	—	1
7.1.3	Hi Vel Type O	Equivocal	II,III	—	1
7.1.4	Hi Vel Recoil NMS	Prom to Estab	II,III	—	1
7.1.5	Hi Vel Recoil Type O	Equivocal	II,III	—	1
7.1.6	Low Velocity NMS	Equiv to Prom	II,III	—	1
7.1.7	Low Velocity Type O	Inv to Equiv	II,III	—	1
	NONSPECIFIC CONTACT				
7.2.1	Mobilization	Established	I,II,III	—	1
	MANUAL FORCE				
7.3.1	Mechanically Assist Drop Piece/Terminal Point NMS	Prom to Estab	III	—	1
7.3.2	Drop Piece/Terminal Point Type O	Inv to Equiv	III (II?)	—	3
7.3.3	Flexion Distraction	Established	II,III	—	2
7.3.4	Pelvic Blocks	Promising	III	—	1
	MECHANICAL FORCE, **MANUALLY ASSISTED**				
7.4.1	Fixed Stylus	Equivocal	III	—	1
7.4.2	Moving Stylus	Prom to Estab	I,II,III	—	1
	MANUAL NONARTICULAR				
7.5.1	Muscle Energy	Promising	II,III	—	1
7.5.2	Neurological Reflex Muscle Relaxation	Equivocal	III	—	1
7.5.3	Other	Investigational	III	—	1
7.5.4	TPT	Established	II,III	—	1
7.5.5	Misc Soft Tissue	Established	II,III	—	1
7.6.1	Neuro Retraining NMS	Equiv to Prom	II,III	—	1
7.6.2	Neuro Retraining Other	Investigational	II,III	—	1
7.6.3	Concep. Mind-Body Approaches	Inappropriate	III	—	1
7.6.4	Surrogate Testing	Inappropriate	III	—	1

	Chapter 7 Modes of Care - Continued				
Rec #	**Recommendation**	**Rating System I**	**Quality of Evidence**	**Strength**	**Consensus Level**
	NON-MANUAL PROCEDURES				
7.7.1	Exercise & Rehab	Prom to Estab	I,II,III	—	1
7.7.2	Strength & Cond	Prom to Estab	I,II,III	—	1
7.7.3	Passive Stretch	Established	I,II,III	—	1
7.8.1	Back School	Prom to Estab	I,II,III	—	1
7.8.2	Wellness & Health Promotion	Prom to Estab	II,III	—	1
7.8.3	Nutritional Counseling	Established	I,II,III	—	1
7.8.4	Bio-Feedback	Prom to Estab	II,III	—	1
7.9.1	Electrical Modalities	Prom to Estab	I,II,III	—	1
7.10.1	Thermal Modalities	Established	I,II,III	—	1
7.11.1	Ultraviolet	Established	II,III	—	1
7.12.1	Ultrasound & Phonophoresis	Established	I,II,III	—	1
7.13.1	Bracing, Casting, etc.	Prom to Estab	II,III	—	2
7.14.1	Traction	Prom to Estab	I,II,III	—	1
7.15.1	Manip.—Sedation/Anesthesia	Equivocal	II,III	—	1
7.16.1	Acupuncture	Promising	I,II,III	—	1
7.17.1	Homeopathic Remedies	Equivocal	II,III	—	1

CHAPTER 8
FREQUENCY AND DURATION OF CARE

Rec #	Recommendation	Rating System I	Quality of Evidence	Strength	Consensus Level
8.1.1	Preconsultation, Duration of Symptoms, Severity of Symptoms, # Previous Episodes, Injury Superimposed on Pre-existing Injury	Promising	II,III	B	1
8.2.1	Tx Care Frequency	Established	II,III	B	1
8.3.1	Patient Cooperation	Promising	II,III	B	1
8.4.1	Failure to Meet Tx, Obj (uncomplicated cases), Acute Disorders, Unresponsive Sub/Chronic, Systematic Interview, Written Tx Goals, Failure-Discharge MMI	Established	I,II,III	A	1
8.5.1	Uncomplicated Cases	Established	I,II,III	A	1
8.6.1	Complicated Cases Signs of Chronicity	Established	I,II,III	A	1
8.6.2	Subacute Episode	Promising	II,III	B	1
8.6.3	Chronic Episodes	Promising	II,III	B	1
8.7.1	Elective Care	Unrated	—	—	—

	CHAPTER 9 REASSESSMENT				
Rec #	Recommendation	Rating System II	Quality of Evidence	Strength	Consensus Level
9.1.1	Integral Component Case Mgt.	Necessary	II,III	—	1
9.2.1	Determined by Pt Response	Necessary	II,III	—	1
9.3.1	ASAP if Worse	Necessary	III	—	1
9.4.1	New Signs/Sx	Necessary	II,III	—	1
9.5.1	By Appropriately Trained Persons	Necessary	II,III	—	1
9.6.1	Same Manner as Initial Assessment	Recommended	I,II,III	—	1
9.7.1	Third Party Interests	Recommended	III	—	1
9.8.1	Interactive Reassessment	Necessary	III	—	1
9.9.1	Periodic Reassessment	Necessary	III	—	1
9.10.1	In Areas of Prior (+) Findings	Necessary	III	—	1

	CHAPTER 10 OUTCOME ASSESSMENT				
Rec #	Recommendation	Rating System I & II	Quality of Evidence	Strength	Consensus Level
10.1.1	Functional Outcome Assessment	Established	I,II,III	—	1
10.2.1	Pain Measurement	Established	I,II,III	—	1
10.2.2	Patient Satisfaction	Established	I,II,III	—	1
10.3.1	General Health	Established	I,II,III	—	1
10.4.1	ROM	Established	I,II,III	—	1
10.4.2	Thermography	Invest to Equiv	II,III	—	3
10.4.3	Muscle Function Inst	Established	I,II,III	—	1
10.4.4	Muscle Function Man	Equivocal	II,III	—	1
10.4.5	Posture	Promising	II,III	—	1
10.5.1	Malposition	Equivocal	II,III	—	1
10.5.2	Abnormal Motion	Equiv to Prom	II,III	—	1
10.5.3	Abnormal X-ray Motion	Investigational	II,III	—	1
10.5.4	Soft Tiss Texture & Tenderness	Promising	I,II,III	—	1
10.5.5	Tone Electrodes	Equivocal	I,II,III	—	1
10.5.6	Tone Scanning	Invest to Equiv	II,III	—	3
10.6.1	Subluxation	Recommended	II,III	—	1
10.6.2	Qualified Individuals	Necessary	II,III	—	1
10.6.3	Consideration	Necessary	II,III	—	1
10.6.4	Appropriate Intervals	Necessary	II,III	—	1
10.6.5	Generic Outcomes	Recommended	II,III	—	1
10.7.1	Thermography	Equivocal		—	Minority Report
10.7.2	Tone Scanning	Equivocal	I,II,III	—	Minority Report

CHAPTER 11
COLLABORATIVE CARE

Rec #	Recommendation	Rating-Mixed	Quality of Evidence	Strength	Consensus Level
11.1.1	Explanation	Necessary	II,III	—	1
11.2.1	Freedom of Choice	Necessary	III	—	1
11.2.2	Informed Decision	Necessary	III	—	1
11.3.1	Familiarity w/Med	Recommended	II,III	—	1
11.3.2	Familiarity w/Alt Hlth	Recommended	III	—	1
11.4.1	Consult or Refer	Necessary	I,II,III	—	1
11.4.2	Accept Referrals	Recommended	III	—	1
11.5.1	Provide Information	Recommended	III	—	1
11.5.2	Post Referral Comm	Recommended	III	—	1
11.5.3	Direct Comm	Recommended	III	—	1
11.5.4	Request for Records	Recommended	III	—	1
11.6.1	Develop Consensus	Recommended	III	—	1
11.6.2	Seek Access	Recommended	III	—	1
11.6.3	Concurrent Care	Recommended	III	—	1
11.6.4	Resolution of Disputes	Recommended	III	—	1
11.6.5	Facilitate Pt Access	Recommended	III	—	1
11.7.1	No Financial Relation	Necessary	III	—	1
11.7.2	Cooperation	Recommended	III	—	1

CHAPTER 12
CONTRAINDICATIONS AND COMPLICATIONS

Rec #	Recommendations	Condition Rating	Quality of Evidence	Strength	Consensus Level
	ARTICULAR DERANGEMENT				
12.1.1	Acute Inflammatory	III	II,III	—	1
12.1.2	Subacute/Chronic	I,II	II,III	—	1
12.1.3	DJD	I,II	II	—	1
12.1.4	Spondylolisthesis	I,II	II	—	1
12.1.5	Fx/Dislocation	III	III	—	1
12.1.6	Os Odontoidum	III	III	—	1
12.1.7	Hypermobility	I,II	II,III	—	1
12.1.8	Postsurgical Jnt	II	III	—	1
12.1.9	Acute Injuries	I,II	I,II	—	1
12.1.10	Scoliosis	I,II	II,III	—	1
	BONE WEAKENING DISORDERS				
12.2.1	Avascular Necrosis	III	III	—	1
12.2.2	Demineralization	II	II,III	—	1
12.2.3	Benign Bone Tumors	II,III	III	—	1
12.2.4	Malignancies	III	II,III	—	1
12.2.5	Infection	III	II	—	1
	CIRCULATORY/CARDIO				
12.3.1	V.B.I.	II,III	I,II,III	—	1
12.3.2	Aneurysm Inv Major Blood Vessel	III	III	—	1
12.3.3	Bleeding	II	III	—	1
12.4.1	Neurological Acute Myelopathy, Cauda Equina	II,III	I,II	—	1

	CHAPTER 13 PREVENTIVE/MAINTENANCE CARE				
Rec #	**Recommendation**	**Rating System I**	**Quality of Evidence**	**Strength**	**Consensus Level**
13.1.1	Disclosure	Established	III	—	1
13.1.2	Chiro Adjustments	Equivocal	III	—	1
13.1.3	Health Screening	Prom to Estab	II,III	—	1
13.1.4	Health Promotion	Established	I,II,III	—	1
13.1.5	Wellness Care Public Health	Equivocal	III	—	1
13.2.1	Community Screening	Promising	II,III	—	1
13.2.2	Public Health Ed	Promising	II,III	—	1

		CHAPTER 14			
	PROFESSIONAL DEVELOPMENT				
Rec #	Recommendation	Rating System II	Quality of Evidence	Strength	Consensus Level
14.1.1	Cont Ed Participation	Necessary	I,II,III	—	1
14.1.2	Ongoing	Recommended	I,II,III	—	1
14.1.3	Assess Outcomes	Recommended	I,II,III	—	1
14.1.4	Variety of Formats	Recommended	II,III	—	1
14.1.5	Critical Reading Postgraduate Ed	Recommended	II,III	—	1
14.2.1	Residency Programs	Recommended	II,III	—	1
14.2.2	Certification Programs	Recommended	II,III	—	1
14.2.3	Encouragement	Discretionary	II,III	—	1
14.2.4	Assess PG Outcomes	Recommended	II,III	—	1
14.2.5	Proprietary Grad Ed	Recommended	II,III	—	1
14.3.1	Encouragement Professional Organz	Discretionary	II,III	—	1
14.4.1	Membership Ethics/Std of Conduct	Recommended	II,III	—	1
14.5.1	Code of Ethics	Necessary	I,II,III	—	1
14.5.2	Advertising Research	Necessary	I,II,III	—	1
14.6.1	Encouragement	Recommended	I,II,III	—	1

Appendix C

Responses to Guidelines

All comments regarding these guidelines should be sent to:

Mercy Center Conference Advisory Committee
P.O. Box 6070
Huntington Beach, CA 92615

Please specify the chapter and specific guideline(s) to be addressed. All responses should be typed and double-spaced to facilitate accurate processing. Whenever possible, responses should include support material and references. Authors should include name, address and telephone number in case additional explanation is required.

Due to the number of responses anticipated, acknowledgment of submissions may not be possible. As future guidelines commissions are established, additional input will be solicited.

Index

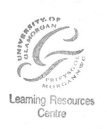